E4

D0413495

the last diet.

SHAHROO IZADI

the
last
diet.

Discover the secret to
losing weight
FOR GOOD

bluebird
books for life

First published 2019 by Bluebird
an imprint of Pan Macmillan
The Smithson, 6 Briset Street, London EC1M 5NR
Associated companies throughout the world
www.panmacmillan.com

ISBN 978-1-5098-8337-0

Copyright © Shahroo Izadi 2019

The right of Shahroo Izadi to be identified as the
author of this work has been asserted by her in accordance
with the Copyright, Designs and Patents Act 1988.

All rights reserved. No part of this publication may be reproduced,
stored in a retrieval system, or transmitted, in any form, or by any means
(electronic, mechanical, photocopying, recording or otherwise)
without the prior written permission of the publisher.

Pan Macmillan does not have any control over, or any responsibility for,
any author or third-party websites referred to in or on this book.

1 3 5 7 9 8 6 4 2

A CIP catalogue record for this book is available from the British Library.

Typeset in Baskerville MT Std and Averta Std by
Palimpsest Book Production Ltd, Falkirk, Stirlingshire

Printed and bound by CPI Group (UK) Ltd, Croydon, CR0 4YY

This book contains the opinions and ideas of its author. It is intended to provide helpful general
information on the subjects that it addresses. It is not in any way a substitute for the advice of the
reader's own physician(s) or other medical professionals based on the reader's own individual
conditions, symptoms, or concerns. If the reader needs personal medical, health, dietary, exercise, or
other assistance or advice, the reader should consult a competent physician and/or other qualified
healthcare professionals. The author and publisher specifically disclaim all responsibility for injury,
damage, or loss that the reader may incur as a direct or indirect consequence of following any
directions or suggestions given in the book or participating in any programmes described in the book.

This book is sold subject to the condition that it shall not, by way of
trade or otherwise, be lent, hired out, or otherwise circulated without
the publisher's prior consent in any form of binding or cover other than
that in which it is published and without a similar condition including
this condition being imposed on the subsequent purchaser.

Visit **www.panmacmillan.com** to read more about all our books
and to buy them. You will also find features, author interviews and
news of any author events, and you can sign up for e-newsletters
so that you're always first to hear about our new releases.

For my mum, who's proof that kindness
and strength go hand in hand.

Contents

introduction

The last time you ever start from scratch again

I'm going to show you how to enjoyably manage your weight for the rest of your life, and I'll do it without telling you what to eat. Because, both from my personal experience of losing eight stone and through my professional experience of working in addiction treatment, I know that telling people how and why they should change is not effective. As a behavioural change specialist in private practice, I help people to achieve their weight-loss goals, whatever they may be, in whatever way best suits their bodies and lives.

I suspect you already know how to literally lose weight, and if you don't, then the briefest of Google searches will bring up all the nutritional information and dietary guidance you need to lose weight sensibly. The basic formulas for safe and effective weight management are widely available and our pool of effective diet options is growing every day.

So, if the problem isn't knowing what you need to do, or knowing how to do it, then why haven't you done it yet? These are the questions that this book is here to help you to answer, and your responses will enable you to create a weight-management plan that is specifically tailored to your needs. One that has your over-all wellbeing in mind.

We often underestimate the amount of thought that is needed in order to create a truly sustainable default 'way of eating' for someone who has always struggled. We make the mistake of think-ing that simply desire, desperation or visible results are enough to keep some people on track.

I imagine that the reason you bought this book is to understand why you even need it. I suspect it's not knowledge of a specific diet you're looking for, but self-knowledge. That's why, when it comes to helping plan the specifics of what you'll be eating or not eating to lose and maintain weight, I won't profess to know what choices are best for your body. Instead I will simply provide the guidance you need to draw out your own wisdom. *The Last Diet* needs you to get on board with the belief that, regardless of why you want to lose weight, how much you want to lose or what practical route you choose to take, your results won't be sustained in a meaningful way unless you commit to:

1. Liking yourself more every day

2. Getting to know yourself better every day

3. Believing in yourself more every day

People often believe that they'll only be capable of doing these things once they've reached a goal weight or size. Quite the oppo-site is true. Starting to be kinder to yourself immediately (regardless of your weight) will make weight-loss goals easier to achieve – although you may have to change your definition of what 'being kinder' means, but we'll come to that later. For many of you, redefining what 'kind decisions' are when it comes to our bodies will bring about the biggest shift in how you see weight loss.

I hope that one day, weight-loss books will simply be evidence-based updates of food and exercise guidance for those who want to literally lose fat from their bodies for whatever reason is important to them. Perhaps because they're prone to putting on weight easily, and they'd just prefer not to, for their own good reasons. As it stands however, almost all of the conversations I have with people about their struggles to shift unwanted weight feature themes like low self-esteem, negative body image and self-sabotage. Luckily though, things seem to be going in the right direction. People are starting to realise what I've seen to be the case over and over again: **believing you're entitled to be happy regardless of your size is actually what helps you to be a size you're happy with.**

So, with that in mind, The Last Diet is a kinder weight-loss plan, that focuses on written exercises designed to increase your self-esteem and self-awareness, not simply physical exercises designed to make you lose fat. This book will help you to design a long-term eating, exercise and wellbeing routine – on purpose. One with self-created guidelines that you're OK with following, even when it's difficult. Because it's much harder to rebel against your diet when you know you created it yourself, and that you put in a lot of work to make sure it's the one with your overall best interests at heart.

Although the word 'diet' gets a bad rap, it needn't only be associated with fads and miracle cures. Of *course* your diet will play a part in the process of you losing weight and keeping it off. The same way it will have played a part in you gaining weight or not being able to keep it off. Your diet is simply a description of things you consume. In this sense, you're always on a diet, it just may not be a predictable one, or one that you've chosen on purpose.

This book is for those who want to create their diet on purpose. Those who have come to realise that without some basic guidelines to follow, their current automatic eating habits will result in their bodies looking and feeling a way they're not happy with. Some people will conclude through the exploratory, preparatory exercises in this book that they can create broad, loose guidelines, while others will decide they need more specific ones.

Some people will never need a book like this. They can't understand how anyone would feel they need to follow self-imposed rules that keep them from enjoying the 'relatively harmless joy and comfort' that food is, whenever they like, and just 'knowing when to stop'. From my experience, these people tend to fall into one of these two categories. Some fall into both. I was always particularly jealous of those people:

1. People who can eat however and whatever they choose, and be content with how those choices make them look and feel

2. People who, regardless of what's going on in their lives, are able to make natural and spontaneous choices for their bodies that are in their best interests long term

You may find it impossible to imagine you could ever belong to one of these categories. But I truly that believe we all can, some of us just need extra help staying in them. I now consider myself to exist in one of those categories most of the time. That said, I still sometimes have to remember that I wasn't always one of those people, and that in order to avoid subtly gaining unwanted weight long term, I'll always need simple default eating guidelines to fall back on.

Throughout this book, I use examples from my own experience of struggling with losing weight and keeping it off. I also draw on the stories of clients I've met through my private practice and habit-change workshops. You will read jargon-free explanations of the approaches I learned working in addiction treatment; motivational concepts that I've seen change people's entire lives for the better. You'll understand why, as soon as I realised the same concepts work for weight loss, I became dedicated to telling everyone about them immediately.

In essence, if you learn the fundamentals of motivation and good planning, you will always feel equipped to understand and change unwanted habits that may emerge around food and exercise, for the rest of your life, without handing yourself over to an 'expert' who needs time to get to know you. The ultimate 'way of eating' you create during this process will eventually become your new normal. But maybe in five years your body or your routine will change, or life circumstances will mean that you can't stick to the same plan anymore. Or you just don't want to. If and when that happens, you can return to the exercises in this book to find everything you need to create a new plan that suits your needs.

For some people, losing weight using this book will be a very simple and practical process of planning things like food choices more consciously and making sure they stay motivated until their new habits can be trusted to their autopilot. Their inability to maintain the weight they want isn't caused by anything much deeper than what they eat and how much they do or don't move around; in other words, their unwanted eating habits aren't wrapped up in strong emotional needs, current or historical. Perhaps they simply associate food with fuel, joy and comfort, but some of the food types and quantities they eat happen to be making them gain or maintain unwanted weight. Perhaps they don't believe any of their value lies in whether they are slim. But it's of course still their prerogative to look how they like, and they just happen to want to be slimmer. Maybe they've never needed to diet in the past but their bodies just aren't playing ball with the status quo anymore.

I was never one of these people. The way I'm made up phys-ically means I've always naturally gained weight very quickly. Still, I always knew that staying overweight was largely due to what I ate, and most importantly why and how I ate it. How much I moved around played a part too, but not such a big one. Throughout my life, there have been a number of reasons why I have eaten in ways that make me gain weight, ranging from:

- Frequent snacking and bingeing on large quantities of unquestionably fattening foods in an attempt to relieve anxiety, stress and low mood

- Loving fattening foods and finding them extremely comforting

- Unconsciously wanting to stay overweight

- Yo-yo dieting and extended bingeing in response to falling off track with restrictive plans

- A childhood spent scheming to get my hands on forbidden 'fattening' foods

- Abusing food to relieve myself from the realisation that I was abusing food

- Never establishing what a healthy, 'normal' way to eat was for my body

How it works

You will use the guidance provided in this book to create a 'normal' way to eat that suits your needs, based on undisputed, common sense principles. Regardless of your current eating style, this process includes the elements we can all agree are a good idea in the short and long term, like:

- Staying hydrated

- Eating vegetables

- Not staying hungry for long

- Eating a variety of foods

- Eating mindfully and enjoying the process of eating

- Not consuming large amounts of sugar

- Not eating in ways that make you feel anxious or in a low mood

- Not eating in ways that make you feel tired or sluggish

- Not eating compulsively

- Eating in ways that give you sustained energy as opposed to a quick 'hit'

- Eating in ways that help you feel focused and energetic

- Eating in ways that give your body a sense of true nourishment

Essentially, The Last Diet is an opportunity to learn how to make choices for your body and mind that you'd want a loved one to make for theirs. That is the most important habit you will develop during this entire process, and one that will make it most meaningful across every area of your life, as well as helping you to achieve your weight-loss goals.

my story

I know you because I am you

The Last Diet was created largely from my experience in two main areas:

1. A lifelong struggle with my weight

2. A career in addiction treatment

There's no denying it, I was a chubby baby. At some point in my childhood, I started realising that my body was causing concern to those around me. When I was around nine years old, my mother began worrying that my weight was becoming an issue. So she started changing what she cooked at home and drawing my attention to the things I ate that I shouldn't eat so much of. She didn't tell me outright that it was because those foods were causing me to gain weight and that gaining weight was a bad thing. And, as a child, I simply picked up on the fact that there was now a new way to be 'good' or 'bad'. This was the first time I realised that some foods were naughty and that eating them would make people unhappy with me.

I had already started to suspect something was up. I remember kids in junior school asking me why I was bigger than them. I remember being in a school uniform shop once when I was about ten and the shop assistant telling my mum that the sizes didn't go up any higher, and that she'd have to start altering my skirts. My mum then started to sew extra panels into the side and, when I went to school, I realised that parts of my skirt were a very slightly different shade to other girls'.

As I became more aware that there was something 'wrong' with me, I became more dependent on behaviours like bingeing and secret eating that would cause me to gain a lot of weight very quickly. As soon as I had a chance to consume the foods that my mother had controlled at home to slow down my weight gain, I would eat them like there was no tomorrow. I would obsess over getting my hands on them and strategise to ensure I could be alone with them. I would lie about how much of them I had eaten. I'm not proud to admit the lengths I'd go to for 'hit' of the forbidden foods. And it was very much a hit, because that's the other force that was embedding my dependency on the forbidden foods: they were very high in sugar and fat. Food addiction was a very real part of my life before I understood what it was or indeed that it even existed.

In a similar way to what happens with many drugs, my tolerance grew and eventually I needed more of those hits more frequently to get my fix. As a result, I continued to gain weight at a rapid pace. By the time I was about twelve, the GP was telling me I was obese, and I had already grown very accustomed to being told by my peers that I was fat (and that being fat was a bad thing).

During secondary school, I started believing that boys didn't fancy fat girls and fat girls aren't popular unless they're funny or have something else to bring to the table. These assumptions began to turn into a self-fulfilling belief, where for example I would choose to stay at home and binge instead of going to a party, because I decided that while I was fat, I wasn't going to have much fun. TV shows and movies didn't help either. It seemed to be a very common storyline that it wasn't until someone lost weight that they became desirable, popular and self-respecting.

Both my relationship with food and with my weight started to become a problem I desperately wanted to deal with. I went to my mum asking for help and, with the best intentions in the world, she started calling for back up. She approached the issue from every angle you could think of. Anything to stop me crying when I'd come home and say someone had made fun of me at school. We'd go to nutritionists, slimming clubs, dieticians, herbalists, hormone specialists and hypnotists. We came at the problem from two angles:

1. Find out what's wrong with my body

2. Find out how not to be fat anymore

My mum would sit there and explain (what she thought was) the whole story to the 'experts' over and over again. What she didn't know was that at this stage I wasn't sure whether it was my secret binges on the forbidden foods that was the issue or if it was a problem with the way my body was working. By this point, I wasn't aware of how much I was already using food as a drug to help me cope with all the social, physical and emotional discomforts of being overweight. Since so many of my impulsive, rebellious, opportunistic eating habits had developed in secret, I didn't register how my actions were spiralling. Plus, I was just a kid!

During the initial consultations and assessments, I was made very aware of how long my weight had been causing concern. I witnessed countless pitches from experts who I realise now could only sell my mum a fix if they concluded that I needed fixing. I became more and more conscious that something was the matter with me and that it was costing those around me time, money and energy to try to fix it (however hard they tried to hide this fact from me). Behind every consultation room door was a new person who would weigh me, prod me, confirm something was wrong with me and offer me a cure.

As a result of many of these appointments, I would adopt various 'expert-recommended' crash diets, and I genuinely wanted them to change my body and my life. But of course, they never did, because every time I fell off the wagon, I would binge. By my mid-teens, I seriously didn't want to be overweight anymore and was prepared to do anything to make that possible. Plus, my mum and I were a team, and although she never put pressure on me, she knew the rules I was meant to be following for each different attempt. Quite naturally, she was disappointed when I couldn't keep up the plans because she knew how desperately I wanted to be slimmer. The problem was that she couldn't really be the team mate she wanted to be because she didn't know the level my dependence on food had reached. Even if I'd wanted to, I didn't have anywhere near enough insight or self-awareness to explain what was going on for me.

So, over and over again I'd fall off track with these plans, become disillusioned and end up heavier than when I started. Any success they brought eventually became a curse, because the diets that gave me quick transformations were the ones I couldn't sustain, the ones that made life miserable. People would applaud me when I was visibly smaller, but they would notice every time I gained weight too. This of course made me feel self-conscious and afraid of being judged, as well as fostering the belief that people preferred me when I wasn't fat.

I reinforced this belief throughout my life, associating not being able to manage my weight with disappointments in other areas. I would look for evidence to confirm my suspicion that being fat was bad. And of course, growing up in the nineties as a girl in the Western world, there was a lot of it flying around.

Since my eating habits became entirely associated with my weight from such a young age, from birth to the time I went to university to study psychology, my 'way of eating' had looked like this:

- Breast milk

- Food my mum knew was healthy for kids in general

- Food my mum knew would help me lose weight + secret binges

- Extreme diet plans

- Extreme diet plans + secret binges

- Food my mum knew would help me lose weight + secret binges

- Extreme diet plans

- Extreme diet plans + secret binges

- Etc.

When my parents dropped me off on campus to live on my own for the first time at university, I was already close to being my heaviest ever. However, I had decided that I would transform while I was there, eventually, by starving myself. And so in the meantime I would eat whatever I wanted, whenever I wanted, however I wanted for the first time in my life. And oh boy, did I go for it. In that first term of university I ate in a way that caused me to gain a lot more weight. I also developed a regular weed smoking habit that didn't help matters. It was a disastrous marriage of substances, joining together to help me avoid and delay emotional discomfort as well as making me want to eat more.

As I grew closer to some of my friends at university, I discovered that they had a very different relationship with food than I did. When we went to the supermarket, they knew which ingredients to buy in order to cook a number of meals that were part of their ordinary way of eating. I, on the other hand, was leaving with shopping bags full of either celery and seeds or chips and trifles. I didn't have a dozen 'meals' in mind because my meals had always consisted of things my mum had cooked and things that were forbidden. Both for cultural reasons and the fact my mum reigned over the kitchen in my house, the only meals I ate regularly were either way too complicated for me to want to learn how to cook, or way too 'healthy' for me to be convinced to cook. A 'big shop' for me often involved picking what I wanted to eat that day and just multiplying it by fourteen to last me two weeks.

I carried on like this into my second year of university, until I got to a point where I was used to waking up feeling lethargic and heavy. It's lucky I wasn't interested in alcohol at that time, as I imagine that would have made the situation much worse. During this time there were of course still attempts to lose weight. Although I told my mum that I was done with all the expert outsourcing, I was still determined to one day be slim. After all, my flawed belief system told me that it wasn't until I had lost weight that I could really go out, take up the space I deserve to and enjoy my life.

I'd got to a stage where if I caught myself starting to feel good or enjoy myself for whatever reason, I would immediately think 'this would be so much better if I wasn't still fat'. Often, I would catch a glimpse of myself and not only realise that I had expanded but also that I had stopped taking pride in my appearance and my surroundings. So, in response, I would punish myself by deciding to embark on another crash diet and life transformation plan. These would commence between one and five times a week, and last for anything between one hour and six weeks. But now they were harder to keep to than when I lived at home, since I didn't have a routine or any supervision. Plus, my addictive eating patterns had a hold on me that made the withdrawals really painful whenever I'd try to rashly deprive myself, thinking that's what I deserved for letting things get to this stage.

I was also able to adopt much more extreme diets, ones that my mum would understandably never have allowed. I started abusing laxatives and taking appetite suppressants from the internet that were essentially amphetamines. I could go days without eating if

I wanted to, without anyone noticing. So not only was university a fertile ground for my food addiction to spiral, it was also the perfect place for my quick-fix, all-or-nothing, lose weight at any cost thinking to get worse.

On one occasion, I continued long after the usual six weeks, and although I used a combination of very unhealthy methods, I managed to lose a lot of weight. I went from a size 20 to a size 8. For the first time in my entire life, I was undeniably thin.

So, I lived as a thin person for a couple of years during my last year of university and the year following it. My hair was thinning and I struggled to focus, but I didn't care because for the first time I was *thin*. Although you will have gathered that this story doesn't end well, I have to admit that it was all that I'd hoped it would be in a lot of ways, but largely because I'd spent my life treating it as the criterion I needed to meet in order to enjoy myself.

I wore the clothes I'd always dreamt of wearing; I went on a holiday and wore a bikini the whole time; I stood up straight and acted more spontaneously. Plus, the world applauded me. And not just because of my achievement, because I was thin. I wish this wasn't true but it was. I knew this because coming into contact with new people as a slim person was an entirely different experience. The suspicions I'd had that fat people weren't treated as well as thin people – at least in the UK – were confirmed. When I met people for the first time as a slim person and told them how much weight I'd lost, they usually reacted to my 'before' pictures with shock and horror. 'That doesn't even look like you!', 'Wow, what an achievement, you looked ten years older then!', 'You look SO much better now', 'Make sure you keep up the good work!', 'It just suits your face more to be thin', 'Boys must be queuing up now . . .' I lapped it up.

Then there were the people who knew and cared for me, who communicated their relief that I was finally thin. They treated my weight loss as a done deal, a solution to a problem that had been low-key concerning everyone for a while, not least because of how much it concerned me. Everything was fixed as far as other people were concerned, and I deserved praise, so they were happy to tell me how much better I looked.

But it wasn't a fix. They didn't know that I hadn't found a long-term solution to staying slim other than things like skipping meals, white knuckling it and abusing appetite suppressants. Plus, every time someone told me how much better I looked now, it made me think they didn't think I looked fine before. Nonetheless, in the short term at least, people reacting positively to my weight loss spurred me on.

Predictably, the combination of not knowing what to eat to maintain my new size and needing constant external validation meant that once the compliments died down and it turned out that all life's problems hadn't disappeared, I subtly started lapsing. I ate to deal with the disappointment of slimness not being the solution to my low self-esteem and also because I was starving all the time. I slipped back into old ways – in that I slipped back into no 'ways', just impulsive, isolated binges – and my weight crept back on until, before I knew it, I wasn't thin anymore. It was like it had all been a dream. I was back where I started and, although it made me desperately sad and disillusioned, it was also strangely comforting in its familiarity and predictability.

Over the next few years, well into my late twenties, I repeated this pattern of losing huge amounts of weight at rapid speeds once I'd hit another 'rock bottom' and then gaining it again. Many had learned to stop commenting on my always fluctuating weight. As an old colleague once said when I walked into a meeting after four months of not seeing her, 'Oh you're thin again! We were all just debating whether we thought you'd be thin or not this time.' I'd say that between the ages of 23 and 30, I spent 20 per cent of the time very slim, 60 per cent very overweight and the other 20 per cent in the transition process.

By this time, I had started living in London. I got my master's degree and when it came to choosing an area of psychology to specialise in, I chose addiction. I started with an unpaid, one-year placement in an NHS service in north-west London, where I was introduced to the world of addiction treatment for the first time. Admittedly, when I walked into the waiting room on the first day for my induction, I remember wondering whether a placement somewhere like this was really going to be worth working two side-jobs for. But just hours into my job there, I knew I'd found my career path for life.

Day after day, I witnessed people's entire lives transform thanks to the help they were getting from my colleagues. I grew obsessed, and gave my role more time and energy than I'd ever given any paid role before. I wanted to learn as much as I could. I soon figured out that one of the best ways to learn was to work on the reception desk. This way I could speak to the patients, hear their stories, help them with forms and make them tea. I learned how to really listen to people and make them feel heard.

As the months passed and my obsession with my role grew evident to my colleagues, I started being given more responsibility. By the end of my placement I was confident that I could go straight into a paid addiction worker role, and that's what I did. My new job was to assess and treat drug addicts using a range of the latest motivational tools, which I was continuously trained in. In contrast to the NHS placement, I was no longer in clinical environments, so most of the approaches I used were focused on motivational exercises, talking therapies and support groups as opposed to prescriptions and risk assessments.

I kept working my way up in the field until eventually I became a consultant and trainer, advising healthcare organisations on the best approaches to use in addiction treatment.

I became knowledgeable in new approaches I had never heard of, and built on what I already knew from my first-hand experience and previous training. I started to travel across the country delivering training to clinical, community and prison staff teams, all of whom wanted additional tools to help them motivate their complex and resistant clients to make lasting changes that they could sustain independently.

The training I delivered would include a lot of written exercises that delegates could try out so that they felt comfortable going back and using them with their own clients. I would mainly guide them to complete 'maps'. This simply involved writing a theme in the middle of a page and scattering ideas around it, as opposed to writing things in a list. In the first few months of delivering training, I'd ask delegates to populate their maps using examples from one of their client's lives. But something kept happening that made me tweak this: people wanted to complete the maps using examples from their own lives, to use the motivational and planning exercises to explore their own unwanted habits. This didn't surprise me, as seeing how effective these tools were at work, I'd also begun to re-approach the ever-looming task of losing weight with more focus on my motivation and personal development.

Although the maps helped me to gain more insight into my behaviours and lose a bit of weight by decreasing the frequency and severity of my binges, I still didn't have a 'way of eating'. I knew from my work across addiction that meaningful change had to be realistic and enjoyable. But I had no idea how to sustain a way of eating that managed my weight and was all of these things at the same time. That's were OA came in.

OA, or Overeaters Anonymous, is a twelve-step programme for people who feel that their behaviours around food have become unmanageable. I came across it when I was doing research for a client on what free support was available. Of course, I had heard of the Alcoholics Anonymous programme, but in order for that to be effective you have to abstain from alcohol entirely. You can't be abstinent from food entirely.

I went to check out OA and learned that some of the same concepts that help us stop doing something altogether can also help us to keep doing it, but differently. I learned that although everyone at OA followed a prescribed twelve-step programme, when it came to the food guidelines they had to follow to be in a state of recovery, everyone's were different. There seemed to be some common themes that ran through people's individual pro-grammes – like trying not to eat refined sugar or starchy carbs, and of course going through the required personal development exercises. But for most, when it came to food, they had different definitions of what lapse and relapse looked like, based on their bodies, their goals and their experience.

Over time, I combined my learning from OA, clinical addiction treatment and training feedback to create an entire personal development plan that enabled me to lose weight gradually, meaningfully and more enjoyably than ever before. I created new maps that focused more on my self-esteem and I designed exercises that helped me find sensible personal definitions for words like 'healthy' and 'moderation'. I kept the weight off this time because I finally realised that there was never anything wrong with me, I just never had the tools, self-awareness or self-belief I needed to make lasting changes.

The Last Diet is a collection of all the tools and knowledge I needed, in the format I needed it, to finally change. It's the book I wish I had twenty years ago.

your story

You're the expert

The Last Diet will give you the tools and guidance you need to write all the next chapters of your story when it comes to how you treat your body.

Regardless of whether you've spent a lifetime struggling to manage your weight or just the past few months, the exercises in this book will enable you to design a plan of change that is most suited to your needs specifically. For them to be effective, however, it's important that you commit to completing them comprehensively and with complete honesty. You should feel that you are taking a much deeper, more exploratory look at what works for you and what habits have brought you to where you are today. Although it will be difficult at times to write down things about your current or previous habits that you're not proud of, this is precisely the kind of investment it's important to make in this process.

When it comes to recording the reasons you want to lose weight, don't worry about what you think you should write: just write what's true. No one will judge you; you're allowed to have whatever motivators you like. Plus, when it comes to gaining momentum in the early stages of change, it's very much a case of 'whatever gets you there'. So if, like me, when you're really honest about what's likely to get you out of bed on a rainy morning to exercise, it's something like 'the thought of feeling great in my favourite jeans as opposed to 'the thought of not getting diabetes', then that's OK. You will find that The Last Diet is not a process of finding yourself, but rather, a process of meeting yourself, and being fine with whoever you meet.

In this book I am going to guide you to the point where you can draw out your own wisdom. I will give you a basic framework in which you can establish and create your own ideal conditions for success.

When I began writing *The Last Diet*, one of the first things I considered was who I was trying to help, and how I could help as many people as possible. So I started by thinking about what we – all of us who have struggled to maintain our weight, whatever the reason – have in common. I scrolled through pages and pages of client notes, and I saw that despite having vastly different stories, those who wanted to lose weight were often saying quite similar things when it came to the changes they wanted to make. I created a top twenty list and, from that, have assumed in writing *The Last Diet* that some or all of these things are true for you:

1. You're tired of making the same resolutions every year (or every Monday)

2. You create meticulous weight-loss plans but can't seem to keep them up

3. You're confused as to why you can't stop behaving a certain way around food, even though you really want to and have all the information you need

4. You feel demoralised and disillusioned after a series of unsuccessful attempts to change

5. You're tired of signing up to miracle plans and quick-fix solutions that aren't sustainable

6. The way you tend to speak to yourself when it comes to weight loss is unkind and self-sabotaging

7. You feel as though you're living life on hold, waiting to achieve your weight-loss goals

8. You believe you'll always be an all-or-nothing person with an 'addictive personality'

9. Your inability to manage your weight is negatively impacting your relationships, social life, professional development or general wellbeing

10. You don't feel you have the self-esteem or self-belief needed to change

11. You struggle to adopt sensible weight-loss plans because slow progress doesn't keep you motivated

12. You're tired of declaring to loved ones that you're making changes, only to have to update them that you've once again fallen off the wagon

13. You want to set your own goals and create habits that fit into your lifestyle, based on what's important to you

14. Your body has changed and so the same weight-management methods that worked before aren't as effective

15. You want to explore healthier ways to deal with stress, worry and boredom than food and/or compulsive eating habits

16. You want to invest in personal development to become more self-aware in general about how you're treating yourself

17. You want to be able to keep your long-term weight-loss goals in mind instead of giving in to immediate temptation when it comes to food choices

18. You feel you don't have an 'off switch' when it comes to engaging in unwanted habits around food

19. You've never found a long-term 'healthy' way of eating that enables you to freely enjoy food and also manage your weight

20. You think you lack the willpower to keep up a plan of change around eating

How your thinking patterns and general behaviours towards your body have developed over time may not be something you stop to consider very often. We're all always engaging in habits, and some will be autopilot ones. Through this process you may well realise that your current 'programming' of autopilot thoughts and behaviours has been influenced by external forces throughout your life; ones you haven't ever stopped to question.

You will continue to eat for the rest of your life whether you give it any thought or you don't. So why not choose to consider it, so that you have more say in the decisions you make instead of being led by self-defeating, unhelpful and unkind beliefs quite possibly carried over from childhood?

If you're a 'quick-fix' kind of person like me, you'll be happy to know you can go through the exercises in this book as quickly as you want and start making positive changes straight away. You can work your own way through to the action plan towards the end and start seeing the visible results soon after. You don't have to wait to book a session with me, turn up for a support group or part with another penny. Plus, the exercises you complete during this process will be ones you can come back to for the rest of your life, as part of a long-term commitment to checking in with yourself and making sure you feel happy about your relationship with food – and with yourself.

In my private practice, I've worked with many clients who have completely changed their relationships with food by using the methods in this book. People who had spent their entire lives never quite finding a way of eating that suits them. People who were demoralised and had lost hope of ever being truly happy with their bodies. People who had lost all the weight they wanted to, only to realise that nothing else in their life had improved at all – a realisation that was making them put the weight back on quickly. They used The Last Diet to take control of their story. And now, so will you.

the last diet

What it's all about

What is it?

The Last Diet is a weight-management programme that takes a deeper approach to changing unwanted eating habits. It's inspired by the motivational approaches that work in drug addiction treatment.

How is it different to other diets?

Instead of just focusing on food and exercise, The Last Diet also considers the self-esteem, self-awareness and self-belief you'll need to sustain your results enjoyably and meaningfully in the long term. Choosing what you eat to lose and to manage your weight will be entirely up to you. I will help you access the information you need to create the plans and goals that are best for you. But I won't presume to know what's best for your body.

The Last Diet assumes that you pretty much know how to lose weight already, but that you need more help understanding why you can't get going or stick to your eating or exercising plan even though you want to.

What will I have to do?

First, you'll work through this book, completing written exercises that I guide you through in order. These are designed to best prepare you for the changes ahead. As soon as you've completed your first written exercise at the end of the next chapter, you can consider yourself 'on' The Last Diet.

Then, when you've finished reading this book, you'll officially activate the more practical eating and exercise elements of your desired weight-loss plan.

(Just in case you're thinking, 'That means I have plenty of time for some last blowouts first', then for now, just try to observe that thought process. Curiously question how much sense it makes. And I don't say this as a professional habit expert, but as a professional excuse-maker.)

Are the exercises hard work?

They're simple to understand and to complete, but they're intended to make you think hard, and in new ways. The intention is that you use the process of reading this book as the first in many opportunities you will now be taking to put time aside for yourself and invest in your wellbeing.

If an exercise in this book requires you to think back to previous failed attempts, for example, it's absolutely worth your time to jog your memory in every way you can. If that means rooting through old calendars and diaries, finding old subscription emails or just taking fifteen extra minutes to sit in silence and really cast your mind back, then it's important that you do it – even if revisiting past failures feels uncomfortable at times. The harder you work on the written exercises, the easier it will feel when it comes to practically changing your eating habits in everyday settings. They need to feel like an investment, to make you feel more accountable and also that you're making truly informed decisions when it comes to creating your bespoke plan of change.

I assume that in buying this book you're acknowledging that it's actually becoming hard work to stay the way you are. If you're anything like I used to be, you're probably spending most of your energy beating yourself up for not having changed yet. I can assure you that none of the exercises in this book are as hard as that.

What's with the maps?

I'll be asking you to complete simple mind maps throughout this process. I have found that it can be very effective to have different thoughts and observations scattered around a page, as opposed to written out as a list. Well populated maps can provide a crucial snapshot of collective ideas, and represent something visually that it is incredibly difficult to recall all at once in our heads, especially when we're feeling like throwing in the towel.

As you work through each chapter, you'll see that some maps will prove useful across all areas of your life, whereas others are only applicable to the specific habits you're focused on changing at that time. When you've completed all the maps in this book, you will have a wealth of visual resources to hand, designed to boost your self-esteem, self-belief and self-awareness.

What's with all the mentions of kindness?

I believe that we all know what kindness looks and feels like, in the context of our relationships with others, both when it comes to giving and receiving it. It's great. The problem is that we're often not very kind to ourselves. And, as I've seen so many times through my work and personal experience, it is those who struggle to be kind to themselves who have the hardest time when they try to make lasting, meaningful changes to their eating habits.

So, what is kindness? A thesaurus search brings up synonyms such as: patience, understanding, consideration, compassion and helpfulness. The Last Diet approach is based on the belief that if we commit to behaving in these ways towards our bodies across every possible area of our lives, then our food choices will follow suit with less effort.

What if my version of kindness is eating chocolate and chips for dinner every night?

In this process you will learn that although kindness is about being gentle with ourselves and enjoying our lives as much as possible overall, when it comes to making difficult changes kindness also means choosing to put ourselves in some manageable short-term discomfort to achieve our most valued goals. It means believing in our ability to do difficult things and challenge our own self-limiting beliefs.

The Last Diet helps you shift your definition of kind behaviours away from being habits that give you instant relief, comfort or distraction, to choices you'll be glad you made for yourself the next day. In many cases, riding out a short-term urge or craving isn't an act of unkindness or depriving yourself, it's an opportunity to show yourself how capable you are. Plus, it's a necessary step to take as many times as possible if the craving is to become less powerful in the long term.

In order to help you act more kindly, this process will require you to first *think* more kindly and not treat it as a punishment or remedy. I've seen many clients fall off track with their plans by thinking that depriving themselves of the things that turn down the volume on unwelcome internal chatter in the short term is a punishment. Often a lapse is prompted by the internal message: 'Its unkind to deprive myself of things that comfort me.' In order to get to where you want to be using The Last Diet, you need to be OK with curiously and consciously listening to your self-sabotaging thoughts and willingly feeling your impulses, instead of impulsively acting on them or pushing them to the back of your mind as soon as they pop up.

If at any point in this process you're unsure about whether the choices you make for your body are kind or not, simply consider whether they're the same choices you'd make for the body of the person you love most in the world.

How will I know what to actually eat?

When you get to the practical planning stages of this book I will ask you to complete a very comprehensive enquiry into what foods and ways of eating are best for you and your body specifically.

Will I have to keep coming back to this book to keep up my results?

Although I will encourage you to reflect on your progress by looking at your maps and taking a keen lifelong interest in your personal development, you will feel progressively less dependent on the written guidance and tools in this book over time. That's because:

- You'll have 'time under your belt' and enjoy results that you'll want to protect and sustain

- You'll have overcome challenging situations that demonstrate how capable you are. This will make you want to keep surprising yourself

- You'll be able to quickly remember why it's important for you to stay on track. This will help you to waste less time entertaining any unhelpful excuses to lapse

- You'll develop a new set of automatic behaviours. Realising you can choose them when it comes to eating habits will get you excited about what other kind habits you can choose for yourself

- The exercises will have helped to increase your self-esteem in an authentic way, so that you don't associate your worth with your weight, and therefore don't fall into the trap of throwing in the towel at the times when your weight invariably plateaus or fluctuates

- You will be less convinced by your own justifications to go off track. The more you practise noticing and questioning them, the less compelling they will become

- The generally kinder landscape of your life will be less accommodating to unkind eating habits

What kinds of people see the best results?

Those who:

- Invest time in getting really clear on why they want to change

- Understand why they haven't changed already

- Change for their own reasons

- Are prepared to own what works for them, even if it means they have to defend it to other people sometimes

- Are completely honest with themselves about why they want to change

- Expect their drive to waver from minute to minute for a while, and put strategies in place to ensure they stay on track when it inevitably dips

- Find a definition for kindness around their eating habits that has their best interests at heart across their entire lives

What beliefs do I need get on board with?

1. You're fine as you are

In order to lose weight with The Last Diet, you're going to have to start believing (or at least wanting to believe) that your body is worthy of kindness regardless of your weight. The process of losing weight will be much easier if you start trying to do all the things you plan to do when you've lost weight as soon as possible. Your weight may well fluctuate throughout your life for a range of reasons. It cannot be a criterion for liking yourself or enjoying your life.

2. Tough love isn't helpful

The Last Diet approach believes that tough love, warnings and scare tactics might get us going initially, but they don't keep us going. To keep pushing through and making kind choices for ourselves in those moments when it's most difficult, we need to focus on what we're moving towards, not what we're moving away from. We need to be given encouragement and positive feedback. Any tough love you think would actually be helpful for you is the kind you can give yourself through the initial exercises in this book.

3. Thoughts and feelings don't have to become actions

When it comes to our eating habits, even when our actions seem impulsive and on autopilot, we are still making a choice to follow our own commands. In order for The Last Diet to be most effective, you need to be willing to slow down your actions and curiously question the thoughts and feelings that drive them. You will need to develop a belief that urges and cravings are 'yoo-hoos' not 'YOU DO . . .'s. They are alerts, not commands.

4. Mental health is physical health

The Last Diet requires you to make your emotional wellbeing and personal development a priority. Not only because poor mental health can negatively impact your ability to take care of your physical health, but also because you may well discover during this process that your current unwanted eating habits are serving as short-term coping strategies for things like stress and anxiety.

5. Rock bottom isn't a prerequisite for change

Many traditional addiction treatment approaches believe that people don't change until things have become truly unbearable. For some, this is the case. I've met people who remember the moment they decided to change their habits and immediately did so without ever looking back.

Most of the time, however, especially when it comes to more day-to-day habits, it's not unusual to have loads of 'rock bottoms'. I can't count the number of times I cried in a changing room where nothing fit me (again) thinking, 'That's it, I never thought things would get this bad. Things are changing TODAY.' Yet despite this, my rock bottoms gradually just kept getting lower, and I eventually normalised them. This was especially the case when it came to numbers on scales.

6. Forewarned is forearmed

Many of us have made the mistake of thinking our desire to change is enough to get us there. As a result, when it comes to creating a plan of action for weight loss, we immediately turn our attention to what we'll eat or not eat. We assume that simply knowing what to do and knowing we want to do it is enough to achieve our goals.

The Last Diet believes that in order to gain momentum with weight loss and maintain it long term, we need to do some far less obvious planning than meal plans and grocery lists. When it comes to ingrained patterns, any change from the status quo can bring physical cravings and urges as well as emotional discomfort, so we need to have a plan for how we'll respond to internal and external triggers. Even if our plan is to do nothing, but on purpose.

Is there anything I won't be allowed to eat again?

No.

that's it

A snapshot of reasons to change

The written exercise at the end of this chapter will mark the first step in starting your Last Diet, and the last time you'll feel you're 'starting from scratch' again. Because this time your goals will be built on foundations of self-knowledge, self-belief and self-care. The plans for change you have tried before probably focused on what foods to eat, how regularly to exercise, what measurements to take, etc. This time will be different. This time you'll work on how you think, act and speak towards yourself before you even consider how you'll eat! And in so doing, you will develop an arsenal of assets and tools that will anchor you and enable you to top up your motivation levels again and again, in a way that simple meal plans and numbers on scales just don't.

Much of the inspiration for the exercises in this chapter came from my time working in substance misuse treatment. In many of the community services I was placed at, there was often a drop-in service, where people could walk in off the street and ask for help. A lot of the time, they would (understandably) expect to be able to speak to someone and get help straight away. Unfortunately, however, this was rarely the case. Due to a shortage of resources, most people could only be assessed that day, and then given a time to return days or weeks later when they could start sessions with a keyworker or attend a support group. Over and over, I would see people for whom things had come to a head walk through the door ready to make changes, only to be told they couldn't start yet.

Very often their decision to come in was a direct result of a 'rock bottom'. Perhaps their addiction had caused them go to lengths they never dreamed they would, or an incident had taken place that shocked them and brought to their attention how important it had become to change. Perhaps they'd finally got to a tipping point where they truly believed in that moment that the negatives of their actions outweighed the positives.

Often people walked in with a sense of urgency. It felt as though they had got to that moment that so many of us do after resolving to make the same changes over and over again: feeling fed up, out of control and ready to do whatever it takes to change the status quo. While this is actually the opposite of the attitude and perspective this book will encourage you to adopt in order to stay motivated in the long run, it's very useful for getting going. In these moments, we have naturally achieved the state that the early exercises in this book are designed to bring about – but in a more meaningful, positive and sustained way. Sometimes when we hit a 'rock bottom', we briefly and organically stumble upon:

- Belief that it's incredibly important and urgent to change the status quo (because of all the negative impacts)

- Belief in our ability to change the status quo (because of our desperation to do so or because we haven't experienced withdrawals yet)

These moments can be absolutely golden when it comes to finding the drive to get us going, but they are often fleeting and temporary. That's why it was so frustrating to see addicts coming in to the drop-in session for help when they'd reached this point but not be able to grasp the opportunity there and then.

What would often happen is that people wouldn't turn up for the future appointment they'd been given. Of course, this could be for a number of reasons, but when I called them to ask why they hadn't come back and try to make another appointment with them, they often sounded considerably less concerned than they did that first time, and definitely less motivated to do something about their unwanted habits. Time had passed and perhaps some of the negative impacts had become more manageable. Bodies had recovered to some extent and levels of desperation to change had decreased. This put me in a tricky position: on the one hand I was happy to hear that things didn't sound as bad as they did before. On the other hand, a big part of me wanted to remind the person on the phone of how bad they told me it had got and all the reasons why it was likely that it would get that bad – or worse – again, if they didn't address their legitimate concerns about their behaviours.

I wanted to warn them, essentially. To stop them from forgetting, to relay back what they'd told me before. To ask them what they thought would be different this time and what made them think everything would be OK, even if they kept repeating the same patterns over and over again. But I couldn't. Partly because good practitioners know that trying to 'save' people doesn't do them any favours. And partly because I knew from my experience with my weight and body struggles that if someone decided it was their job to remind me of what I should be doing and what's best for me, I'd become defensive, and feel more inclined to engage in the behaviours that made things worse (I would eat to distract from anger and annoyance and to demonstrate that I can do whatever the hell I like with my body). Plus, I would always assume that they had misunderstood my needs and struggles.

I'd spent a few months witnessing people come in to drug treatment services ready to change and then not coming back, when a colleague from another drug service taught me something they had implemented that was really helping. When people came in asking for help, as well as assessing them, practitioners asked them to write themselves a little note, in their own handwriting, that gave a snapshot of why they had chosen to come in to ask for help. Then, if they didn't come back for a second appointment, the service would post that note to them. This meant that people would be presented with something they couldn't push back against: a snapshot of themselves, by themselves and for themselves.

This small change had made a huge difference to how many people decided to come back and ask for help again. And the great thing was, they didn't need to feel as awful as they did on that first day to want to come back, they just needed to remember how bad things had been. Often they could recognise that what they had written to themselves was a description of the kind of day that was becoming more and more frequent, even if it wasn't how they felt the day they received it.

The exercise you will complete in this chapter will help you to capture those same moments: the ones when it's clear to you why it's important for you to change. It's an opportunity to write all the negatives in one place and show yourself that although motivation and importance will waver from day to day, overall, the negatives are outweighing the positives and you do want to change.

Things will present themselves every single day that will make you minimise, trivialise and normalise the behaviours that on other days come together and make things feel unmanageable and out of control. For example, when I was trying to lose weight, I could often trace a binge back to an experience of deciding that my goals weren't important in that moment. This could be something like a great evening out with friends a few weeks into a weight-loss diet, eating whatever I liked and genuinely enjoying myself. The next day I'd wake up and my all-or-nothing thinking patterns would mean all I could do was fixate on all the other things I wished I could eat since I'd already been so 'bad.'

Trivialising overeating, bingeing and eating mindlessly over and over again would always leave me in the same place: more unhappy in how my body felt and looked. In that moment, when I would tell myself that I should have fun and treat food like a joy, I wasn't able to remember that I didn't know how to do that yet, for one reason or another, even if other people could. I couldn't (and didn't want to) recall all the times I hadn't managed to do it before when the circumstances had been identical. I couldn't (and didn't want to) focus my attention on how I'd feel in a day or week, when history would dictate that I'd still be in a cycle of bingeing and self-loathing. I told myself I was 'living in the moment' and 'eating intuitively'. In theory of course, this is great. It's how I live now much of the time. But it's something that, for people like me, needs to be learned and practised and understood. I couldn't wing it yet.

Another method of trivialising my desire to lose weight was by berating myself about how silly my problems were compared to those of others. Working in substance misuse treatment, this wasn't difficult to do. I would meet people who had problems I couldn't even imagine dealing with. I heard accounts of extreme trauma and abuse. I saw people's immense gratitude for things I took for granted every day. Then I would go home at the end of the day (usually hungry and tired) and when it came to trying not to order a take-out, I'd think, 'Who cares about my weight? I have a roof over my head, legs that get me from A to B and a supportive family. I need to get some perspective . . . and also three pizzas and a tub of ice cream.'

Yes, the issues my clients were facing were far more urgent and serious than my waistline. They were also more important than me learning to speak to myself less horribly every day, and dragging around a tired, uncared-for body. But there is room for them both to matter. And, more importantly, they in fact have nothing to do with each other. Exercises like the ones you'll complete in this book showed me that I was always quick to find an 'out' by trivialising my relationship with food and my body because:

- Hearing disturbing stories all day was making me want immediate emotional relief from things like sugar to make me feel a bit better

- The fact I was already in a cycle of eating that left me craving unhealthy foods meant I was looking for any excuse to relieve myself from the sensation of physical withdrawal when trying to eat healthier ones

- I was looking for confirmation wherever I could find it that my body wasn't as worthy as everyone else's of being taken care of, and my problems were not as important

When you get to the section towards the end of this book which asks you to design and activate a practical plan of change, you will be starting something difficult, because it will be a change. You will face internal and external challenge. Even if every single meal you eat is delicious and healthy; even if you love completing the written exercises; even when you start to see results. There will still be moments when you tell yourself it's not as important to change as you thought it was that day when you swore you had to make changes once and for all.

At the end of this chapter, I am going to ask you to write a letter to yourself describing why things need to change. In this 'That's It' letter, you'll list as many reasons as you can think of why you want this to be last time you ever 'start again'. It'll be for your eyes only, so when it comes to completing it, be as honest as you can, and give importance to whatever you want. If, like me, you think that vanity will spur you on more than fear of heart disease, then that's absolutely fine. You're allowed to have whatever motivations you like, even if you're not proud of them. Plus, bear in mind, these won't be the same motivators that keep you going long term. Moving away from negative impacts just gets us going. It's the moving towards positive ones that keeps us going.

There's another reason why complete honesty and vulnerability with yourself is key here: we need a reliable baseline. I often mention how difficult it can be for even the most skilled, non-judgemental and compassionate therapists to create an environment in which people feel comfortable to tell the whole truth about the stuff they're not proud of straight away, without first building rapport. To give an honest and accurate picture of where they're starting from and how bad things can really get on the worst days. For obvious reasons (especially in my line of work that involved stigmatised and illegal activities), we often don't want to tell a complete stranger our true reasons for wanting to change or where our habits have taken us. But this also means that the therapist doesn't collect reliable information at the starting point, and therefore can't accurately measure our progress. Many smokers will be familiar with this. Clients have often told me that they've forgotten how much they downplayed the number of cigarettes they smoke per day to the GP during the last appointment. They forget their own lie. Then, even if they have cut down by the next appointment and report truthfully, their notes might say that they're smoking more than last time!

Moments of pride

Since you're doing this process on your own, you will be depriving yourself of a much-deserved pat on the back and celebration of milestones if you're not completely honest in this first exercise about things you're not happy with. For this process to work, you need to feel worthy. For that, you need to feel capable and strong.

To feel capable enough to face the challenges in this process and stay motivated, you'll need to be reflecting on and collecting examples of having felt proud of yourself. To feel authentically proud of yourself, you'll need to recognise when an accomplishment is truly an accomplishment for you personally. For that, you need to be completely honest about where you started.

When I look back on my own 'That's It' exercise, I still can't believe how many years I spent accepting and normalising all the tiny ways I was needlessly suffering every day. Seeing what I'd written at the start of this process reminded me that for most of my life, from the second I'd wake up in the morning, my weight was at the forefont of my thoughts. From how I felt as soon as I opened my eyes (anyone who is familiar with the late-night binge will tell you that this can cause a serious hangover), to what I said to myself when I looked in the mirror, to what clothes I chose to wear, to what assumptions I made about other people's responses and judgements towards me throughout the day, to my plan of whether to be 'good' or 'bad' with every single food choice. It was exhausting and constant and relentless.

While writing this book, I took a train journey that resulted in me going back and adding something I'd forgotten to add all those years ago to my 'That's It' letter:

So much of my brain space is taken up by how much physical space I'm taking up in lifts, on benches and cars.

I got on a tube line recently that I haven't taken for years, one where the seats don't have separators, and I saw one available next to the window. I simply walked through some people and over some bags, and sat down. This may sound ridiculous, but a few years ago, there's absolutely no way I would have done that. Even if my legs were aching and I had fifteen stops to take home. Why? Because this seemingly simple act of taking a seat would make me think this:

'All these other people will be looking at me scrambling around over them trying to get to that seat. They have nothing else to look at on this train so they'll be judging the hot and flustered giant fat woman wearing clothes that are too tight. The person I'd be sitting next to will be annoyed about all the space I'm taking up, plus my body will be pressed against theirs and they'll feel all my rolls. I won't be able to eat my sandwich because people will be thinking, "She shouldn't be eating that", and what if I have to get off the train before they do, which means I have to do that all over again?! Not worth it. I'll stand.'

I feel a mixture of sympathy for my former self and pride in my accomplishments when I notice that simple but grinding daily worries like whether to take a tube seat are things of the past. So, when highly personal realisations like this one come about, I go back to the exercise you'll do in this chapter and write down my observations. While I'm there, I glance at the other things too, just to help me remember to remember how far I've come. (And by the way, these days, even if for some reason I was three times the size I was at my heaviest, I would absolutely still push through everyone and take the tube seat with great joy. I know now that my lunch-needing, tax-paying, hard-working body deserves to sit down if it wants to – regardless of its size.)

The 'That's It' exercise in this chapter is the first of many to encourage you to think about how your relationship with your body and or eating habits is impacting various different areas of your life, and how these things might be inter-related. When people are completing this exercise, they commonly begin by thinking of the more obvious things they're not happy with, such as feeling unfit, uncomfortable or unattractive, or feeling out of control and emotionally, compulsively dependent on food. But I also ask that you consider the more subtle ones, such as the impact your diet has on your mental health and general sense of wellbeing, and what that means for your moods, and what your moods mean for your relationships with others, etc.

Applying this new kinder, more self-aware approach to weight management and body positivity involves getting really good at forward thinking. But I don't mean in terms of food choices. By forward thinking, I mean making decisions based on how we are likely to feel about them the next day, or week or month. To do this effectively, we need to understand how our habits impact each other. Sometimes we discover that habits we didn't even think were related to our eating patterns and body image are partly responsible for them.

Many of my clients realised after doing exercises like the one in this chapter that when choosing what to eat and drink in order to achieve the weight they want, they would have to limit their alcohol intake, not only for calorie reasons but also for resolve-lowering reasons. That's definitely something that was true for me – good luck getting me to look at a letter I wrote myself about why I want to lose weight when I'd had three glasses of wine and spotted a

McDonalds. Plus, drinking heavily made me wake up craving the kinds of foods that made me feel sluggish, anxious, bloated, disappointed – and wanting more.

By taking time to really capture how things are at their 'worst' for you in this exercise, you will create a powerful motivational tool to refer to when you feel challenged in the early stages of change, when the novelty of getting going may have worn off a bit. The letter you will write is to be written by past (and current you), for future you. While writing, try to visualise all times when you felt that you desperately want to change for good, when you've thought 'I never thought it would get to this stage. Something has to change once and for all.'

While I certainly don't want you to be feeling at your most fed up right at this second, it is those moments we want to capture for this exercise. For me, writing this letter involved thinking about crying in changing rooms, feeling too self-conscious and sweaty to dance at a wedding and walking home from the GP.

'That's It' Letter

I'd like you to now grab a notebook and write your own 'That's It' letter. Copy out and build on any of the following cues I've listed that makes sense for you personally. The more you write, the better. If you find yourself writing pages and pages, and going off on different branches from the first cue, go with it and see where it takes you! Don't feel under pressure to work through this or any of the other exercises in this book like a tick-box process or a questionnaire. They are designed to draw out wisdom you already have – not tell you exactly what to do.

They're here to help you be your own therapist and client at the same time. Let's go!

It's [insert date],

I've decided to try The Last Diet because . . .

I'm frustrated that . . .

Not making changes is negatively impacting my life in ways like . . .

Once and for all it's time to . . .

By now I thought I would have . . .

I know it would make me happier if I stopped . . .

Carrying on like this will mean that . . .

I would currently describe my relationship with food as . . .

I would currently describe my relationship with my body as . . .

I would currently describe my self-esteem as being . . .

At the moment my body feels . . .

Some of my reasons for wanting to change are things I don't want to share with anyone else. Things I'm not proud of. It's time to be honest with myself and admit that these include . . .

If, over the next weeks, I'm tempted to trivialise how important it is for me to change, I need to remember that . . .

I never thought I'd get to the stage where I'm . . .

If I start finding it harder than I expected, I want to remember it's important to push through because . . .

I need to take this seriously because . . .

There are other, related habits I'll need to change as well, these are things like . . .

I want to feel like I'm . . .

There are so many things that maintaining the status quo is holding me back from doing, like . . .

That's it!

[*Signature*]

Congratulations! You've started on your process of change! To mark the day you started The Last Diet, I suggest that you commit to introducing one tiny self-care ritual into your morning routine as of tomorrow. I mean tiny, and it needn't obviously have anything to do with losing weight. Anything that makes your body feel cared for and reminds you that things have changed as of today. It can be anything from setting a reminder alarm to stretch for one minute before you get in the shower, deciding to brew fresh coffee for yourself instead of grabbing the instant, or putting on music while you get ready for work. Something that reminds you that things have started to change for the better and you've embarked on a mission.

Ritual declaration

As of tomorrow I will _____ every day, just to make my life a little more pleasant. I'll remind myself to do it by _____.

no more mondays

Creating urgency to get going

I often hear people say, 'I know what I need to do, I just can't seem to get going.' I can absolutely relate to this. Especially when it comes to starting plans of change around eating habits and general self-care.

Until a few years ago, my life was essentially a cycle of full-bellied, well-intentioned, meticulously planned Sunday night resolutions, followed by deprived and emotional Mondays and finally compulsive, impulsive binges on foods I had deemed 'forbidden' by Tuesday night. That would continue on a loop until Sunday came around again. And of course, the Sundays kept coming around, and those binges added up over time to make me feel more weak, tired, out of control and disconnected from my body. The goals I set for myself were unrealistic, not suited to my body and didn't take into consideration that I'd wake up on Monday feeling hungry and lacking in emotional and physical resilience after another week of treating myself unkindly.

Often it took something as obvious as New Year's Eve or a birthday, or receiving an email from a boot camp I signed up to twenty-five Sunday nights ago to make me realise that with every week I said 'I'll start again on Monday', I was moving myself further away from having the relationship with my body that I ultimately wanted.

The mapping exercises later in this chapter are designed to help you bring about an urgency to change – that spark to 'get going'. They will involve you choosing a date in the future and mapping out two possible outcomes for yourself. Writing that date down will remind you that it's coming around whether you commit to making changes or not. First though, it is important to get excited about the future and remind yourself that this time around you're going to be considering how you can improve your wellbeing and prioritise self-care in every aspect of how you treat your body. That's what these next preparatory exercises will help you to do.

Written Exercise: No More Mondays: Part 1

For this first written exercise, answer the following question in as much detail as you can. Take time to paint a clear picture in your response, taking into consideration all the different life areas that you hope will have changed for the better:

> In six months' time, if I asked the people closest to you what they've noticed has changed in terms of how you look and how you treat yourself, what would you like them to say?

_____

_____

_____

Let's now zoom in a little bit and start to get a clearer idea of your long-term goals in a nutshell, by using the following cues. Try to finish as many of these sentences as you can, depending on which are most relevant to you, and include as many different changes that come to mind.

Written Exercise: No More Mondays: Part 2

In six months' time, I want to be doing more . . .

_____

_____

_____

In six months' time, I want to be doing less . . .

_____

_____

_____

In six months' time, I want to be more . . .

_____

_____

_____

In six months' time, I want to be less . . .

_____

_____

_____

In six months' time, I want to feel more in control of . . .

_____

_____

_____

In six months' time, I want to have started . . .

_____

_____

_____

In six months' time, I want to have stopped . . .

_____

_____

_____

Briefly put, I'll know I've achieved my goals when I've:

_____

_____

_____

E.g. *changed my relationship with food, lost weight and started treating myself more kindly*

Map: No More Mondays: Part 3

Now, get out your notebook and in the middle of a blank page, write 'If I haven't . . .' followed by your final response in the part 2 exercise you just completed. Then write a date in the future underneath and draw a circle around them both together. When it comes to choosing what date to write, for the purpose of this exercise, I recommend six to twelve months from the date you wrote your 'That's It' letter.

If you're anything like me, this suggestion will immediately annoy you because it sounds like you won't be able to see results for ages. Worry not, when it comes to making practical changes to bring about any desired weight loss, you can go at whatever speed keeps you feeling strong and happy. Provided how you're eating helps your body to feel energetic, balanced and comfortable, you can design whatever eating habits are going to work for you and start losing weight immediately.

However, when it comes to addressing things that challenge the sustainability of your changes in the long term – like negative self-talk, self-sabotage and low self-esteem – there's no way around it: a deeper, more forward-thinking approach needs to be taken. One that considers all areas of your life and how you engage with the world around you as well as how you feel about your body. Irritating as it is, The Last Diet is the opposite of a crash diet, and there aren't any shortcuts. And while I'm already throwing around clichés about weight loss that used to annoy the hell out of me, I may as well share something I've observed in a lot of people trying to keep off lost weight: the quicker you lose it, the quicker you put it back on. Just my two cents.

Back to your map. Around the title and date you've already written, make notes to describe:

- How you are likely to be looking and feeling in your body if you haven't made changes

- The kinds of things you are likely to be saying to yourself and others about your body

- The kinds of things you are likely to be saying to yourself and others about how capable you are

- How your social life is likely to be looking

- How your relationships have been directly or indirectly impacted

- What the impact on your self-esteem is likely to be

- Ways you might have proven others – or yourself – right

- Ways your other habits may have changed as well

- Feedback you might be getting from those around you

- How you are likely to be spending your time, money and energy

- How you'll be feeling in general

When you're finished, put that map to one side for a moment.

Map: No More Mondays: Part 4

Now, on a new page, I'd like you to recreate the structure of the last map, writing down the same future date you chose before. The only difference is that you write 'If I have . . .' and again insert the same following sentence as before in the centre of the page, and draw a circle around it.

A note before you begin: try not to fall into the trap of simply populating this map with the opposite of what you wrote on the first map – in fact, put that map somewhere you can't see it. Think creatively about the many differences you might experience. Be ambitious for yourself; go into detail describing what this more favourable outcome would look and feel like for you across every possible life area. Describe:

- How you are likely to be looking and feeling in your body if you have made changes

- The kinds of things you are likely to be saying to yourself and others about your body

- The kinds of things you are likely to be saying to yourself and others about how capable you are

- How your social life is likely to be looking

- How your relationships have been directly or indirectly impacted

- What the impact on your self-esteem is likely to be

- Ways you might have proven others – or yourself – wrong

- Ways your other habits may have changed as well

- Feedback you might be getting from those around you

- How you're likely to be spending your time, money and energy

- How you'll be feeling in general

Reflection: No More Mondays: Part 5

Now, hold the last two maps side by side and compare the different outcomes. Note how it makes you feel to see the difference between them.

Although this exercise should bring about a sense of urgency to begin and stay on track, it will only be truly effective during this early part of the process, where I am assuming a few things may be the case:

- You're currently basing some or all of your worthiness to enjoy life on your body and/or your relationship with food

- You don't speak in a kind or encouraging manner towards yourself when you're not happy with how your body looks or how you've eaten

- You're highly alert to how other people may be judging your body or eating habits and still sensitive to what they think. Perhaps their voices or those of the media seem louder than yours, even when it comes to what choices you make for your body

- During times when you are neglecting or abusing your body in terms of food and exercise, you are taking an all-or-nothing and perhaps self-sabotaging approach to other areas of your life too

- You currently think that not looking how you want to look means you can't truly enjoy yourself in various settings

- You live life 'on hold' and still assume that there are certain things you can't do/wear/see/experience unless you've achieved weight-loss goals

From the next chapter onwards, the exercises I'm going to ask you to do will be focused on changing all of these beliefs about who you are, what you're capable of and what kind of life you deserve. That's why, soon, the comparison exercise you just did won't work quite as well again. Because by the end of this process you will have committed to disassociating your worthiness for joy, self-care and self-compassion from how you look or what you eat.

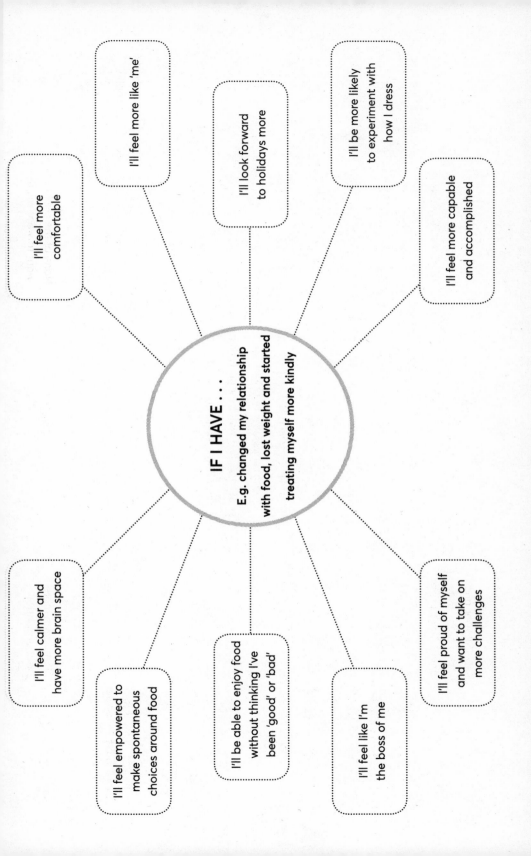

IF I HAVE...

E.g. changed my relationship with food, lost weight and started treating myself more kindly

I'll feel more comfortable

I'll feel more like 'me'

I'll look forward to holidays more

I'll be more likely to experiment with how I dress

I'll feel more capable and accomplished

I'll feel calmer and have more brain space

I'll feel empowered to make spontaneous choices around food

I'll be able to enjoy food without thinking I've been 'good' or 'bad'

I'll feel like I'm the boss of me

I'll feel proud of myself and want to take on more challenges

your body can

Losing weight is the least of what you're capable of

For many years, the only time I felt proud of my body was when it was managing to achieve a weight I was happy with, and look slim. I didn't acknowledge it in any other way – for example, when it managed to recover quickly after an operation. I didn't think the hair on its head deserved to be given care and attention unless it was growing out of the top of a slim face. If you asked me how much of my opinion of my body being attractive or healthy was tied up in my weight, for most of my life I would have said at least 90 per cent.

I've learned through my work that a lot of people can relate to feeling their opinion of their body is determined by their thoughts on what size they are. Most of us don't really stop to think about what our bodies have accomplished unless something is put in place to bring it to our attention. Perhaps giving birth or maybe a challenging physical expedition.

In the past, whenever I reached a goal weight, I'd feel temporarily euphoric. That day I would be on cloud nine. I wasn't at risk of succumbing to temptations. I felt strong because I was proud of myself and my body. Before long though, this would wear off and I wouldn't experience that powerful and euphoric feeling again until the next time the scales showed I'd lost weight.

I want to help you to change how you speak to your body about all it's capable of in addition to losing weight, so you can recreate that feeling of pride and therefore resilience every day. Think about the times when you talk to yourself and others about your body's abilities. How much of it is concerned with how it is serving you versus how it's not?

Naturally, this is partly because we take for granted our body's ability to complete basic functions. Many of us only come to acknowledge our bodies' power when it's brought to our attention how many people aren't as lucky. And when we go to the GP, it's remedial, it's to identify what's wrong, not what's strong. We're reminded every time we catch a common cold how debilitating and horrible it can be, yet when we're well we don't walk around saying, 'I'm really glad I don't have a cold today.'

This chapter is designed to help you realise that your body is more than capable of achieving your weight-loss goals, whatever they may be, and it provides an opportunity for you to record the amazing things your body has managed to accomplish in the past. Completing the 'My Body Can' map will mark the first step towards achieving the ultimate goal of shifting your thoughts so they focus on your assets more than your perceived deficits. It will remind you of how strong, resilient and useful your body is – and has always been.

Focusing on that evidence will help you to achieve your weight-loss goals far more effectively than focusing on what you wish your body didn't do, feel or look like. By shifting the focus from what you think your body can't do to what it can do, you will draw your attention to the unique combination of assets and resources you already possess. Some of which will play a direct role in you losing weight.

You will also learn to draw your attention more easily to all of your body's assets that are worthy of acknowledgment and care. Regardless of your size, your skin weathers tough conditions and deserves to be treated with care. Regardless of your weight, your spine deserves a stretching routine since it allows you to sit at a computer all day without having back problems. When you realise that your body has been your friend, and that all parts of it deserve to be treated well in every way, then what and how you eat becomes just one of those many ways.

One way to repay the favours your body has done (and to keep them coming) is to demonstrate more gratitude towards it across all areas of your life, and not just when it manages not to eat a second dessert or drag itself to the gym, but every day all day as it helps you navigate life.

Developing a kind attitude towards your whole body, one that takes the spotlight *off* your weight specifically, will actually help you to lose weight and keep it off. That's because the practice of identifying as many reasons as possible to treat all of your body well creates loads of opportunities to adopt a new range of kind habits. Ones that may not seem to have much to do with keeping off unwanted weight, but absolutely do. I believe that paying long-term attention to more subtle, seemingly unrelated self-care habits is what creates the stable foundation on which to maintain a weight you're happy with.

My process of successfully learning to care for my body regardless of its size has relied heavily on regularly bringing to my daily attention the ways in which I'm capable already. That's what the map in this chapter will help you to do for yourself. It's essentially a collection of ways your body has demonstrated that it's able to do difficult things.

Once you commit to regularly looking at and developing this map, you'll gradually notice a shift: what you're writing and reading about yourself will start to influence how you're thinking and feeling and behaving towards yourself. That's why, years from now, you'll only use this map as an ongoing record of your achievements and a motivational boost. You'll no longer need to refer to it immediately at times when your body feels challenged; you won't need regular visual reminders because you'll have developed a strong enough belief in your body to withstand short-term discomfort. You'll have developed a new habit of challenging your own self-doubting thoughts and beliefs by being able to quickly draw on recent and varied examples that disprove them. Examples of things your body has already achieved, survived and overcome. The times it's done you a favour without asking for much in return.

Map: My Body Can

I would like you to give this map a theme, by writing 'My Body Can' in the middle of a blank page, with a circle drawn around it. Then, note down your answers to the following questions anywhere you'd like on the page, drawing circles around each one of them as you go.

- What has your body managed to survive/endure/recover from over the years?

- What has your body helped/allowed you to accomplish?

- What has your body done to demonstrate how strong, resilient and capable it is?

- What does your body enable you to do on a daily basis?

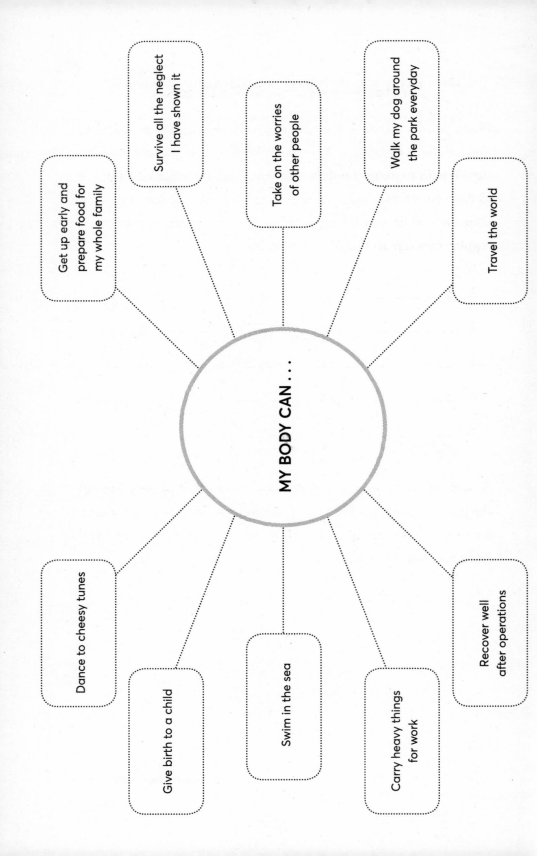

Written Exercise: My Body Deserves

Once you've acknowledged what your body is capable of, note down some suggestions of new self-care habits you could adopt to treat it with more gratitude. Ones that may not be directly related to diet or exercise. Anything from deciding to play music to please your ears while you do household chores to booking yourself a regular massage to thank your muscles.

1. _____

2. _____

3. _____

4. _____

5. _____

As with all of the exercises in this book, this one is intended to get the juices flowing. Ideally you will feel you are always on the search for new and practical ways to treat your body with the care and consideration it needs and deserves.

your body has

Focusing on your strengths

Now it's time to look at all the amazing things about your body; the purpose of this chapter is to apply this same principle to increasing your self-esteem by drawing your attention to the things you like about yourself. I will help you to create a collection of positive qualities that your body possesses. Learning to like yourself more will then help in convincing you that you're deserving of being treated with care, consideration and respect.

I often ask my clients to tell me how they think someone who really likes themselves and is happy in their body behaves on a daily basis. They often respond with suggestions like, 'They drink lots of water, they sit up straight, they take pride in their appearance, they're confident, they take vitamins, they are active and energetic, and eat things like vegetables and fish.'

This answer tells us two interesting things:

1. That whether or not they know how to keep it up, my clients already know what to do to practically lose weight. So even if they just *pretended* they were someone who liked themselves more, they'd probably manage to do that

2. That they believe being worthy of acting kindly towards their body in general is dependent on the weight and size of it at any given time. I know this because they automatically assume the person I'm asking them to describe in my question (the one who likes their body) is slim. I believe that in order to achieve long-term, sustained and meaningful weight loss, this belief needs to change

At some stage of our lives, for many different reasons, some of us started believing that being able to like our bodies was dependent on the size or weight of them. I won't patronise you by explaining why that's sad. But it's often why many people have a lot of unlearning to do when it comes to separating body weight and size from body likeability and worthiness. Years of ingrained habits will of course mean that there is often emotional and physical resistance and delay. For many of us, it is not as simple as adopting all the habits of a slim person. A deeper, more considered approach is needed to change how we think about our bodies.

But I don't want my clients and readers to have to wait until they've done loads of mindset shifting before they can get going with the actual weight loss. So I don't ask them to act like the person they *wish* they were. I simply ask them to immediately start realising and acting like the person they already are. I help them to do this by asking them to list all the things they like about all the different parts of their body, as you'll do later in this chapter.

One challenge faced by many clients who have learned to associate liking their bodies with being slim is that they struggle to identify positive qualities, especially at the times when they're not at a weight they want to be. They forget that their bodies are made up of eyebrows, skin, the shape of their forearms, their ankles, their toes, hair, muscles and other completely unique and beautiful features. Not to mention the qualities that have enabled them to accomplish the things they wrote on their 'My Body Can' map.

The idea is that when you look at a collection of positive qualities you already possess and things your body has managed to do, you can start to think, 'That is a person who deserves to be treated well. That is a person I imagine has a lot of self-esteem. That is a person who is totally capable and worthy of achieving any goal they like.' In this way, you can start to see the contrast between the person you actually already are, and the person you treat your body as though you are. When you focus on the qualities you don't possess, you're more likely to make the day-to-day choices of someone who doesn't feel worthy of aspiring to and achieving ambitious goals.

So this isn't just an 'it's nice to be nice' exercise. While you're busy creating tiny new habits that treat all of your body with the kindness it already deserves, you'll start to naturally enjoy the benefits you don't think it deserves (yet). Your body and mind can start taking care of the weight loss while you're busy taking care of your body and mind.

This idea of embodying who I already am was one of the earliest and most important shifts that helped me to lose weight both quickly and meaningfully. It came as a result of a therapy session I had when I was at one of my heaviest stages. I was once again telling the counsellor about all the things I intended to do when I was slim. Things like wearing nice jewellery and heels, going on dates, jogging in the park. And she asked me a question that really angered me: 'What if you're never slim?'

I can't tell you how much this suggestion enraged me. So much so that I drafted break-up messages during the days after this session. Not losing weight was simply not an option that had ever crossed my mind. For as long as I could remember, I believed that I could only truly enjoy my life when I was slim, and that during the stages when I wasn't slim, my main focus had to be getting slim again so I could enjoy my life again.

Once the anger subsided, I started realising that my way of thinking had resulted in me living huge chunks of my life completely 'on hold', not least since my slim phases were always very brief. By 'on hold', I don't even mean just not going out much because clothes didn't fit. I mean not lighting candles, not using nice face creams, not drinking nice bottles of wine, not listening to music. By assuming that these were only things people who liked themselves (because they were thin) did, I was depriving myself of so much self-care, enjoyment and motivation.

Many times when I was very overweight, I would buy clothes that were three sizes too small for me and hang them around my flat as a reminder of what I wanted to achieve. Any time spent not being slim was time spent planning to get slim again, without any consideration for the parts of my body that weren't directly related to losing weight.

So I made a list of the things I was waiting until I was slim to do, and really asked myself whether being able or worthy of doing them was dependent on my size. Turns out none of it was. I started doing the things on that list. It turned out that a lot of the habits I developed with the period of living life 'on hold' were actually contributing to my weight gain. Habits like being at home by myself for long periods either snacking mindlessly or starving while I browsed online for a dress I could maybe wear in four months' time if I stayed hungry until then.

Once I stopped living my life on hold, not only did I enjoy it more, but I lost weight more quickly than I had before. Embracing the kind habits I deserved, regardless of my size, across every possible aspect of my life actually made it difficult for the unkind food habits to fit in anymore. I noticed that when I lit those candles, put on that music, picked out that jumper I was keeping for a special 'thin' occasion or meditated for ten minutes, the environment wasn't so welcoming to unkind food habits. I discovered I could pepper my day with so much self-care that my stubborn unwanted eating habits – like eating compulsively out of anger or sadness – started looking and feeling out of place.

Here are some of the self-care habits that work for me at the time of writing this book. I change them every few months, as my routine and needs change or I discover something new I want to add.

When I wake up in the morning, I purposefully abstain from looking at my phone, and instead put out a yoga mat to have a stretch. I quite often consciously take a couple minutes more in the shower than I need to, just enjoy it. I try to make sure I eat some fruit, I moisturise my body well, use my favourite mug for coffee and take pride in my clothing choices – it then just doesn't feel right to eat three croissants mindlessly on the tube. It's like every time I make even the smallest kind choice for myself, it impacts the next one, and the one after that. It just so happens that over the course of every day, some of my choices involve food and exercise. They're just mixed in with all the kindness.

There's less resistance to change when you've made it easy to slot new eating habits into an established self-care framework. The following exercise will help you feel more deserving and motivated to create that framework.

Map: My Body Has

First I'd like you to write 'My Body Has' in the middle of the page with a circle drawn around it. Then simply start noting down all the things you like about any and every aspect of your body, drawing circles around each one of those as you go. What bits of it do you like and why? Which would you not like to change and why? Try to keep your entries as brief as possible on this map. No more than a few words for each one.

Note: When you start writing these down, notice any caveats that pop up. Do you feel resistance when you try to believe you really possess positive qualities? Perhaps you went to write 'beautiful hair' and immediately thought, 'Well it could be better, it does need a cut, it's never been as shiny as my sister's.' All I ask for now is that you notice that, and write down the positive quality nonetheless.

Learning to own and believe in our positive qualities is a hugely important part of this process. Firstly of course because we deserve to focus on what we like about ourselves and it makes for a nicer life. But also because when we feel totally secure in the knowledge that we possess loads of indisputably positive qualities, we can take on useful advice and criticism more easily without becoming defensive. In my experience, the people who are most willing to consider how they could change for the better are the ones who feel very clear in why they like themselves whether or not they change.

When you've completed this map you'll have a collection of your body's self-identified positive qualities. The idea is that glancing at this will help you want to create more self-care habits – at moments when you want to neglect or do a disservice to your body's needs in any way, I want you to look at it and think, 'That's a body worth treating well.'

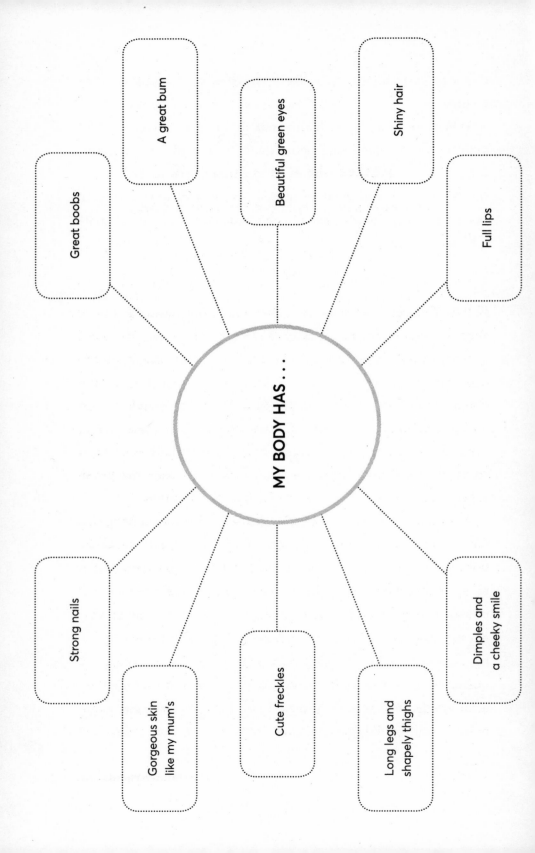

your soundtrack

Turning urges from commands into alerts

People often come to me because their behaviour around food and abuse of their bodies has made them feel out of control. They feel they are trapped in a cycle of behaving in ways they don't want to and that they can't withstand the short-term physical and emotional discomfort of making changes for long enough to see meaningful and lasting results. Clients often describe their urgent, compulsive and impulsive actions towards their bodies when it comes to eating habits as being very reactionary: when the physical craving or emotional need arises they feel powerless.

A big part of adopting The Last Diet effectively is realising that our actions are determined by internal commands and conversations that we have with ourselves. Ultimately, we decide whether to act in a certain way. It doesn't matter how hungry we are and how delicious something we're trying to avoid looks, that craving doesn't physically force our hands to pick it up and eat it. What happens is, we tell ourselves a story about the situation, and about ourselves. This often happens very quickly, and so it isn't until we acknowledge that it is happening, look at our patterns and externalise what's going on that we can start to slow down the decision-making process when it comes to how we act towards our bodies. We can commit to turning a physical or emotional craving into an alert as opposed to a command. We do this by compassionately and curiously examining what those commands are and where they came from, before practising ways to catch them, change them and create new ones.

When I began to look consciously at my internal commands, I found the shift that it brought about to be life changing. By doing exercises like the ones in this book to change the conversations I have with my body, I have changed how I speak to myself about everything. That's the thing with The Last Diet; as soon as you really commit to practising the self-awareness and self-esteem tools, you find yourself using them in every other possible area of your life.

Through working with clients to change their habits around food, I have come to realise that we all have a very unique internal soundtrack playing most of the time. One that's made up of assumptions and beliefs about ourselves, others and the situations we're in. One that ultimately dictates how we act. When we're faced with the decision of how to react to a challenging situation or feeling, that soundtrack becomes very important.

Despite how long we've spent beating ourselves up for it, I have been very pleasantly surprised at how quickly myself, and my clients who want to lose weight, have been able to change years of negative self-talk. I think that may be because, when working with issues of weight, we have so many opportunities to practise throughout the day! Being challenged with constant food choices turns up the volume on our soundtrack; it helps us to listen in on our commands more clearly and notice the same unhelpful ones popping up over and over again. If you have spent a lifetime listening to a negative soundtrack about your body and eating habits, you'll have many opportunities throughout the day to listen in on what it is telling you to do.

Applying The Last Diet to change your commands about food will of course help you to lose as much weight as you'd like. To keep it off however, you need to feel capable. For that to feel authentic, you need evidence of having survived physical cravings and self-doubt and come out the other side unharmed. Since short-term discomfort is a volume-increaser on our internal commands, one way to gather new evidence of how resilient you are in general is this:

1. Pick a habit you want to change

2. Identify the challenges you're most sceptical about being able to overcome when trying to change

3. Decide that you'll now be consciously facing these challenges head on, and putting yourself in that discomfort on purpose. Not for something as basic as losing weight, but so that you can do a check-in on the current unhelpful commands you have about them

Challenges turn up the volume and give us invaluable insight into why we're finding it so difficult to change. We just have to choose to tune in on purpose and with purpose. The smallest tweaks to the status quo can be used to turn up those conversations you have with yourself and draw out the wisdom you need to change your commands.

One of my clients recently described how she noticed her internal dialogue change as a result of applying just two of my suggestions to her daily routine: 1) First thing in the morning, look in the mirror and acknowledge one thing you like about your body out loud. 2) When 4pm comes around, have three fingers of KitKat instead of all four as you usually would.

I received an email from this client one week after our first session, reporting her findings:

Hi Shahroo,

So, I tried out the mirror and KitKat missions. To be honest, when I left our session I thought they sounded too easy. Then I tried them and was shocked to discover what I did.

When I tried to stand in front of the mirror and say out loud just one thing I liked about my body, I heard:

This is so stupid.

Who are you kidding? This self-love stuff isn't for you. Just stop eating so much.

This is actually making me notice more things I don't like about myself.

Eurgh, I feel gross, I don't want to do this.

I'm just going to say whatever. My eyebrows. Although my aunt always used to say they were an odd shape.

You already look awful, who cares what you put in your body.

When I tried to leave one finger of KitKat in the afternoon, I heard:

You're not the kind of person who can just leave it. You never have been.

People are starving in the world, just eat it.

This is stupid, you can start tomorrow.

You need it, you're stressed.

You should eat it, you're already being bad for eating KitKats at all.

As you can see, the commands I'm giving myself don't have my best interests at heart. They don't have much faith in me at all.

For this client, it was incredibly impactful to realise that her internal dialogue was making the process of change so much more difficult than it needed to be. After the initial shock of how unhelpful she'd been to herself in her soundtrack, she resolved to create tiny tweaks across various areas of her life, just to turn up the volume and check in with what she'd been telling herself she could do or could not do without even realising.

How you speak to yourself in general will determine whether you get back on track – and stay there – in the event that you deviate from your weight-loss plan. Let's say for example you've stuck to an eating plan that you're really happy with. You've been following your own guidelines for two weeks – so long enough to feel proud of yourself, but not long enough to have addressed and changed all-or-nothing thinking patterns and self-sabotaging messages about food and your relationship with it. You get invited to a dinner party at someone's house and when you get there, you realise that eating anything they've cooked would mean you went off-plan. You don't say anything, and decide you have no choice but to eat it. You know, logically, rationally speaking, that this one evening will not derail all of your efforts to date. You know that one meal will not be responsible for weight gain. What *will* be responsible for it is what you do after that meal. The twenty meals you choose to have after it will depend on the conversation you have with yourself; what you tell yourself that one meal meant about you and the situation you were in.

There will come a point in this process when you will need to identify more practically, clearly and in detail what eating plan you would like to implement in order to lose weight. As you will have gathered by now, I believe it's no business of mine what you decide to eat or not eat and how many times (if any) you decide to exercise in order to reach your goals. My focus will be on helping you to identify which of these three conditions you are in in relation to your chosen 'way of eating' at any given time:

1. On track

2. Lapse

3. Relapse

Later on, you will have more clarity on what each of these conditions looks like for you. Broadly speaking, being 'on track' means that you're keeping to whatever eating, exercise and personal development plan you've assigned for yourself. Lapsing is a deviation from this plan and relapsing is when you've fully returned to old, unwanted habits.

The conversation we have with ourselves determines whether a lapse turns into a relapse. In this process, mastering lapse management by changing your internal commands will enable you to master weight management and still enjoy the more fattening foods you love. I now manage my weight practically speaking, by spending about 70 per cent of the time sticking to whatever my 'on track' is and 30 per cent lapsing at will, safe in the knowledge I'll immediately get back on track.

Since my internal dialogue no longer tells me to lapse again immediately (and even if it does, I've demonstrated it's not the boss of me), my weight isn't affected. By using the exercises in this book, I've learned to 'listen in' on my commands and self-doubting thoughts, and challenge them with genuine facts; I've developed a bullshit filter for all-or-nothing, self-sabotaging thinking. I still hear it now and then, but it just doesn't put forward a compelling argument. Just because I had one meal and woke up predictably craving sugar doesn't mean I am forced to not get back on track immediately.

In the next exercise, you shine a light on how you've been speaking to yourself in those moments when the script is most important. This will in turn help you understand the kinds of commands you'll be giving yourself about what the next step should be after a lapse. Resist the temptation to downplay any parts of your internal conversation because it causes you discomfort when you see it all written down. One of the unfortunate realities of making meaningful shifts by becoming more self-aware is that sometimes things have to get a tiny bit harder before they get a whole lot easier.

Map: My Soundtrack: Part 1

Start by writing 'My Soundtrack' in the middle of a blank page with a circle around it. Now, think back to times when you've attempted to change your eating and exercise habits but failed to keep it up. What kinds of things did you say to yourself in those moments when you realised you'd 'failed' at keeping up your plan? Write down the messages you give yourself in those moments and draw a circle around each one as you go.

Next, move on to the things you say to yourself in general when you're finding something more difficult than you think you should, or you feel you've let yourself down in some way. For example, if you make a mistake at work, or snap at a loved one and later feel guilty about it.

Finally, write down the things you say about your body specifically when you don't manage to stick to a weight-loss or exercise plan.

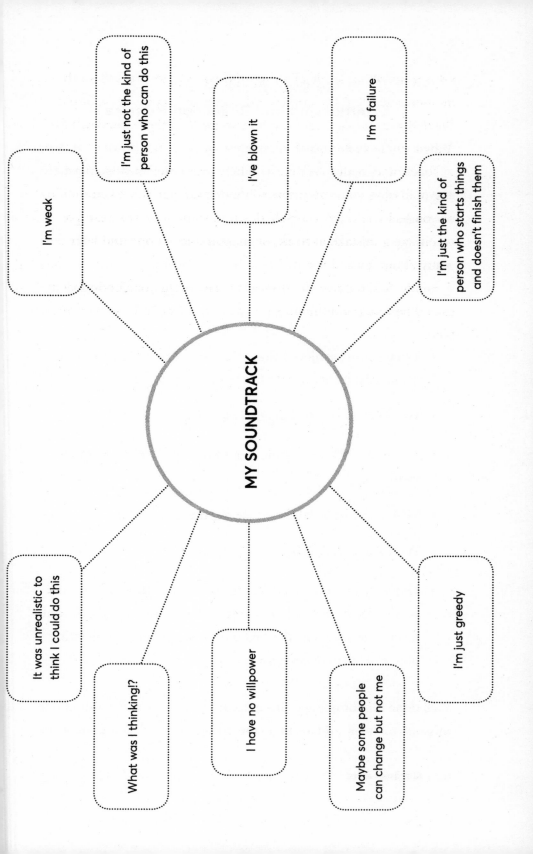

My Soundtrack: Part 2 – Externalising and Reflection Exercise

When you feel like you've completed the map, put down your pen, sit back and really look at it. Then, read out loud (somewhere private) what you've written. Consider how it feels to hear these messages.

Now, go through each message again, and ask yourself the following questions about it. Make notes as you go on any of your answers that provide new insight on why you've developed the soundtrack that you have.

- What have I achieved that challenges this and proves that it's at least partly unfair, false or exaggerated?

- Would I say this to someone else? If not, why not?

- Is it useful? Does hearing it get me any closer to where I want to be?

- When and why did I start saying this to myself?

- Who else's voice does this sound like?

- Did someone else make me think this was true? If so, who was it? When was it? Do I respect their opinion? Do I want to live the way they do? Should their opinions be dictating how I behave towards myself?

Well done for completing this map. It's not an easy one, but in our mission to hear and change the soundtrack of commands for good, we've got to first understand what we're up against – and that's often years of outdated, unhelpful, untrue yet truly compelling core beliefs about ourselves and what we're capable of. Finishing this chapter is a good opportunity to acknowledge that you no longer want to speak to yourself unkindly. That you realise now it's unhelpful in every possible way. That you will commit to observing then questioning any cruel or unfair assumptions about how capable you are of achieving even your most ambitious weight-loss goals. And that you will reframe tiny challenges throughout your day as opportunities to choose to check in with how you're speaking to yourself.

cheerleading

Becoming your own motivational coach

When it comes to supporting the people we care about, most of us think we know how to give decent advice and that we recognise what kinds of messages make people feel strong, empowered, resilient and able to overcome a hurdle. But for various reasons some of us developed a habit of not applying that same wisdom when it came to supporting ourselves. We became skilled at being able to sit in front of our loved ones and tell them that they are capable and strong and worthy of achieving ambitious goals, all the while showing ourselves in how we behave towards our own bodies that we don't think we are capable or strong or worthy of doing the same.

I often ask my clients how they would react if someone they loved and respected was beating themselves up about having behaved in a way they weren't happy with. Without fail, everyone responds that they would say things like 'Don't worry about it! You didn't set out to do it! These things happen, don't beat yourself up about it! Worrying won't change anything, everyone makes mistakes, this doesn't deserve to ruin your day.' And yet very few people can recall the last time they spoke to themselves like this when they had a blip and lapsed from a healthy eating plan, forgot someone's birthday or made a blunder at work.

Making changes is hard, especially in the early stages. Your motivation to stay on track will waver and you will need pep talks. You'll need reminders of why you're doing this and why it's important, as well as why you're capable of withstanding short-term discomfort to achieve your long-term goals. Essentially, you'll need a wise, protective, enthusiastic coach who has every faith in you and keeps you motivated around the clock. Since you're the only person who's with you twenty-four hours a day (plus you're the only one who truly knows all of your most private of motivations) you're the best candidate for the job.

Before you can start though, you'll need a script. Because you may well have discovered in the last chapter that your current script won't motivate anyone to do anything for long. You'll also need to hand yourself over to the process a little bit, and push through the initial discomfort of how unnatural it feels to encourage and motivate yourself. You may well find it difficult to feel that you deserve to be supported and championed in the same way that someone you love deserves to be supported and championed. So, to get around that possible stumbling block, we're now going to draw that motivating script out of you – the one you already know.

Map: Cheerleading: Part 1

First, think of someone you love dearly. Someone you really believe in and for whom you wish nothing but success. A person you would be prepared to help in any way they needed if it meant they could be happier. Write their name down in the centre of a blank page in your notebook and draw a circle around it.

Then, imagine this person comes to you and says that they're struggling to lose weight and it's really upsetting them. They don't think they're capable of achieving their goals and don't feel like they deserve success. They tell you that they don't have the strength to stay on track and feel disappointed in themselves for lapsing so often. Imagine your task is to help them get back on track and believe in themselves as quickly as possible. Write down everything you would say to them, and what you'd advise them to do. Draw a circle around each statement as you go along.

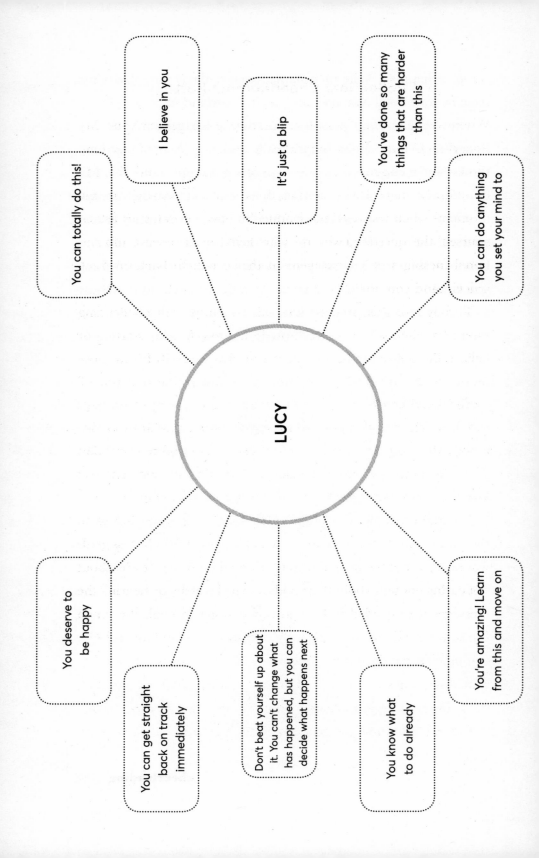

Reflection: Cheerleading: Part 2

When you've finished your 'Cheerleading' map, get out your 'My Soundtrack' map and compare the two. The Cheerleading map shows the messages you believe motivate people and the My Soundtrack map shows the messages you give yourself in the moments when you need motivating. So now you can start asking yourself the question, why do your loved ones deserve motivational messages of encouragement that get them back on track quickly, and you don't?

Throughout this process, you will be faced with challenging moments when you want to throw in the towel, delay starting or believe the self-doubting messages you give yourself. It's in those moments that it's most important that you step into that role of motivational coach. Where you decide you're going to be your own best friend and choose new messages and commands to give a body that you are learning to love and respect more every day. The good news is you already know how to motivate someone you love. You have the script there on your Cheerleading map.

For many people, reflecting on these two exercises brings to their attention that their inability to achieve their weight-loss goals was never about being unable to motivate themselves. It was about not caring enough about their bodies to feel worthy of hearing the messages they needed to hear in order to get through the tough times. It was about unconsciously obeying all-or-nothing, self-defeating commands and framing a lapse as a failure as opposed to something that can be learned from, engaged in consciously and, most importantly, immediately bounced back to 'on track' from.

I have found time and time again that the simplest way to start helping people treat and speak to themselves with more kindness all day and in every way is to pretend they are living in the body of someone they love.

One of my clients was a single father who worked long hours and found it difficult to manage the stress of day-to-day life without taking comfort in convenient fast food, even though he felt it was making him feel sluggish and irritable with his children and his colleagues. His food choices were causing him to gain unwanted weight. He would snack throughout the day on the same stuff; mainly foods that gave him a quick hit but then caused his energy levels to slump. He would eat mindlessly and on the go, not taking time to present his meals in a way that made them look appealing. He wanted to lose weight in order to feel more mobile when playing with his children and to set a good example for them, so he came to me for help.

I noticed during our first conversation that many of his reasons to change involved giving his children the best possible quality of life. He knew that taking better care of his body was the way to be able to do that long term, but when it came to his day-to-day choices for himself, his own needs were always last when it came to the smallest acts of kindness, respect and consideration.

So I set him this mission: imagine one of your daughters is living on her own for the first time. She's setting a precedent and creating a new 'normal' for how she will treat her body and what kind of routine she will have when no one is there to supervise her anymore. This includes how often she exercises or gets some fresh air; what choices she makes when she wants a snack; how she consumes alcohol and sugar; how much time and consideration she takes choosing ingredients for the meals she makes. Imagine her sitting down eating a meal at dinnertime. How would you like to think her food would be presented, and how would she be eating it? Would it be in a rushed manner, grabbing whatever she can get that gives her a quick fix? Or in a mindful way where she can show her body respect?

Once he had imagined it in detail, I asked the client to simply resolve to spend the next week treating himself as he'd like his daughter to treat herself when it came to food, exercise and general wellbeing decisions. I asked that whenever he went to buy an unhealthy snack, he considered whether he'd want his daughter to make that same choice for her body. I asked that when it came to deciding whether to put in the extra time and effort to prepare a meal from scratch for himself (one that he knew would be better for his body and mind than one that took two minutes to make), he made the same decision he'd want his daughter to make for herself.

After three weeks or so, I heard back from this client and he told me he was still doing the exercise every day. He said that it helped him open his eyes to all the healthier substitutes there were available when he wanted a snack – he had just needed to give it a bit more thought. And he hadn't realised quite how little he cared for his body until he saw how many times a day he was treating it extremely differently to how he'd want someone he loved to treat theirs. Naturally he'd also lost weight, but as is the case with all of my clients, achieving the goals they initially set out to achieve quickly becomes a bonus, a by-product of learning to treat themselves more kindly in every possible way throughout the day.

not your bag

Acknowledging the approaches that don't work for you

I don't know about you, but I feel extremely overwhelmed with how much conflicting advice is going around when it comes to the healthiest way to lose and manage weight. The majority of clients who come to me for help with weight loss are like me in that they've spent many years trying out different methods. They're always keen to hear about a new miracle diet or exercise programme. All of my clients, regardless of whatever has proven successful in helping them to lose weight in the past, share one thing in common: they haven't yet found a 'normal', 'healthy' way of eating long term that enables them to maintain weight loss while also enjoying the more fattening foods that they love.

Whenever I ask clients why they think past plans failed to keep them at a weight they were happy with, they describe different elements of each plan that simply weren't realistic, sustainable or appealing. In other words, keeping up their new 'healthier' habits involved continuing to hand themselves over to a prescriptive plan, some elements of which they could get on board with long term and others that they couldn't. But they never stopped to consider whether they could pick and choose the parts of these plans that they liked, not based on what they were told about them, but based on how they had responded to them time and time again.

There have been so many occasions throughout my life when I've sat at a laptop, or at a notebook with different coloured pens, planning meticulously how I'd wake up at 7am, go for a run, then make a fresh grapefruit juice (because I read when I was twelve that it burns fat). How I'll then have a warm glass of water with lemon followed by whichever breakfast made with nine different expensive ingredients (seven of which I don't even like) is required by the diet I'm following right now.

I've since learned that when attempting to design the most pain-less and enjoyable weight-loss plan possible for ourselves, the answers lie in the wisdom we've developed from past experience. Some plans will have made us feel bored after a while, others may have left us lethargic, or often feeling like we had to isolate our-selves and avoid socialising to keep it up.

This next exercise is the one I did right before I created the eating and exercise plan that finally helped me lose weight once and for all. First I made a list of all the diets I'd tried in the past, and then, next to each one, I wrote down why I thought I didn't manage to keep it up.

I decided that, for once, instead of thinking there was something wrong with me and presuming I'd one day transform into someone else, I would be honest with myself about who I was today. And who I have demonstrated myself to be when it comes to trying to change my relationship with food and my body in the past. I entertained the possibility that maybe I didn't need to change to accommodate the plan, but that the plan needed to change to accommodate me.

This is the list I initially made of the kinds of plans that hadn't worked for me in the past, with some of my reasons why. I simply based these reasons on who I was at the time of starting, and how I'd always shown myself to behave and react prior to that.

Things that I discovered weren't my bag:

- Eating plans that suggested I cut out a lot of the foods that I loved forever if I wanted to maintain my weight loss

- Having to measure and weigh my food

- Anything that stopped me going out to eat at restaurants

- Plans that didn't involve eating solid food

- Diets that required me to purchase specific bars and sachets and supplements

- Exercise classes that required me to wake up early in the morning

- Meal plans that required me to cook complicated things

- Plans that didn't let me drink coffee

- Plans that didn't let me drink alcohol

- Diet plans that technically allowed me to consume huge amounts of things that you don't have to be a nutritionist to know isn't right (I've been known to snack on canisters of whipped cream because it's permitted)

- Diets that focus so much on not combining certain foods that I'm made to feel one wrong decision will ruin the whole thing (I didn't need to be adopting approaches that reinforce my all-or-nothing thinking)

- Plans that permitted me to still eat my usual binge foods daily and expected me to miraculously be able to eat them in more moderate quantities

- Plans that said I had to stop eating many hours before I go to bed (going to bed hungry bothers me so much that it has genuinely been known to make me emotional)

- Having to measure myself with a measuring tape (I'd always lose them, plus I have the kind of body that can sometimes look seven months pregnant for a few hours after even an undisputedly healthy meal. Wrongly timed measuring could be demoralising)

- Having to eat the same thing over and over again (I still can't really be around cabbage soup without feeling sick)

- Having to report to someone for a public weigh-in (this reinforced my inclination to want to binge straight after being weighed, safe in the knowledge I wouldn't be monitored again for another six days)

I can't stress enough that I haven't shared this list in the hope you will use the same ones. I simply want to show you an example of how a plan of eating can be designed from a place of honest self-acceptance, with your bespoke needs in mind. Losing weight and finding a routine that keeps it off is difficult enough, the last thing you need is for your plan to include things that experience has regularly shown don't work for you.

It's also important to note that I wrote this list very early on, when I had not yet developed an ability to challenge all-or-nothing thinking, or the tools to motivate myself to go out to exercise even if it's cold. I also didn't appreciate the value of waking up earlier. These are things I feel much more able to do now, but I'm still so glad that, back when I made the list, I gave myself the best possible chance at getting through the difficult initial stages of change by facing up to the things that don't work for me, and accepting myself just as I was.

Recently, I had a consultation with a new client. She came in (as most clients do) feeling very clear on what her goals were. She wanted to lose three stone as quickly as possible so she could feel her best for her upcoming fortieth birthday party. She said, 'I read that you help people who already know what they want to do and how they want to do it. So, all I need from you is to help me understand why I can't keep up this eating and exercise plan. I always get to day thirteen and give up. I need you to help me understand how to be less weak so I can do this.'

I looked at the plan she had written down in her notebook. It included eating different meals to the ones she prepared for the rest of her family, missing breakfast despite having extremely busy mornings that required her to be focused at work, snacks that sounded as appealing as cardboard and so on. I asked her where she had got this plan from and she replied that it had always been her go-to plan to shed a few pounds since she was fifteen years old. Not only had the landscape of her life changed since then, but the needs of her body had too. She was beating herself up for not being able to keep up a regime that was already challenging when she had no bills to pay, no children to care for and very little to make her want to throw in the towel other than hunger on a day-to-day basis.

So I asked her why she kept going back to the same plan despite having totally different needs (and it clearly not working in a sustainable way to begin with). Her response: 'I was weaker then, it wasn't the right time to change, I didn't want it badly enough. Now I feel like I can really focus on this because I want to lose weight so badly.'

Instead of thinking there was something wrong with the plan, she thought there was something wrong with her. Plus, she assumed that increased desire, desperation and urgency were enough to keep her on track this time, despite it never working before. I invited her to start again. To consider that her weight-loss plan choices could be the ones that create the path of least resistance and make the journey less difficult.

I asked her when she needed to be more energetic, when she felt at her most resilient against temptation in the day, what foods she absolutely didn't want to cut out so she could enjoy her life and not fixate on them, how her body and tastes had changed over the years. What we created together was a plan that not only looked much kinder than her outdated, restrictive one based on generic guidelines, but that also helped her lose weight more effortlessly than she had ever imagined. It was bespoke and it worked for her – not the other way around.

The 'Not My Bag' list that you will now create in map form should take into consideration your inclinations and unique set of life circumstances – even if this includes things about yourself and your life that you ultimately want to change as well. For now, just accept the current situation so you can get going with a plan of action that yields results as soon as possible. Perhaps you have children, and so diets that require you to prepare separate meals aren't your bag. Maybe the industry you work in will always require you to attend a lot of late dinners, so a plan that demands you always know what is in your food and how it has been prepared might not be your bag – at least for as long as you have that job.

The exercise you complete now will invite you to reflect on previous attempts to lose weight or make changes to your relationship with food and your body. Think about what hasn't worked in the past and honestly ask yourself what things you simply don't want featuring in the eating, exercising and personal development plan you are going to design to help you lose and keep off weight.

Map: Not My Bag

First, write 'Not My Bag' in the centre of a blank page and draw a circle around it. Then think back to previous attempts and write why you don't think they worked for you long term.

To get the juices flowing and jog your memory, you may find it useful to ask yourself these questions:

- What elements of it weren't suited to my lifestyle?

- What was unrealistic about it?

- What aspects of it didn't suit my body?

- What aspects of it didn't suit my personality?

- What circumstances or events led up to me going off track eventually?

- How come I didn't get back on track when things started going wrong?

When you've taken time to note down all the things that aren't your bag, you will have a collection of personal wisdom that you can apply when it comes to formulating the best weight-loss and maintenance plan for you specifically. When creating your plan of least resistance, you'll already know what elements just aren't going to work for you, so you either rule them out or find an alternative. You'll create the plan it's most difficult to rebel against, since it's truly bespoke and based on self-knowledge and internal wisdom.

your style

Creating a plan of least resistance

Now that we've considered what doesn't work for you when it comes to losing and keeping off weight, we're going to look at what does. We'll do this by thinking about what kinds of plans tend to get you excited and make you want to keep them up across all areas of your life. The unique combination of circumstances to give you the best chance of achieving your weight-loss and maintenance goals.

Some people find it useful to declare their plans to others as this keeps them feeling accountable. Others find that this creates an added pressure and deprives them of the empowering feeling of being on something of a secret mission. When it comes to food, some people like to graze all day; others know it's best for them to eat three proper meals. Some people find that ramping up the exercise at the beginning of a new eating plan is an effective added motivator; others want to stay away from Lycra, mirrors and feeling out of breath until they've got past the initial adjustment stages of changing how they eat.

In this chapter you will start to think about what you'd like 'your style' to be when it comes to how you change and maintain your weight. The 'My Style' exercise you complete will not simply be a case of noting down the opposite of what you wrote on your 'Not My Bag' map. It will go further by asking you to consider the conditions you have shown yourself to thrive in across all areas of your life in the past. It will invite you to reflect on all of your proudest accomplishments to date – particularly the things that required you to push through (some of which you will have written on your 'My Body Can' map) – and think about what supports and resources you had in place at the time, both internally and externally.

What was it that made you stay on track in those moments when you wanted to give up? Did you have a deadline to work towards? Or someone else you were doing it for? Was it that you were organised and spent time planning properly, or perhaps that you were checking in with some kind of support network? How did you feel in yourself; did you have a self-care routine? Did you have any routine at all? Or do you feel at your most productive and motivated when free to make more spontaneous decisions? Did your most productive times happen to occur when something in particular was going on in a seemingly unrelated area of your life? Perhaps when you think back to your most productive and motivated periods they were during times when you were also taking more pride in your appearance and your surroundings.

I certainly find that the times when I'm feeling most resilient generally coincide with periods when my home environment is organised and aesthetically pleasing to me. I know that my enjoyment of seeing flowers in my flat first thing in the morning plays an indirect role in helping me to make kind decisions in my food choices later that day. How much time I take to brew my coffee so it's really delicious and do my hair so I like how it looks also play a role in the decisions I make regarding my eating habits and how I speak to my body once I've left the house. That's because these tiny acts of self-care are signals reminding me that I am worthy of taking care of in every way. That my quality of life matters. That my body is worthy of feeling its best, and therefore also eating in ways that makes it feel strong, happy, energetic and calm.

In taking time to consider what you'd like 'your style' to be when it comes to eating and exercise, you are also giving yourself an opportunity to consider what activities and conditions make you feel positive and resilient in general, so you can bring about the ones that are in your control and strive to create as many new ones as possible. When it comes to maintaining the resilience we need to change ingrained habits around food and resist temptation, especially during the early stages of change, trying to feel good in every possible way is an incredibly effective motivational tool for staying on track.

I can't help but notice that when it comes to weight-loss plans, almost all of my clients find it absurd if I suggest they start on Sunday as opposed to Monday. I understand, since I used to be like this too. It makes sense, because usually Monday is when our routines start up again and when we are less likely to feel idle and prone to mindless eating. Plus we associate the weekends with comfort and lack of restrictions, so why would we embark on the first day of a difficult plan when we're meant to be doing whatever we like?

The thing is, we know that we're better at doing difficult things when we're feeling strong, positive and energetic. Now, some people will feel this way on a Monday morning, and so it would make sense to embark on day one of a challenging eating plan then. For many people, however, Monday morning is associated with feeling sluggish, accompanied by a desire to ease back into the working week as gently as possible. So now I don't ask clients what day or time they'd like to start their plan. I simply ask them to tell me the day when they think they'll feel most positive, energetic and resilient. Their response is what I use to assign their day one.

Throughout this process, difficult choices will present themselves, often out of nowhere. The best you can do to prepare for them is to believe in your ability to overcome unforeseen challenges while doing what you can to create a practical plan of least resistance for you personally. The next exercise will help you to do that.

Map: My Style

First, write 'My Style' in the centre of a blank page, with a circle drawn around it. Then start to write down answers to these questions and cues, drawing circles around each response as you go:

- Think back to the periods when you've stuck to a difficult task in order to achieve a long-term goal. Write down the factors that you feel kept you on track

- Think back to the times you've been 'in the zone' with a weight-loss plan. Write a description of how things looked for you, internally and externally, that meant you could succeed, at least for a while

- Consider if there are any types of exercise you've not minded sticking to for a while in the past, and why you think that was

- Write down some delicious meals that you consider healthy. Ones you believe you can enjoy eating while still losing weight

- Write down your personal tastes when it comes to food choices. Is it important for you to eat something sweet after dinner? Are you someone who wants a diet that is heavy in meat?

- Think back to a time in your life when you've felt really capable for an extended period of time. Note down what it was about the activity that made you feel accomplished and proud of yourself

Once you've completed this exercise, the map in front of you will look like a random collection of foods, quirks, preferences, characteristics and conditions that are unique to you. Identifying these factors will enable you to create a more specific, personal weight-loss plan, one that you'll know you've put together by taking 'your style' into consideration.

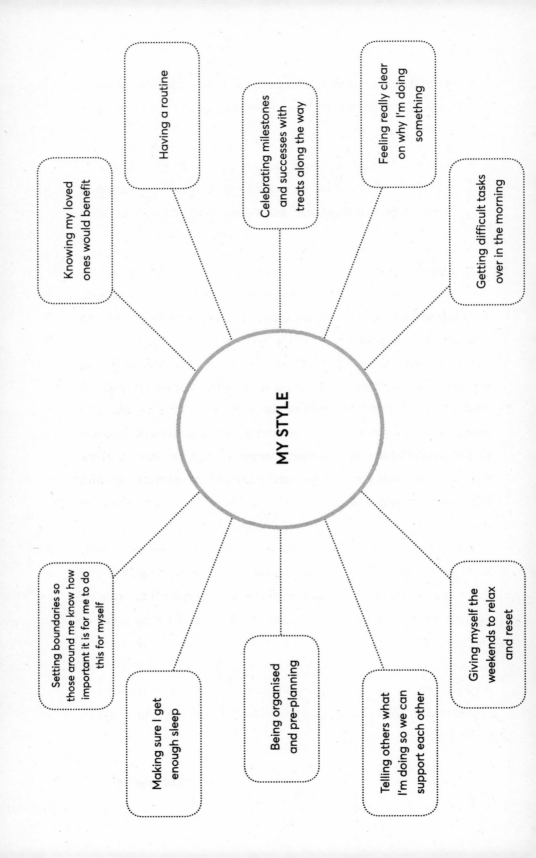

what's good

Reframing problems as solutions

At the beginning of this process, I asked you to write a letter to yourself detailing all the things you don't like about not being where you want to be when it comes to your relationship with food and your body. I asked that you consider the negatives, which I imagine was relatively simple to do, since the thing people who come to me tend to have in common is that the negative impacts of their habits have, on balance, come to outweigh the positives. On many occasions, clients have come to me saying that they can't think of a single thing that could make them want to continue as they are, and that at this stage there are no positives.

Having delivered countless workshops during which I ask people to share the negatives associated with their habits, I can tell you that when it comes to weight loss, these tend to roll off the tongue and are pretty predictable. People explain that their inability to change makes them feel weak or out of control, that the foods they eat and the ways they eat them are causing their bodies to feel tired and unfit, that their self-esteem is suffering as a result of their body image. They express anxiety that their lifestyle choices will result in illness.

However, when I then ask people to share some possible *positives* of staying the way they are, responses take time and answers vary wildly. And often become personal, reflective, revealing and therefore very useful for the purpose of changing and replacing habits. That's because understanding what is keeping you as you are helps you to identify a need your current habit is fulfilling, or once fulfilled. What you see as a problem now was once – and may still be – a solution. If you take that solution away and the problem it was solving still exists, then you'll need to deal with the problem some other way. If you expect that to be the case, you can prepare for it, and put an alternative coping mechanism in place. In this chapter, you're going to uncover what's 'good' about your unwanted status quo, so that you can understand why you haven't been able to change already and put strategies in place for the needs that will crop up when you disrupt it.

I believe that any life change becomes easier to implement and sustain when we shift our focus from negative to positive in every possible way. We've already started to do this in previous chapters – for example, by shifting the focus from what your body can't do and hasn't done to what it can do and has done, you have been able to uncover useful motivational resources that you may have overlooked before. In this chapter, I will invite you to take this idea one step further. Following The Last Diet effectively involves treating yourself with forgiveness and getting to know yourself better. If you can understand why and how your unwanted patterns developed, you can take a more informed, understanding and compassionate approach to weight loss and address the very personal relationship you've developed with your body on your own terms, for the reasons that are most important to you personally.

Over the years when I was at my heaviest, a lot of people tried to remind me of the negative impacts of my eating behaviours, since bringing my attention to how 'bad' things had got was what they genuinely believed would spur me to change. Usually they would remind me about health risks, inform me of how many calories were in something I was about to eat, and remind me of how unhappy I'd told them I was with my size, as if these weren't things I already knew. I have no doubt that they were well intentioned, but the 'intervention' approach just never worked, because instead of motivating me to make positive changes, it made me:

- Self-conscious, because I felt exposed and observed

- Shameful and dishonest, because I felt judged

- Rebellious, because I'll change when I'm good and ready

- Defensive and patronised, because I'd been researching diets my whole life

- Disappointed in myself for still having this obvious issue that everyone could literally see, from my body size, was getting worse

- Hopeless, because even when I tried my hardest I couldn't imagine other people's suggestions actually working for me long term

- More convinced that people's main take-away about who I am was based on the size of my body

• Sad, and hungry for large quantities of foods that helped me escape that sadness as quickly as possible

As you can see, this combination of responses was not conducive to me getting motivated to like myself and find a viable long-term solution. I must admit that sometimes the odd scary lecture about my weight did cause me to lose some weight, but because it caused me to initially binge, then immediately starve myself for three days – losing maybe three pounds, nearly faint, and then binge again. As we discussed at the beginning of the book, I now know that things like spite, fear, revenge, anger and resentment towards ourselves or other people can get us going, but they don't keep us going. The same goes for changing for other people's reasons.

After years of listening to other people patronise me and tell me what's wrong with me, I now believe that even if it's someone's job to warn people about health risks, any advice should begin with things like, 'I imagine you already know this,' before saying things like 'you are dangerously overweight' or 'obesity is not healthy' or 'vegetables are good and biscuits are bad'. I just can't imagine anyone has ever gained the bespoke personal insight and motivation they needed to lose weight and finally keep it off after years of complex struggle by focusing on generic and obvious negatives.

Those who have spent years trying and failing to change their habits are more aware of the negatives than anyone else. They are living with those negatives twenty-four hours a day. They're constantly on high alert, listening out for possible options to get rid of those negatives. They've done the research, they have access to all the same information everyone else does.

Admittedly, there were some occasions when I was trying to lose weight or feeling particularly unhappy with my body, when I would go to people asking for practical weight-loss advice. Before I had the tools to gain proper insight into my own behaviours, I sometimes invited other people to tell me what they thought I should do. This was usually people I didn't know very well, probably because I hadn't had time to develop resentment around the content and delivery of their advice. I noticed that the people I struck off most quickly tended to do two things.

The first was to come straight in with patronising advice without asking for any backstory. They didn't ask what I'd already tried or wonder why I hadn't been able to maintain a weight I was happy with on my own.

It's a bit like spending four hours at home alone desperately trying to fix a laptop that's broken down. You've spent all afternoon frantically Googling every possible solution, called helplines, insurers and manufacturers, tried all the suggestions and nothing's worked. You've cried over lost work, been through a rollercoaster of hope and despair, and checked your bank balance to see if you've got enough to buy a new one. You've tried to see if you can borrow one from a friend in order to meet an important deadline and read all the forums and instruction manuals.

Just then, your partner casually arrives home, gathers there's a broken laptop situation and, without wanting more details, immediately assumes they can fix it. They sit down and smugly offer their miracle solution: pressing the reset button. While waiting for something to happen, they also take the opportunity to explain that you're in this position because you don't take care of things properly and remind you that you'll only damage it more if you don't change your ways.

They sit there, waiting for the laptop to come to life, genuinely expecting to have cracked it, and therefore completely believing that you've not yet considered this most basic of possible solutions. Because they never asked, they are oblivious to the fact that they walked in on you half an hour away from essentially graduating from laptop repair school. Does that sound like the kind of motivational support you needed, or the kind of support that makes you want to cry, eat a cake, and then cry again because the laptop's still not fixed?

The other kind of advice that eventually started making me switch off came from people who offered weight-loss plans that weren't sustainable long term because they didn't consider my mental health. They didn't care that I'd have to feel crap during and after the process in order to lose weight. The promise of feeling better as a result relied entirely on me being delighted about being slim. These plans were offered up by people who assumed that just losing weight would be enough to give me more self-esteem and sustain the resilience I needed to make considered choices with food for the rest of my life.

But I knew from experience that losing weight wasn't going to be enough to make me a happier person overall. It had never authentically increased my self-esteem in the past, so I had started to realise I needed something different. Experience had also shown me that unless I started feeling happier overall, I wouldn't be motivated to keep up any plan of change. Feeling miserable made me want to eat in ways that made me gain weight.

So, having established that we all know the negatives, I'm going to invite you to complete this next exercise either once or twice, depending on which approach makes sense for you. I needed to complete it twice – the first time to explore how it served me to eat the way I did, and again to explore how it served me to keep a layer of fat around me. It wasn't until relatively recently that I discovered there weren't only positives for me in how I was eating, but there were positives in staying overweight too!

This was a complete revelation to me. I discovered through the second optional exercise in this chapter that I had associated being overweight with getting attention from my parents from a very young age – even if it was attention because they thought something in me needed fixing. Staying overweight then became my excuse for delaying living life and avoiding taking risks and facing rejection; I'd decided that slimness was a prerequisite for these things, so that ruled me out. Before this realisation, if you had ever told me that staying overweight was serving me in any way, I wouldn't have believed you. That's the beauty of these exercises, they can help us to uncover the more subtle factors that drive our beliefs and actions when it comes to our bodies.

What's Good: Part 1

First, I'd like you to make a quick list of the main eating habits (or absence of eating habits) you believe are holding you back from losing and maintaining your weight. The general things you're doing or not doing with food that are making it difficult for you to achieve your goals:

1. _____

2. _____

3. _____

4. _____

5. _____

E.g. Snacking mindlessly in front of the TV, eating sugar when I'm stressed, prolonged bingeing after periods of restricting myself

Map: What's Good: Part 2

Now, in the centre of a blank page, write 'What's Good' and draw a circle around it. Then go to the first habit on the list you just wrote and ask yourself the following list of questions about it. On your map, write answers to any of the following questions that make sense for you, drawing a circle around each one as you go:

- What kind of comfort does it give you/did it once give you?

- What kinds of things does it allow you to do/has it allowed you to do in the past?

- What does it help you to avoid/has it helped you to avoid in the past?

- What does it make easier for you/has it made easier for you in the past?

- What does it protect you from/has it protected you from in the past?

- What parts of your life does it make easier to cope with/ has it made easier to cope with in the past?

- What does it help you feel more in control of/has it helped you feel more in control of in the past?

- What do you enjoy about it/have you enjoyed about it in the past?

- How does it connect you with others/has it connected you with others in the past?

- How does it benefit your relationships/has it benefited your relationships in the past?

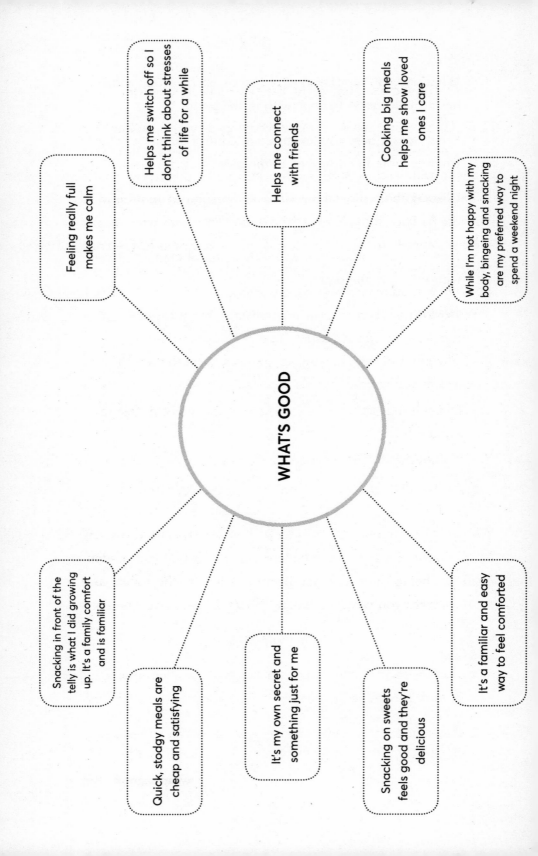

WHAT'S GOOD

Feeling really full makes me calm

Helps me switch off so I don't think about stresses of life for a while

Helps me connect with friends

Cooking big meals helps me show loved ones I care

While I'm not happy with my body, bingeing and snacking are my preferred way to spend a weekend night

Snacking in front of the telly is what I did growing up. It's a family comfort and is familiar

Quick, stodgy meals are cheap and satisfying

It's my own secret and something just for me

Snacking on sweets feels good and they're delicious

It's a familiar and easy way to feel comforted

What's Good: Optional Written Exercise: Part 3

If, like I did, you want to explore whether the forces pulling you to stay the same are multi-layered, then you can repeat this exercise with a different theme. In the centre of a black page, write 'What's good about staying this size?' and draw a circle around it. Then go to back to the first of the main habits you wrote down and ask yourself the following list of questions about it. On your map, write answers to the questions that make sense for you, drawing a circle around each one as you go.

Write down:

- The kinds of comfort it gives you to remain the size or weight you're currently at
- Difficult things that staying your current size helps you to avoid
- Things that staying overweight helps you to do
- Any comfort that being physically bigger gives you

When you've completed one or both of these maps, what you will have in front of you is a collection of the needs that you've identified are being (or have once been) fulfilled by the habits and circumstances you want to change. Now you have two questions to ask yourself:

1. Has staying the same way been solving a problem that doesn't need solving anymore?

2. Are your current habits solving a problem that still exists?

The people who will find this process the easiest are those who discover through the exercises in this chapter that they don't need their unwanted habits anymore. That they've outgrown their need for them as a coping mechanism; they simply hadn't stopped to acknowledge that before. A simple example is picking up the habit of eating a box of chocolates every night while getting over the sadness of a break-up. It's comforting and it serves a purpose in that moment. But then, over time, boxes of chocolate have found their way on to your grocery list, and you're still eating one an evening. It has subtly turned into a part of your routine, which brings with it associations and physical alerts and cravings. Then, before you know it, you're still eating break-up chocolate even though you're not heartbroken anymore.

If this sounds like you, then maintaining your weight loss will be much easier than it will be for many others. You can focus on simply repeating new habits as frequently as possible until they become your new norm, with minimal forces pulling you to maintain the status quo other than things like fear of change and short-term physical withdrawal.

If, however, you are in the category of people for whom their current eating habits are still serving a purpose, then there will be more commitment required to adopting new effective 'solution-habits'. The following exercise is designed to help you do that.

What's Good: Written Exercise: Part 4

In a notebook, copy out these sentences and complete them in as much detail as you can.

I see now that there are various understandable reasons I'm finding it difficult to change. These include . . .

_____

_____

_____

Staying as I am helps me fulfil some important needs, like . . .

_____

_____

_____

I'd prefer to be fulfilling these needs long term by doing things like . . .

_____

_____

_____

In the short term, I could distract myself from the discomfort of not having these needs met by . . .

_____

_____

_____

I hope that this chapter has given you any insight you may have needed to believe that you are not weak and there is nothing wrong with you. Your habits have developed for a reason, and whether you need them anymore or not, they're not 'bad' and neither are you.

testing times

Removing surprise where possible

It's time to start considering what, other than core beliefs from childhood, may contribute to the soundtrack of commands that tells you to go off track when trying to stick to a practical weight-loss plan. Forewarned is forearmed when it comes to triggers. So, we will now take time to reflect on the kinds of things that increase your desire to fulfil the needs you identified in the last chapter. If, for example, you identified that your current eating habits help you to deal with stress, then we need to assume going into a new plan that you will find it hardest not to eat in those ways in moments when you feel stressed.

Taking surprise out of the equation can help us to behave in a calm and considered manner when we're triggered. Later on in this chapter, you will complete a 'Testing Times' exercise which asks you to write down all the situations, states and conditions you suspect will make it difficult for you, specifically, to stick to a weight-loss plan.

We have explored some of the conversations we have with ourselves that can derail us. Many people, when they complete reflective exercises like those in this book, realise that it's quite a predictable set of conditions that trigger them to want to convince themselves to give up on their weight-loss plans. In the early stages of change, you will need to use past experience to pre-empt what might throw you off track and make you want to revert to the comfortable status quo.

Although I will encourage you to consider new reactions to challenging situations, you will no doubt be glad to hear that it will start happening naturally as soon as you begin to realise how predictable your patterns are. You don't need to have loads of tools at your disposal to be able to ride out short-term discomfort. The trick to responding in a way you're proud of is very often simply just expecting it. Expect the discomfort: expect physical cravings; expect to want to give up; expect to hear sabotaging self-talk and expect it to be difficult and scary sometimes – even if just for the simple reason that it's a change. If you can't avoid discomfort, then don't fight it. The important thing is to save your energy to withstand short-term discomfort, all the time reminding yourself why you're voluntarily choosing to withstand it. Ultimately, I want to show you how to welcome these feeling as an opportunity to practise getting through them without treating your body unkindly in response. Because once you have, you'll realise your own strength and find it much easier to stick to your plan.

Some of the feelings that will arise during this time you'll be able to predict, though some will seem to come out of nowhere. But the thing to bear in mind is that, inevitably, before your new habits have had the chance to become automatic, unavoidable and unforeseen circumstances will present themselves that make you feel like it's too difficult to stay on track. Although many of our triggers are out of our hands, how we react towards our bodies in response to them isn't.

When I am helping clients to stick to their weight-loss plans, I ask them to identify their high-risk scenarios, and I have noticed a few themes that keep coming up. Here's a list of day-to-day triggers that tend to directly or indirectly put people in high-risk scenarios where they feel more likely to lapse, especially during the early stages of change:

- Hunger

- Anxiety and stress

- Complacency

- Mountain-to-climb thinking

- Self-defeating, self-doubting thoughts

- Resentment – of others and the process

- Low mood

- Mindless use of smartphones

- Impatience and disappointment

Keep in mind, often we can overcome these in ways we're happy with when we're just dealing with one or two. However, when they pile up and present themselves all at once, we can find ourselves feeling very challenged indeed. That's why it's important to keep an eye on the levels of these things in general. To help us to feel like we still have resilience reserves in those moments when new things challenge us that we hadn't expected.

One of my clients described a situation recently where high-risk factors multiplied out of the blue, at an unprecedented rate, causing him to go from having no problem dealing with discomfort to going off track in a matter of minutes. He had gone to the supermarket after work to buy dinner and noticed that, having missed lunch, he was really tired and hungry. He recognised that the combination of how he was feeling and where he was meant he was in a high-risk situation. However, he told himself that he would use it as an opportunity to practise noticing the urge and pushing through it. So he focused on buying fresh ingredients as opposed to grabbing a family bag of crisps and eating them while he shopped. It had only been a couple of weeks since he started his weight-loss plan, but in that moment he felt in control and proud of himself in a way he hadn't experienced before. Almost smugly, he thought to himself 'I don't think shopping hungry is ever going to be a problem for me again.'

Just then, he got a call from his wife telling him that they'd be entertaining last-minute guests, who he happened not to be very fond of. This would mean he'd have to think of something else to cook because of their dietary requirements. He agreed and started thinking of options he could eat as well that would still keep him on track with his weight-loss plan. Before he had time to put his phone back in his pocket, he saw an email had popped up, informing him that he'd made a big error in a piece of work earlier that day, meaning he'd have to work into the night after the guests had left.

He put his phone in his pocket, looked up and saw someone who was slim happily working their way through a huge pack of crisps. He remembered that he hadn't lost any weight the previous week and started getting annoyed about the fact he had to have a plan at all; why wasn't he the kind of person who could just be naturally slim? Finally, he glanced at the lengthy queue at the tills and that was it. He called his wife and told her they'd be ordering take-out for everyone.

My client proceeded to spend the evening, following morning and week after that eating in ways that he'd identified as unkind and responsible for weight gain when he created his plan in the first place. His all-or-nothing thinking also meant that he neglected all the other habits he'd just started to get used to, having been on track for three weeks.

Now, I'm not saying he couldn't have still stuck to his plan. If he'd been further along in the change process, he may well have learned to say to himself, 'Yes, these things all make me feel like I want to go off-plan but they're not making me, so I'm choosing to disobey the commands they're giving me and hand myself over the version of myself that wants the best for me, the one who wrote the plan in the first place. Life will continue to look like this, it's up to me what I do to my body in response to it.'

But as it was so early in the process of becoming more self-aware about his patterns (plus he was in a supermarket), I'm not surprised the craving to relieve what began as just hunger went from manageable to unbearable in a matter of minutes.

Let's go back to our list of triggers and look at them more closely:

Hunger

This might seem obvious, but never underestimate the power of hunger. It can come on suddenly and lower resolve around food in a way you never imagined. It has a selective memory for how certain foods make your body feel. The commands it is able to create can be much louder than any of the helpful ones in your soundtrack. Hunger is highly skilled in convincing you that your plans are stupid. If you choose to create a plan that involves you being hungry at any point then, during the early stages of change, try to avoid taking that hunger to places that are filled with opportunities to go off-plan. Or at least take the edge off before. I've eaten many an apple en route to a dinner so that when it comes to giving the waiter my side order, I've lowered my chances of blurting out 'cheesy chips' when I genuinely intended to say 'salad'.

Another point on hunger is that it can cause us to forget how little it will take to make it go away and get us thinking rationally again. There were many occasions in the past when, shopping in the supermarket while hungry, I decided for one reason or another that I was going to lapse from a strict weight-loss plan, and because my commands were coming from hunger (and all-or-nothing thinking), I'd then purchase a buffet of foods to binge on. Enough to last me three days (thus creating an excuse to eat those foods for three more days so as to not waste them). It's wasn't until I'd take a couple of bites out of the first item in my bursting shopping bags that I'd realise how quickly my hunger was relieved, and that a healthier snack would have taken the edge off just as sufficiently – i.e. enough for me to start thinking rationally about what I was doing. At this stage I had the option of nipping my lapse in the bud after just a couple of bites and getting straight back on track. But a combination of never having seen myself be able to do that before and a passenger's seat full of all the foods I'd already bought meant that logic never stood a chance.

Anxiety and stress

Many of us experience stress and anxious thinking patterns to varying degrees at different times. Despite this, I have noticed that most of my clients come to me having never developed go-to coping strategies for them that can be used on the spot. Quite often, through exercises like the 'What's Good' map, clients discover that the habits that are holding them back from achieving their weight-loss goals are the ones that help them to deal most effectively with things like general anxiety and stress, so removing these presents them with some important needs that will still need fulfilling.

These days, I don't often tend to eat foods that are very high in sugar. That said, when I do eat them, I am immediately reminded how good they are at doing their job in that moment. If I'm feeling low, there is no denying that a delicious cupcake is going to give me a boost. That's fine. That's why, sometimes in response to feeling low, I choose to eat a cupcake.

But the cupcake isn't the only thing I can turn to. I can decide to listen to the ten-minute guided meditation app I have ready on my phone, or revisit a written exercise or run myself a bath. Now I know what you're thinking, none of these things are as effective as a cupcake. I agree, they're not as immediately effective, but they remain effective long term. They may not make you feel as good straight away, but they keep you feeling good for longer.

When an unwanted habit does a very important job for us, like relieve daily stress and worry, it's imperative that we respect that and acknowledge it for doing that, even if we want to change it. The kind way to create change for yourself is not to take away all the things that relieve you at once. Instead, start trying to reduce the number of times you go to those old habits for relief while increasing the number of times you turn to a new range of habits. Make sure your new habits are ones that you'd be proud to think of as your coping strategies for stress and anxiety in five years' time.

If you've identified daily stress and worry as resilience-lowering factors that have held you back from achieving your long-term weight-loss goals in the past, you may wish to complete the following exercise when met with them.

Optional Stress Exercise

Things that tend to cause me stress:

_____

How I tend to cope with this stress:

_____

How I'd like to be coping with stress in five years' time:

_____

Things I can start doing on a day-to-day basis that will help me get there:

_____

Things that tend to cause me to worry:

_____

How I tend to cope with worry:

_____

How I'd like to be coping with worry in five years' time:

_____

Things I can start doing on a day-to-day basis that will
help me get there:

_____

Like many of my clients, I have struggled a lot with anxiety in the past, and the most effective coping mechanism I have found is doing exercises, both physical and the written exercises in this book. In fact, completing the written exercises often determines whether I do the physical exercises.

After years of catastrophising and long periods of relieving stress with food, I have learned to feel much more in control of my actions when even the faintest signal of anxiety creeps in. A large part of that is due to learning that when I take the worry out of my head and take a second to write down the actual facts, I feel immediately calmer. Don't get me wrong, as much as I wish it could, I'm not suggesting that the following optional exercise I use on myself will 'cure' feelings of general, day-to-day anxiety. What it will do, however, is help you to collect factual data that you can't contest, which will show you how frequently you are spending energy worrying about things you can't change or don't need to.

Optional Anxiety Exercise

As soon as you feel anxious or notice that you've been in a cycle of worrying about the same thing for a period of time, stop, and make some quick observation notes, use your phone if that's easiest. The idea is that you quickly take a snapshot of what you think is going on in that moment and how you're feeling about it. Then, you put it away. It's effective for four reasons:

1. Having to stop for a moment and externalise can help you slow things down, focus your thoughts and give you a different perspective on the situation so you feel more in control of your response

2. The act of choosing to complete this exercise instead of responding as usual will remind you that you're investing in yourself and practising new ways of coping

3. Creating an ever-growing database of moments when you've felt overwhelmed allows you to revisit them – say a week later – to see how much needless, resilience-lowering worry you engage in

4. Over time, you will notice yourself making fewer entries because you've learned to 'cut to the end'. For example, when a familiar anxious thinking pattern crops up that

you've seen written down over and over again, you'll be more able to tell yourself things like 'I've worried about this a million times before and always landed on the realisation that worrying is not a useful way to spend my energy'

To try it out, simply commit to writing down your responses to these questions in the moments you feel anxious:

• What do I think is happening right now?

• What am I worried is going to happen?

Then, put your answers away and carry on as you were.

Over time, as your list gets longer and features some repeats, set a reminder in your calendar to check your worry exercise once a month for a couple of minutes, whenever you like. In that time, briefly reflect on your past entries. For each one, ask yourself with hindsight, 'Does my description of what was going on reflect the reality of what was really going on? And were my fears realised? If they were, was I better equipped to deal with them because I worried?'

Complacency

It might sound strange, but success can be a trigger for a lapse. I have seen people be caught out by it time and time again when it comes to sustaining new habits.

Often, I will spend a session with a new client discussing a particular event that they have coming up. One that is far enough away that they'd like to have started making changes by then, but not so far away that they will feel able to make instinctive food choices without going off track with their relatively new plan.

We will often play out high-risk scenarios and establish a plan of action. This in turn helps them to feel like they're going in prepared and that they've done the motivational groundwork to make decisions they will feel proud of after the event. I always warn my clients that creating a goal out of an event is only effective if you have considered how you will feel post-event. Sometimes after we achieve something difficult, we have a renewed motivation and resilience against the next challenge. Other times we feel we should be rewarded – often with the kinds of foods and behaviours that we were trying to change.

In other cases, clients fall into the trap of thinking that because they've found the first three weeks of their plan easier than they thought, when they have an event coming up, they don't need to give any prior thought to their food choices. That even if they eat something off-plan they've changed so much they'll be able to wake up the next day and be straight back on plan (even though that's never happened in the past). These clients tend to come back to me reporting that they had become complacent and completely underestimated the forces they were working against.

This process is designed to help you shift the way you think and behave in your everyday life in as many ways as possible, starting straight away. Plus, it's meant to make you feel better than before. But it's not a miracle cure, so however exciting and novel it is to be experiencing positive change across your life, don't forget that, when it comes to your body, you are trying to replace years and years of old habits. It's going to take a while for you to feel like you can do that without deliberately taking time to remember how important it is to stay on your own plan of change.

Mountain-to-climb thinking

This will be relevant to those who feel they want to lose large amounts of weight, or for whom it will take a longer period of time to reach their weight-loss goals, for whatever reasons.

I can't tell you the number of times I have thrown myself off track with otherwise successful weight-loss plans upon realising how far I still was from my ultimate goal. I've had people telling me I should do something about my weight seven months into very much doing something about my weight. Looking at a BMI chart and realising that despite weeks of hard work I was still months away from just about not being obese resulted in many a hopeless binge and quick return to old ways.

The most effective shift in thinking I have found to help with mountain-to-climb thinking is this: however many steps it takes to reach my goal, I'm going to have to take all of them at some point. So then it's up to me whether I want to take any of them more than once.

If it gets to week seven and you think, 'I've still got fifty weeks to go, what's the point?', then it can help to have the response ready: 'I want to lose weight eventually, and whether I get through week seven now or in three months, week seven is going to need to get done.'

Self-defeating, self-doubting internal dialogue and commands

We've covered this in previous chapters and we'll go on to look at all-or-nothing thinking patterns in the next chapter. If you feel that unhelpful inner dialogue plays a big part in you not achieving your weight-loss goals, then in addition to reflecting on and developing the 'My Soundtrack' and 'Cheerleading' maps, you may find it helpful to bring affirmations into your daily routine. A lot of people find the idea of this hard to get on board with, however, everyone I know of who's given it a proper chance for a few weeks has reported that it was genuinely helpful. For many who haven't done much personal development before, trying out this exercise will involve pushing past the cringe, going through the motions and seeing it as a harmless experiment. It still works even if you're sceptical while you do it.

First, choose a statement that directly challenges a common self-defeating thought you regularly have. One that you believe makes it harder for you to achieve your goals. You may want to refer to your 'My Body Can' and 'My Body Has' maps for inspiration here. Now, choose a short statement that firmly contradicts this self-defeating thought. To give you an example, if you're used to saying to yourself, 'I have no willpower and will probably end up failing at this plan as well,' then the statement you choose may be something as simple as 'I'm strong and committed.'

Then, you commit to saying this statement to yourself ten times every morning – privately, but out loud. (It can help when trying to make this practice a part of your routine to attach it to an existing daily habit. For example, you could do it in the bathroom right before you brush your teeth.)

'I'm strong and committed.'
'I'm strong and committed.'
'I'm strong and committed.'
'I'm strong and committed.'
'I'm strong and committed.'
'I'm strong and committed.'
'I'm strong and committed.'
'I'm strong and committed.'
'I'm strong and committed.'
'I'm strong and committed.'

While you do it, notice if any self-doubting thoughts or unhelpful dialogue creep in. You might start thinking 'this is silly' or be trying to think of all the times you've not demonstrated yourself to be strong or committed. That's OK, just notice what's happening and, if you feel you can, try to shift your focus to the times that have proven this statement to be true. The times on your 'My Body Can' map.

Different people experience different benefits from doing affirmations. The most effective role it has played for me is in helping to set something of a concrete intention for the day when it comes to how I speak to myself. So, if and when self-doubting thoughts come in, I'm reminded that I set time aside this morning as part of a mission to help me deal with this exact thing. It helps me remember that I can hand over to the version of me who wanted to try out the affirmation thing, the one who knows me the best today and wants the best for me tomorrow.

Resentment – of others and the process

For many years, when it came to eating, my mantra was 'I would rather be the kind of person who can eat whatever they like without gaining weight than win the lottery.' I spent my childhood wondering why other children my age stayed slim and I was getting bigger every day, when we were essentially doing and eating the same things. Like an angry stalker, I have observed the bellies of people who can consume huge amounts of food and continue to feel comfortable in their jeans. For various reasons, many of which I discuss in this book and many of which are out of my control, my body and mind did not develop in a way that resulted in me being able to naturally maintain a weight I was happy with. But some other people did. That would sometimes make me feel very resentful. And this in turn used to make me think, 'Why am I the only one having to worry about this? I should just face it: however hard I try this will never become easy for me. Maybe I'm just wired to be this way. This is pointless; I should just give up.'

Realising that, in the past, resentment had always moved me further away from achieving my goals helped me decide I would stop falling at this hurdle once and for all. Everyone has their challenges to deal with, this is just mine. And I'm lucky, because it's something I have the ability to change.

Gratitude can play a big role in helping with feelings of resentment too. Working in drug treatment, I've seen daily gratitude lists help people enormously with shifting the focus from what they wish they had to what they already do have across their entire lives on a daily basis. So I created my own version of a gratitude practice that many of my clients have turned into a very enjoyable annual ritual.

What I do is keep a jar next to my couch, filled with little strips of blank paper and a pen. When I think of something new I am grateful for – something that had happened that day, or as a result of something I'd seen in the news, for example – I grab a blank strip from my jar and note down it down. Then I just throw it back in the jar and forget about it. Provided I keep the jar in the right place, they collect without me thinking.

The positioning of the jar is very important. It needs to be somewhere visible and somewhere that you tend to be when you can spare (or be bothered to spare) thirty seconds to write something down. For me, this is next to the couch right alongside where I always place my mug of tea while I watch TV in the evenings. That way, when faced with the option of watching another advert or writing something nice on a strip of paper that's within reaching distance, I sometimes pick the paper.

Finally, on New Year's Eve, I tip out the jar and read through all the things I am thankful for that year. It's certainly a pleasant change from the many New Year's Eves spent focusing on what I don't have.

Low mood

Other than wanting you to feel as good as possible in every possible way because everyone deserves to, I want you to feel as good as possible, so that this process is as easy as possible for you. Creating your path of least resistance when it comes to achieving weight-loss goals involves considering everything you can independently be doing to feel more positive about yourself and your life.

When it comes to creating your practical plan of action, it is important that you factor in ways to take care of your mental wellbeing in general. It can be anything from including an action point to get more fresh air or connect with your friends more, to finally arranging a GP appointment for a counselling referral. Remember, change is difficult and it's a lot easier to do difficult things when you feel good.

Mindless use of smartphones

Many of us have got into the habit of looking at our phones to check emails, social media and the news before we've even got out of bed in the morning. This can leave us feeling overwhelmed and get our day started on an urgent, not very mindful note. Clients often tell me that viewing certain kinds of images on Instagram or being bombarded with WhatsApp notifications first thing in the morning can set them up to make less than kind decisions about how they speak to and treat themselves for the rest of the day. We are far better placed to behave in ways we're proud of towards ourselves and others when we feel we are on the best footing emotionally and physically. With this in mind, it can be helpful to try not to look at your phone until you've got out of bed, had a shower and eaten breakfast, for example.

Smartphone use is something that I discuss with a lot of clients when it comes to triggers. I have countless examples of clients tracing back steps to the beginning of a lapse and discovering it was triggered by something they saw on their phones.

I'm not saying that smartphones aren't incredibly useful. I suggest several times in this book that you can use your phone as a motivational aid. That said, many of us have developed a relationship with our phones that is not having a positive impact on how we speak to and treat our bodies throughout the day. It's often subtle and indirect, but it's real and I'm noticing it become more and more common.

Whether it's looking at unrealistic bodies and lifestyles on Instagram, reading harrowing news stories and angry threads on Twitter, getting absorbed in emails the second they've arrived in the inbox, feeling overwhelmed with bridesmaid group chat messages on WhatsApp, or developing an expensive online shopping habit, more and more clients come to see me intending to talk about food and leave realising they've spent most of the session talking about the things that happen on their phones.

If you feel that your relationship with your smartphone is distracting you from how you're really feeling, or that what you're looking at on it makes you feel less resilient or positive in any way, then it may be an idea to use your weight-loss action plan as an opportunity to introduce a new approach when it comes to your smartphone habits. The following exercise is one that my clients and I have found to be extremely effective. For those who have grown used to checking their phones last thing in the evening and first thing in the morning, this experiment may well provide a shocking surprise. The guidelines are simple: **Don't look at your phone for the first fifteen minutes of the day.**

By not looking at your phone for those first minutes of the day, you are deciding what you will expose yourself to. You're actively choosing not to start your day by exposing yourself to unhelpful content and messages that can get your day started on a negative foot. That first part of the day is your first opportunity to have a say in what kind of day you're going to have. Please don't voluntarily hand that power to literally everyone else in the entire world but yourself.

Some people will find this morning phone exercise much more difficult than others, not least because it involves keeping your phone completely silent and somewhere you can't see it overnight. Therefore, they can't fall asleep looking at it. Plus, the realisation that they're finding this exercise so difficult brings to people's attention how dependent they've become on their phones.

Persevering with this practice and collecting reliable data on how many times nothing bad happened as a result of you not looking at your phone is also useful in learning that many situations no longer need to be treated as an emergency. This shift in thinking of course becomes a transferrable skill when it comes to making challenging decisions around food.

Impatience and disappointment

We all want quick results when it comes achieving any goal that's important to us. When it comes to weight loss specifically, we are able to measure our progress in numbers and how we look. The problem comes when we measure our progress entirely on these things, because they are prone to fluctuate, and we don't want to base how motivated we feel on numbers. Plus, how proud of yourself you feel on a daily basis shouldn't depend on your body size or how much you weigh.

That's why, when you create a weight-loss plan, food and

exercise are just two elements of a much bigger objective: to treat your body with more kindness. That way, if you happen to weigh yourself one week and see that despite doing all the 'right' things you haven't lost any weight, you know that you're still making progress with your self-care and self-esteem routine and your personal development. All of your other habits are still moving you in the direction of weight loss, it's just a matter of continuing what you're doing until numbers on the scales catch up again.

I can think back to so many experiences when I've been totally on track until I made the mistake of weighing myself at the wrong time of the day (and month) and being left feeling disappointed and hopeless as a result. Feeling like this would often then lead to a binge (via a conversation with myself I didn't yet know I was having that went something like, 'My plan obviously isn't working, what's the point in going to all this effort, I'm basically in the same place I was a week ago, I may as well binge on everything I've managed not to eat, since evidently it makes no difference anyway.').

It can help to simply accept that your literal weight-loss process will, predictably, include boring periods of plateau during which it will be difficult to justify continuing to put yourself in challenging situations. At times your body will not do what you want it to as quickly as you want it to. Commit to remembering that so that when those moments do come around, you maintain an awareness that they were always going to, and that you've already decided you're going to push through them.

In my experience, it's soon after you push through the most stagnant sections of weight loss that you stumble upon the most rapid.

It's important to expect this process to be difficult. Exciting, positive, novel, but also difficult. Remember that you knew it would be hard and you've chosen to do it anyway. All the foods you may choose not to eat for a while are always there. Nothing is forbidden, you're just deciding to do this for yourself for a bit and see how it works out for you.

If, right at the beginning, I had asked you, 'How many points in the weight-loss process do you imagine are going be boring or difficult to push through?' I imagine you would have said quite a few. Remembering this can help you in those moments when it feels like you're not getting the results you wanted yet. If you'd have guessed that twenty out of sixty days would really challenge you, then when day five of challenge presents itself, you can think 'I expected this, and there's still more to come. I knew that it was going to be an inevitable part of achieving a truly meaningful goal.'

At the end of this chapter I will invite you to complete a map where you write down all of the situations, feelings, thoughts and circumstances that you feel directly or indirectly make it harder for you to stick to your weight-loss plan. First though, I'd like to introduce you to an exercise that you will be doing every morning. Stay with me, it's extremely effective and in total only requires five minutes of your time.

I started using this exercise to help me with weight loss, but I now use it every day to help me manage my behaviours in all areas of my life. It's become my version of a journal, and I spend just five minutes on it in the morning. I believe that this exercise was largely responsible for helping me push through in those weeks when I hadn't lost weight and wanted to throw in the towel, since it enabled me to realise that not losing weight was one of the predictable excuses I'd give myself to throw in the towel. It is based on the belief that simply expecting to be presented with a challenge is enough to stop you reacting to it in a way you later regret. It's also based on the assumption that you tend to fall at the same hurdles. Finally, it assumes that we all have moments when we look back on how we reacted to feeling internally or externally challenged and wish we'd handled it differently.

During the initial stages of implementing a plan of change, my clients often say that they wish we could start every day with a quick coaching session. Aside from this being unrealistic, it also goes against the spirit of handing over tools that people can use on themselves. But often it's not more tools that these clients want, it's a sense of accountability, a reminder that they've committed to something, and an opportunity to externalise their observations on how they're changing.

I believe that if you commit to completing the next exercise every day, and integrating it permanently into your routine, you will be able to provide this for yourself. When it comes to formulating your plan of change, you will be in charge of deciding what and how to eat and exercise. But I will insist that you include this daily exercise and treat it as seriously – if not more seriously – than the new food and exercise choices you make. It is designed to increase your moment-to-moment awareness of how you're feeling and become more aware of triggers, so that you can feel more in control of how you respond to them.

AM Check-in: Compulsory Daily Exercise

First, choose a time every morning (as soon as possible after you've woken up) when you know you can assign yourself five minutes to make some quick notes. Ideally, try to pick a time that you can add on to something you already know you do every single morning. That way you can create a new association. For example, the five-minute slot you may choose could be right after you get out of the shower, while you're drying off in a towel. I do my five minutes while I'm making and drinking my first coffee of the day. Make sure that you have some paper and a pen that works close to hand, so you don't waste any time or get deterred from completing it in the morning rush. If it's absolutely impossible for you to complete this on paper first thing in the morning, then it can be done on your phone during a commute, or even recorded out loud in the car as a voice note. The most important thing is that you repeat it every day and make it such a part of your routine that you notice when you haven't done it. At times when you want to skip it, instead get into the habit of saying to yourself, 'I deserve five minutes a day to check-in with myself.'

You are going to compile a list of the things that, if you had to put money on it, would directly or indirectly lead to you wanting to go off track with your weight-loss plan. All the circumstances and situations you're likely to face on that specific day that may test you. Anything from knowing there will be cake in the office for someone's birthday to expecting sugar cravings because you didn't get a decent night's sleep. That way, if and when those things present themselves, you've removed the element of surprise and feel more prepared to react in a way you're still of proud the next day. Sometimes, of course, this will involve not reacting at all. In these cases, the simple realisation of its predictability will help you to feel more in control.

So, from tomorrow, using the template below, start to spend that allocated five minutes thinking about as many possible triggers as you like, using whatever language is quickest and most comfortable for you. Once my list is complete, I take a quick photograph of it on my phone and then throw away the original – for added privacy and also so I have it to hand if I want to glance at it during the course of the day.

What might make it difficult to stay on track with my weight-loss plan today? e.g. Lunch with a colleague who always makes comments about my weight. Usually come away from those feeling crap and wanting to binge.

How I will respond: e.g. Remind myself that her comments aren't worth undoing all my plans for and make sure I look at the photo I took of my 'My Body Has' map for a boost on the way back from lunch. Remember that she doesn't mean badly and I'll regret it if I snap at her or get triggered.

What might make it difficult to stay on track with my weight-loss plan today? e.g. Leaving party at work, cake everywhere. Will be drinking so resolve around food likely to be low. Plus, I'll probably be hungry which never helps matters.

How I will respond: e.g. Eat a substantial lunch a little bit later so I'm not drinking on an empty stomach, stick to two glasses and remind myself that cake is available everywhere, I can have it whenever I want. I'm not forced to eat it because a colleague is leaving.

What might make it difficult to stay on track with my weight-loss plan today? e.g. I have to have a difficult conversation with someone and I feel really anxious about. Not sure breathing exercises and maps are going to take the edge off like a cheeseburger could.

How I will respond: e.g. Remind myself that this is an opportunity to practise my new skill of being able to watch the urge pass. I need examples of having dealt with this in new, kinder ways, and today can be one of them. I'll listen to myself want the cheeseburger and decide to let it just play in the background while I patiently wait for the discomfort to pass.

What might make it difficult to stay on track with my weight-loss plan today? e.g. When I have a slump as I always do at about 3.30pm and tell myself the only way to fix it is to eat chocolate at my desk.

How I will respond: e.g. Remind myself that it's never worked before and any boost that the chocolate gives me will be fleeting, leaving me feeling even more sluggish than I did before. If I do decide I really want some chocolate, reframe this trigger as a challenge to see if I can eat half the amount I usually would.

Once you feel more familiar with the check-in exercise, you'll find that you don't need such prescriptive questions. You may choose to extend the exercise to different areas of your life. So, in addition to pre-empting the things that make you want to eat in ways you're not happy with, you might also choose to pre-empt the things that tend to make you snap at a loved one or smoke cigarettes. Remember, pre-empting and externalising won't make the feeling of being triggered disappear, it will allow you to observe it as opposed to be driven by it. You will be able to collect examples of how discomfort also passes and evidence of how well you know your body and how predictable it is. Then, more and more often, for the rest of your life, when you feel discomfort, you begin to believe that it will pass and that you can endure it without adding to it by responding in ways you later regret.

My final word on the AM check-in exercise: I cannot stress enough how beneficial it is to commit to this practice every day. My clients who successfully incorporate it into their lives start seeing transformations in their behaviour more quickly than they could ever have expected. When it comes to keeping up weight-loss plans, they find themselves effortlessly jumping over hurdles that they fell at in the past. Trust me, if there's just one way you change your life as a result of reading this book, let it be that you make this check-in exercise a part of your daily routine.

Map: Testing Times

The time has come for you to create your own collection of internal and external high-risk scenarios, to enable you to become more aware of the warning signs and how they can pile on top of each other to create seemingly unmanageable situations.

First, write 'Testing Times' in the middle of a blank page with a circle drawn around it. Then write down the things that generally cause you have unhelpful, self-limiting and self-sabotaging conversations with yourself. Draw a circle around each one as you go. It may help to use some of these cues:

- Thinking . . .

- Doing . . .

- Seeing . . .

- Feeling . . .

- Discovering . . .

- Realising . . .

- Being exposed to . . .

- Smelling . . .

- Touching . . .

- Remembering . . .

- Convincing myself that...

- Saying . . .

- Hearing . . .

- Meeting . . .

A few final notes on triggers:

1. Everyone has their own triggers

2. New triggers will pop up throughout life, it's unavoidable

3. Triggers are important to be aware of when it comes to changing habits

4. Triggers can negatively impact how motivated you feel, physically and psychologically

5. Triggers do not control how you act towards your body – only you do

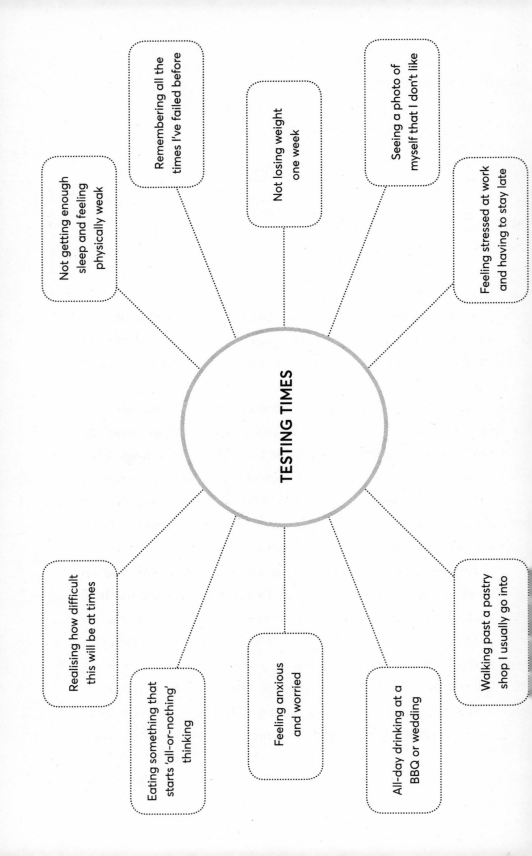

TESTING TIMES

Not getting enough sleep and feeling physically weak

Remembering all the times I've failed before

Not losing weight one week

Seeing a photo of myself that I don't like

Feeling stressed at work and having to stay late

Realising how difficult this will be at times

Eating something that starts 'all-or-nothing' thinking

Feeling anxious and worried

All-day drinking at a BBQ or wedding

Walking past a pastry shop I usually go into

gig's up

Don't insult your own intelligence

The excuses we make to delay starting something difficult and keeping it up can look irrational, illogical, even absurd when written down. Yet when they're just in our heads, they can compel and convince us.

We've discussed how we can throw ourselves off track with our plans by coming up with excuses that we use to sabotage ourselves. Self-sabotage happens for a number of reasons. These range from deeper things – like not feeling worthy of achieving success or subconsciously wanting to remain overweight for protection – to simply wanting to put off experiencing the initial period of physical withdrawal associated with changing your diet.

Regardless of why it's happening, sabotaging our own progress by allowing ourselves to be led by flawed internal logic has held back me and many of my clients from keeping up plans of change in the past. In this chapter, you will look at the common excuses that you make to justify going off track with your plans when things get difficult. We will build on the last chapter, where we looked at high-risk scenarios for going off track, but this time focus in on the stories we tell ourselves about the weight-loss process that don't help us and sometimes just don't make any sense. By starting to write them down, you will get into the habit of noticing – and challenging – their validity more frequently.

With hindsight, many of my clients identify that they fully relapsed with their weight-loss plans because two things happened to them in a moment when they felt challenged:

1. First, they believed illogical internal reasons and justification to go off-plan on one occasion

2. Then they threw the rest of the plan out of the window because of illogical, all-or-nothing thinking

All-or-nothing thinking is something I am very familiar with, but it wasn't until I started writing down examples of it in my own patterns that I realised how much I was letting it affect me. I've always liked to consider myself intelligent, yet when I saw the flawed logic behind the justifications I was allowing to guide my choices, I felt like a fool. When I did the exercise that you will complete in this chapter, I realised that six-day binges had begun with two thoughts that sounded something like: *It's raining so I deserve to 'cheat' tonight. That's ruined everything now, and the only day I can start again is Monday.*

I don't need to tell you that rain has nothing to do with what I eat; deviation from an eating plan does not 'ruin' the whole thing, and Monday is not the only day available for starting again. Yet I was guided by this kind of nonsense logic for years. If you feel that you too are readily suspending your disbelief for the self-limiting fictions you tell yourself, this exercise may help.

The next time you hear yourself making an excuse to neglect, change or ignore an element of your weight-loss plan, imagine the most intelligent person you know is standing in front of you. Choose someone whom you respect, someone whom nothing gets past, who is sharp and doesn't suffer fools gladly. Assume that they know how important it is for you to stick to your plan and they have your best interests at heart. Then, imagine justifying to them why you think you should go off-plan on this occasion, using your excuse as the 'pitch'. You will most likely conclude when you do this exercise that your excuse doesn't make as much sense as you once thought. Remember, you are also an intelligent person who is discerning and worthy of respect. You shouldn't suffer your own foolishness.

This exercise saved me in a moment when, despite being quite far into my weight-loss process, I was caught off guard by how suddenly tempted I was to follow a pretty ridiculous all-or-nothing internal command. I had ordered a take-out that I considered on-plan for me and my weight loss, which included a bottle of Diet Coke. They incorrectly gave me a bottle of Coke, in addition to a free starter and dessert that would have been off-plan. I put those foods to one side, but decided that since I was looking forward to a fizzy drink, it couldn't hurt to have one glass of full-fat Coke with my otherwise healthy meal. I had barely finished half my glass before I started telling myself that by drinking the full-fat Coke, I had ruined everything and that now I may as well eat the starter and dessert, which rather unhelpfully, had started to look more appetising than my meal.

However, having already done some self-awareness and mindfulness work, I caught my flawed logic in motion this time. I started thinking, 'Why does half a glass of Coke have to equal a binge? Do I really believe that is true?' If someone else came to me and said, 'I drank half a glass of Coke and someone told me it meant I had to sabotage myself with every choice I made after that for a while,' I would tell them not to listen to that person as they clearly don't understand even the basics of weight loss.

So, I decided to speak to myself out loud, and pretend I was talking to someone I know who has a very finely tuned bullshit detector, my old boss Ray Jenkins. I'd actually say things like, 'Hi Ray, so you know I'm trying to lose weight, well, I want to run something by you. I reckon I have no choice but to eat loads of fattening things tonight – and probably tomorrow, if I'm honest. The reason I have no choice is because I just drank half a glass of Coca-Cola. You'd agree that that's a good enough reason, right?'

Frankly, hearing myself made me laugh and feel a little bit embarrassed. Don't get me wrong, there are some foods that make you crave more of them physically, and that is a very real current to swim against sometimes. But in my experience, provided the all-or-nothing thinking is caught and curbed early, then any damage done in the process requires minimal effort to bounce back from.

In the past, I was most guilty of falling into the trap of believing my own excuses in the very first few days of starting a practical weight-loss plan. I've learned that this was also the case for many of my clients. What we shared was the habit of justifying going off track by telling ourselves it was still such early days that we may as well just start again tomorrow – i.e. nothing is squandered because we haven't lost any weight yet. Needless to say, this kind of thinking resulted in a succession of false starts that chipped away at our self-belief over time. All because we were so desperate to maintain the status quo and delay having to experience the discomforts of changing, we were prepared to believe stories that made no sense.

Committing to demystifying and myth-busting your all-or-nothing thinking can benefit you in many life areas, not least when it comes to maintaining your weight loss long term. That is because, treating your body well in every possible way will create conditions in which it simply doesn't feel right anymore to abuse it with unkind behaviour. That just doesn't fit in the new, kinder, day-to-day experience you've created for your body. This eventually makes it effortless to instinctively make better food decisions – i.e. the ones that help you maintain the weight that makes you feel most strong, attractive and healthy.

In order to create an environment in which unkind food and body choices simply don't have a place, you need to have lots of fingers in lots of self-care pies – just two of which are how you eat and how you move around. You can then challenge the kind of all-or-nothing thinking that reinforces an idea that your body isn't worthy of care, respect and enjoyment unless it is a certain weight or size.

If and when you fall off track with your eating or exercise plans, it will feel so much more natural to slip back into the new 'normal' you have created, not least because it's a nice place. It's a supportive place full of kindness, where you forgive yourself and continue to treat yourself nicely regardless of what you have or have not eaten. The bonus is that that this place of kindness just so happens to be one that gives you most resilience against all-or-nothing thinking and short-term physical cravings, which is of course what we need in order to limit any deviations from eating plans to harmless, enjoyable, intentional blips as opposed to catastrophes.

This myth-busting approach to the stories we tell ourselves can really help those who feel that they are living life 'on hold'. If you find yourself thinking things like, 'I'll pay attention to how I dress when I'm thinner' or 'I can't possibly start dating until I've lost weight' or 'I can't apply for that promotion until I'm a smaller size', then consider whether these things make any sense and whether debunking them is in fact a perfect opportunity to practise disassociating any of your value from your weight. Plus, doing things like taking pride in your appearance, placing importance on your social life and being ambitious in your professional life involves you doing the same kinds of things that create your kinder framework in which your kinder eating habits will comfortably sit.

Map: Gig's Up

We're now going to consider some of your own excuses and delay tactics. The ones that have, in the past, derailed your plans. Ones that make perfect sense at the time, but maybe not so much when you have to explain the thinking process behind them. First, write 'Gig's Up' in the centre of a blank page, with a circle around it. Then, write down:

- The excuses and delaying tactics you've allowed to work in the past to go off-plan with weight-loss diets when things got tough

- The excuses and delaying tactics you're already thinking of for this plan

- The excuses you're most likely to make to justify lapsing from your plan during the periods when you're not seeing fast results

- The excuses you're likely to make to justify neglecting the other self-care and self-development aspects of this process, like the written exercises and self-esteem building practices

You may find it helpful to finish some of the following sentences as a way to get the juices flowing. Although I still encourage you to think hard about your own collection of common excuses and stories, as they can be very creative and unique to you. (In the past, I used to justify a random binge when I was finding a weight-loss diet difficult because somewhere along the way I convinced myself this would actually speed up my metabolism by shocking my body out of a plateau and into weight loss.)

'Now isn't the right time to do this because . . .'

'It's not actually that important to do this because . . .'

'I should be able to make exceptions when it comes to things like . . . '

'_____ makes it impossible for me to change right now'

When you've finished, reflect on the collection of excuses that are currently clogging up your soundtrack when you try to make changes. Decide whether they look as convincing when they're written down. Even if some of them are reasonable, ask yourself whether it makes sense to let them impact your thought processes so much that you move further away from your weight-loss goals.

In the case of the excuses that make no sense, resolve not only to prevent them working specifically, but also not to let variations of them work either. I say this because when you start telling yourself that some excuses are no longer available to you, your mind may start to find loopholes, like, 'I lapsed because it was snowing, not raining. I never said anything about snow.' Commit to not insulting your own intelligence anymore.

the plan

The time has come to plan what you'll
actually be doing to achieve your goals.

First, you will identify the 'off-track' behaviours and foods that you already know are currently contributing to weight gain or making it difficult to maintain a weight you're happy with.

Then you'll establish your 'gateway' foods, i.e. the foods that might even be undisputedly healthy but that you don't seem to be able to eat in moderation. You will decide whether you have faith in your ability to start behaving differently around these challenging foods or if – as part of this process – you will temporarily abstain from your 'gateway' foods as well as your 'off-track' foods. This can be revised and you may realise (as a result of your regular three-week check-ins) that you would like to cut these things out for a time, perhaps down the line, if not at first.

Later, you'll reintroduce all of the foods you want to eat in a planned, considered and mindful way, until you feel confident that you've developed new go-to habits. The idea is to make things as simple as possible in the short term and then create new habits to help you unlearn any core beliefs around some foods being 'bad' and others 'good.' Most importantly, you'll stop thinking you are being 'bad' or 'good' depending on what you choose to eat.

Once you've used the guidance in this chapter to create your first plan, you will get into the habit of reviewing it every three weeks until eventually you don't feel you need to tweak and reflect anymore.

The vast majority of clients I work with feel that they *do* need some eating guidelines in order to ultimately decide on a plan they can stick to without thinking about it too much anymore. They are tired of diets that are purely focused on losing weight as opposed to maintaining it, and want to create a bespoke, realistic 'way of eating', based on how their body specifically responds to tweaks in their diet over time. They are prepared to treat the process as an ongoing investigation until they've landed on something that works for them.

Temporary 'abstinence'

Perhaps you don't trust in your ability to eat smaller amounts of your off-track or gateway foods yet, because historically you haven't been able to. Or, the thought of not having to make any decisions about some foods at all for a while sounds freeing. Maybe you've been meaning to cut them out of your diet for good for a while. Perhaps, knowing yourself as you do, you'd prefer to avoid listening to the usual internal negotiations around certain foods for the time being and relearn how to eat them later down the line, once you have some practice under your belt, positive results and more self-belief.

Note: I know we've been told for years that it's not a good idea to cut anything out altogether, and I'm certainly not a nutritionist. I'm pretty sure though, that if someone decided they really wanted to stop consuming gummy bears or Coca-Cola for a couple of months – or indeed forever – they'd be fine.

Creating your plan

I believe that you already know what food choices are making your body gain or maintain unwanted weight, either because of what you're eating, how you're eating it or how frequently you're eating it. So first, I'm going to ask that you make a list of the foods you already know are making it difficult for you to lose weight. This can be for any reason, from the nutritional value they contain, what quantities of them you're used to eating, whether they're tied up in childhood associations or habitual patterns like snacking in front of the TV, how your body happens to respond to them, or any unkind, unhelpful internal dialogue they currently bring about.

I'm not simply asking you to make a list of objectively 'unhealthy' foods to cut out. It should also be a list of any foods that cause you to have illogical, self-limiting or unkind conversations with yourself. The foods that, for one reason or another, bring about guilt, all-or-nothing thinking and flawed reasoning which historically, goes on to dictate that your next food choice is an unwanted one. The foods that, when it comes to weight loss, for one reason or another, make you think 'I've blown it' when you eat them.

When it came to creating my own list of off-track foods to cut out in the short term, there were of course many obvious (and delicious) ones that I'd just never been able to eat in moderation or without feeling guilty and out of control. These were things like pizza, crisps, nuts, refined sugar and bagels. But there were also much less obvious foods that only applied to me, because of my unique relationship with them and therefore the specific unhelpful conversation they caused me to have with myself that threw me off track. For example, one of the foods I listed as off track in my first plan, without hesitation, was bananas. At some point during one of my many impractical dieting stints over the years, I apparently picked up the belief that bananas were a rebellious, 'bad' fruit that wasn't helpful for rapid weight-loss. I had only ever learned to associate them with eating five or six at a time, as they were often the food I'd initially lapse from a strict diet plan with in the past. So, when it came to creating an initial weight-loss plan for myself, I cut out bananas for a few months to keep it simple, and decided I'd reintroduce them when I felt ready to teach myself how to eat them using common sense.

Here's what the plan I'll be guiding you through will be comprised of. Once you've written it all out, you'll be ready to get going. You'll then keep reviewing this plan every three weeks and spending about ten minutes reflecting on how you got on with it. That's how you'll continually make sure it's moving you closer to your goals. If it's not, you'll work out why not and tweak and add to it until it is. Your plan table will be the basis of your three-week reviews and cover the following:

- Off-track foods and drinks

- Gateway foods and drinks

- On-track options (for breakfast, lunch, dinner, daytime and evening snacks, drinks - alcoholic or otherwise, take-out and restaurant choices)

- Quantity and frequency guidelines

- Feedback on internal shifts noticed, weight loss results, how you feel in your clothes, changes in internal conversations, general observations and any tweaks required to stay on track for the next three weeks

- Review date in three weeks' time (put it in your calendar)

After trialling various options with myself and my clients, I found three weeks to be the optimum time to review. It offers enough time to still see results (even if blips took place) plus it helps people avoid becoming obsessive with frequent weigh-ins. Ten minutes of feedback was enough time to notice weight-loss results, internal shifts, general observations about changes in the conversations happening internally and any tweaks required to stay on track for the next three weeks.

When I made my first plan, I made a really simple list in a table much like this one and eventually all the foods were in the right column.

OFF TRACK	GATEWAY	ON TRACK
Foods that I can't eat in moderation	Foods that make me tell myself I should eat the foods I can't eat in moderation	Foods that I can eat freely and feel I'm on track with weight loss

It took me eighteen months in total to lose eight stone. I spent the first four months losing weight quickly, mainly by staying away from off-track foods. I had fewer blips than I'd ever had before, and they were inconsequential thanks to my AM check-ins, excuse-busting motivational tools and, frankly, visible results. At around the five-month mark, I started noticing myself craving my gateway and off-track foods more frequently. Although I could manage the cravings, they were making me feel uneasy. After all, I'd never experienced losing weight while eating these foods. I worried that even tasting them again would derail me as it always had in the past.

So I decided to try reintroducing a couple of the foods that I was craving in a planned way. I chose the ones I felt had the least hold on me personally. I reframed the reintroduction of gateway foods as an exercise in busting myths about who I am and what I'm capable of. It became an exercise in creating a new relationship with an old friend. One in which I needed to establish – and adjust to – new boundaries and norms by being consistent in how I imposed them.

Admittedly, my first attempts at reintroducing gateway foods didn't go well. On a few occasions, I ended up eating a lot more than I'd intended and even *gaining* back a bit of lost weight due to gateway experiments gone wrong. But I quickly got back on track after each blip because I knew the experiments were responsible for the sudden weight gain – something that had never happened before.

Then something really amazing happened. When it came to reflecting on and reviewing the first plan that included the reintro-duction of gateway foods, I found myself feeling really positive about my progress overall! My main take-away was that I felt incredibly proud of myself and that I was noticing great shifts in my all-or-nothing thinking. Weight gain and experiment 'failure' or not, this was the first time I had ever demonstrated that I could get back on track after a blip. It was big for me! Over that three weeks of falling off track and getting back on without days, weeks or months of spiralling, I finally understood the power that my kinder internal dialogue had in helping me make decisions that move me back in the direction I wanted to be going. In the past, the combination of blips, lost momentum and weight gain after four months of steady results would have been more than enough to make me throw in the towel.

For the first time in my life, I cared more about how I felt about myself than how much I weighed. As a result, I felt worthy of giving myself the same advice I'd give a loved one: disregard the weight gain, tweak the plan so it's easier, refer to the 'My Body Can' map and stop weighing yourself so frequently. And that's what I did.

Logic and self-compassion had finally started to prevail. I couldn't believe that weight gain hadn't made me like myself less or beat myself up. I finally saw the process for what it was (a little food experiment that had caused a human body to gain a few pounds) instead of seeing it as evidence I was a weak person, failing and spiralling needlessly out of control. I genuinely didn't feel compelled to abandon all my other new acts of self-care because of numbers on scales. I realised that I knew too much about myself and about how motivating people works to go back. In the aftermath of each blip, I watched myself naturally want to do the opposite of what I would have done before. I actually *wanted* to practise forgiving myself quickly. I wanted to show myself that I could get back on track immediately. The work I'd done on developing my self-care, self-esteem and self-compassion in every area of my life had made it impossible to believe that I wasn't capable or worthy.

This realisation was enough to make the next few weeks far easier and the fact I didn't feel the need to eat away any feelings of shame or guilt around my weight gain certainly helped in a practical sense. I decided to keep the gateway foods in and try again. I kept trying and tweaking until eventually they didn't feel like gateway foods anymore. My usual patterns around them became predictable, manageable and eventually non-existent. I started transferring them to the category of 'on-track' foods. I simply learned, that if I did consume them, I should expect to want to eat more even past feeling full. I could expect to tell myself I could ride out unhelpful urges and become more and more conscious of how much I was eating of them – and how frequently I could eat them – in order to maintain a weight I'm happy with.

After some time experimenting with myself this way it was very smooth sailing to lose the rest of my unwanted weight. I'd started mastering the art of seeing a challenging situation around food as an opportunity for personal development. As I became more confident in my ability to choose how I speak to and behave towards myself, I was able to overcome bigger and bigger challenges with ease. By month eleven, when it came to creating a new three-week plan, I was in the habit of moving four or five off-track foods into my on-track plan each time. Usually I wouldn't even choose to eat them despite 'allowing' myself to, as I now had so many new options that I enjoyed more and made my body feel better. When

I did choose to eat previously off-track foods, whatever they were, I stuck to each new set of guidelines without trying too hard. That's because all the kinder, bullshit-detecting, impulse control skills I'd been practising throughout this process were transferrable to every food and every circumstance. I was now convinced of my own abilities and there was no turning back.

By around month fourteen, I stopped needing to do check-ins or weigh-ins as frequently. I noticed that I seemed to be able to effortlessly, consistently and spontaneously make decisions that ultimately aligned with my long-term goals. I just made sure I kept doing my daily AM check-ins and applying my self-kindness tools at every opportunity. As I started approaching the end of my weight loss, I had developed a habit of treating lapses or blips as enjoyable experiences. I'd stopped regretting them, even if they were unplanned. All the three-week plans I reviewed and created had eventually come together to create my 'way of eating', my Last Diet. Thanks to my experiences with gateway and off-track food experiments as well as the new curious, respectful and compassionate approach I'd adapted to my body's needs, I found myself instinctively knowing how much of certain foods I could generally 'afford' to eat and how frequently I could afford to eat them.

Table: Populating Your Plan

Choosing your off-track foods

First you'll establish what you won't be eating at all, at least for the first three weeks of your weight-loss plan. Think about the foods you've never been able to eat in moderate quantities. Next, think of the foods you currently eat that you know for sure are contributing to weight gain, because of how frequently you eat them and how your body responds to them. There might only be a few foods and drinks that you choose to list, or you might start with more and review them as you go along.

In a notebook, write the heading 'OFF TRACK', and under it, make a list of the foods that, for whatever reason, you don't currently think you're able to enjoy while being able to lose weight.

Choosing your gateway foods and drinks

When we're used to all-or-nothing thinking and believing our own internal negotiations, it's not uncommon to go off-plan as a result of a technically harmless decision that eventually turns into a lapse onto the foods we're trying to avoid all together. For example, as I mentioned earlier when I was populating the gateway foods section of my plan, that you are about to fill out, too, it included bananas. Not because I thought they were contributing to my weight gain as obviously as things like pastries and pasta binges, but because I still considered them 'bad'. My ingrained crash diet, all-or-nothing thinking associated them with being off track. They'd never been allowed on my usual extreme diets, so I knew that if I consumed them, I'd start thinking 'I've blown it' and convince myself that I should eat the off-plan foods while I'm there.

With the exception of foods that specifically make us crave others, gateway foods are very personal because they're often based in our associations rather than with common sense principles of nutrition and weight loss.

By choosing to adopt The Last Diet, you're acknowledging that you're choosing to start losing weight but you haven't yet truly addressed the issue of not being able to make common sense decisions around some foods.

Now, write the heading 'GATEWAY FOODS AND DRINKS' and under it, list the foods you think cause you to have self-sabotaging conversations or crave off-track foods.

Choosing your on-track foods, meals and drinks

To do this, first consider your realistic needs. Perhaps refer to previous maps you've completed that remind you of what sort of plan works for you.

If you're a person who likes to snack throughout the day, and don't want to change this habit now – or ever – then cool. Just reflect on what points in the day you usually snack and list possible alternatives that you believe are more helpful in helping you lose weight. If you can't think of any, put aside twenty minutes and do some online research.

About 90 per cent of my clients and workshop attendees don't find they need to do any initial research to get going on their first few three-week plans. Seasoned dieters have a lot of knowledge, both about their bodies and the healthier alternatives that they don't mind substituting their unhelpful snacks with, provided they just give it a bit of thought. If you don't trust that you'll eat them in reasonable amounts, then set yourself a simple quantity guideline.

Even if you have a lot of experience and knowledge, I strongly encourage you to make an ongoing habit of looking out for new foods and recipes that you consider on track. Ones you can imagine wanting to eat when your task is to maintain your lost weight. The ultimate 'way of eating' you eventually create will need to be realistic, enjoyable and varied. So, even if you can manage to lose weight for six weeks with only two snack options on your eating plan, it's worth anticipating boredom. Commit to keeping your plan interesting, not least as it's an investment in establishing how you want to be typically eating in the future. When it comes to reviewing your plan every three weeks, consider whether all the food options you gave yourself were appealing enough and whether you're growing bored of them yet. If you are, commit to some research and consider yourself on a mission to create the most varied list of options you can.

Apply exactly the same thinking to breakfast, lunch, dinner, take-out and restaurant options. Take some time to list all the options you have available to you as on-track foods and meals. Ones you know you can enjoy and still feel like you're moving towards weight loss. Think back to any previous weight-loss attempts that worked, at least for a while, and write down any of the meals you enjoyed cooking and eating as part of them. Write down all the possible options you can think of. Again, if experience of dieting and your body's usual responses to foods isn't enough, then absolutely do some research for undisputedly healthy recipe options. If experience has taught you that low-carb diets tend to make you feel good, then research which one of those seems most sensible and look at the food options there. If the basic formula of calories in and out has served you in the past, then research what low-calorie recipes seem appealing. If you know you don't want – or don't have time in the morning to eat a substantial breakfast – then look online to see if there's a healthy smoothie you can make.

Ultimately, I can give you all the guidance and templates in the world. But in order to make realistic changes to your current 'way of eating' that you can sustain, you'll need to view this process as an experiment for a while. Practically speaking, the thing that makes this your Last Diet is that you're conducting an ongoing and comprehensive enquiry into what choices make your body specifically gain and lose weight. I believe that the vast majority of people reading and relating to this book already know what general type of diet tends to suit their bodies, and what they'd need to Google for recipe options that enable them to lose weight.

Setting quantity and frequency guidelines

If you think that things like portion size or the frequency with which you tend to eat on-track foods could still contribute to you gaining weight, you can create some additional guidelines. You might find it helpful to create your own rules, like 'only on weekends' or 'half the amount I usually eat' or 'not if I've had pasta for lunch'. If you think this would be helpful for you then either add your 'rules' after each on-track option, or in a new column of your table.

Note: although we want to keep internal negotiation at bay with a few clear rules on how much you intend to eat, being able to follow general, default eating guidelines spontaneously is the ultimate goal. You may feel that you initially need more specific non-negotiable rules around what quantities of certain foods you're allowed to eat. That's fine.

Three-week reviews

Every three weeks, spend ten minutes feeding back on your plan. Reflect on how things have gone and record your progress so you know what updates you might need to consider. If you haven't achieved the results you expected, use this time to write down why you think that may have been the case. Identify the choices you made over the last three weeks that you suspect are responsible for this, and decide what tweaks to make. Perhaps you could look at adjusting the portion sizes of some foods you know are technically healthy, but that you suspect aren't helping you with weight loss goals. You may change the frequency with which you're allowing yourself snacks, and consider researching more weight-loss friendly alternatives.

If you realise your first plan was too difficult, just tweak it! Compassionately and curiously observe why the plan didn't work for you and go again, this time creating more manageable guidelines to start with. You should feel that every three weeks, no matter what you weigh, you're embarking on new experiments with enthusiasm. That's because you know that this time, instead of investing in a quick fix, you're completing a total mind and body audit. You're investing in understanding your specific needs and what choices are best for your body at this stage in your life.

When you're finished recording your progress, add the date of your next three-week review to your calendar.

From abstinence to moderation and mindfulness

There may be some foods you've cut out that you don't want to eat again. That's your call. Most of the people I've seen lose weight successfully don't like the thought of never eating their off-track foods again. That said, after weeks, months or even years of not consuming those foods at all, they're very apprehensive about trying to eat them again, for fear it will slow down their weight loss or cause them to gain unwanted weight. This is very rarely due to the calories, fat or carbs they fear these foods contain. It's almost always because they still don't have specific evidence of having eaten these foods in ways that still enable them to lose or maintain weight. Even if they've seen great shifts in their mindset and ability to choose common sense principles in challenging moments, they've not practically seen themselves undo their all-or-nothing ways when it comes to certain foods. Abstinence has taught them how to not do something. It hasn't taught them how to do it differently.

For that, you need to see evidence of having done it the new way over and over again consecutively, until it gradually gets easier and eventually becomes your default way. How long this takes to happen will vary enormously from person to person, depending on anything from how things look for them when they start this process to how many opportunities they have to practise undoing old habits.

My clients tend to want to reintroduce off-track foods when one or all of these things happen:

1. They've achieved their weight-loss goals and feel ready to maintain their weight

2. They miss their off-track foods and want to reintroduce them in a controlled way

3. Regardless of where they are in the process, due to a boost in their self-belief and the priority of finding a long-term 'way of eating', they feel ready to start practising new ways, even if it means they risk slowing down their progress in the short term.

Creating your reintroduction plan

The next time you're due a three-week review, simply choose a couple of your gateway foods, and add them to your list of 'on-track' foods. When it comes to deciding what quantity of them you'll be attempting to eat and how frequently, create guidelines that you imagine you'll have to follow in order to maintain your weight once you've lost it.

This approach works even if you're reintroducing gateway and off-track foods before you've lost all the weight you intend to lose. That's because, as your three-week reviews will have shown you, as you lose weight, your body will require tweaks to your plan in order to keep losing it. In this way, one of the simplest ways to define your ideal quantity and frequency guidelines when it comes to reintroducing gateway and off-track foods is to start making the decisions of someone who is tasked with maintaining a lower weight. Essentially, when you set guidelines for what new habits you want to create around challenging foods, you'll be taking a guess. You'll base this guess on how you suspect this food will need to need to feature in your life if it's to stay around in some capacity, but not cause you to gain unwanted weight.

When it comes to your AM check-ins, make sure that you focus your contingency plans around attempts to reintroduce these new foods. However motivated you may feel, remind yourself that now more than ever, it's important to commit to expecting things to get difficult and reminding yourself that you're capable of doing difficult things.

When you get to the next three-week review, reflect on how things went, just as you've done before. Make notes on your progress in your ten-minute feedback exercise.

If you managed to stick to your new habits around previous gateway foods, but still gained weight or didn't continue to lose weight as you'd hoped, ask yourself why you think it was. Do you suspect the guidelines around them need to be tweaked so that you're consuming less of them or eating them less frequently? If you're keen to keep enjoying and practising on these foods in particular, would it make sense to tweak the guidelines on some of your other on-track foods? If you've reintroduced chocolate twice a week, it may be an idea to take the take-aways down from twice to once a week. Again, it's all a process of experimenting with your choices and capabilities and observing how your body and mind respond with compassion and curiosity.

If you didn't manage to stick to your new guidelines around gateway foods, or you found it more challenging than you feel ready for, then either simply try again or move them back into the off-track category again for now. I suggest you base the decision of whether to move a gateway food back into the off-track category on how many consecutive times you managed to behave differently around it. You're the only one who can really judge when you're ready to test yourself, so if you feel like you're getting closer to being able to keep up the new guidelines consecutively for three weeks, then go again! Carry them over. I know this may feel like a risk, but, the way I see it, if you adopt the principles of The Last Diet and believe in your ability to get back on track however the experiment goes, you can afford to take risks. You can willingly put yourself in front of consecutive challenges in a conscious effort to make them less challenging.

The idea is that you continue reviewing this same template every three weeks until you've found your new 'way of eating'. How long that takes will depend on how much weight you want to lose, how much of this process you embrace and a range of other factors. The most important part in making sure this is a long-term sustainable new 'way of being' is that you notice shifts in your self-belief and self-esteem.

You continue to gradually introduce gateway foods at three-week reviews, until your list is more varied and you've grown skilled at adjusting quantities and frequencies so that your overall food intake balances out to help you achieve your goal of losing or maintaining weight. When you feel more comfortable around all your gateway foods, you will start introducing your off-track foods and keep applying the same tweaking review process. So you include them as on-track foods and set yourself guidelines based on how you logically guess you're going to need to be eating them in the future if you're to maintain a lower weight.

Committing to AM check-ins

When you know what your off-track foods and food-specific new challenges are going to be, you can make your five-minute AM check-ins more specific. You can spend that five minutes guessing what kinds of things will make you want to eat off-track foods that day and deciding how you'll respond if and when you're met with that challenge.

I strongly believe that when it comes to building the self-awareness, self-belief and internal bullshit-filter you'll need to make changes that last, the daily AM check-in is the most effective and useful habit you can adopt.

Physical exercise

I don't profess to know much about fitness, but when it comes to acknowledging the benefits of moving my body around, not only to manage my weight but also to feel good in every way, we're in no-brainer territory.

That said, I think it's important to make an admission in the spirit of complete honesty – though I hope you will not let it influence your decision if you are in a different position to the one I was in when I lost weight. The thing is, I really hated exercise. I hated being out of breath, every minute feeling like it was lasting a lifetime – and actually every single thing about it from the mirrors to the running shoes to the Lycra to the yoga mats to the 'burn' and the elusive 'zone' everyone kept going on about. I was not an active child, or teen, or young adult, or adult-adult, and I had never found a way of moving my body on purpose that I enjoyed. The fact that it was usually either in a state of extremely full or extremely starving certainly didn't help matters.

I discovered in hindsight, having completed exercises like the ones in this book, that I could trace the source of many of my unsuccessful false starts in part to starting to exercise as soon as I started changing what I was eating. It appealed to my all-or-nothing, dramatic-transformation-wanting thinking style at the time. Plus, it made sense, since exercise aids weight loss both in a literal sense and through things like effectively relieving the stress and anxiety that can lead to unkind food choices.

The problem was that, for me, in the initial stages, exercise was a trigger to want to behave in ways that threw me off track with my eating choices, and therefore actually delayed me from achieving my weight-loss goals overall. To make matters worse, since I only associated exercise with feeling uncomfortable, embarrassed and disappointed, not to mention physically exhausted, I used to use exercise as an excuse to go off track with my eating plan for weight loss. I often fell into one of two thinking patterns:

1. I've done exercise, that means I've been good and so I deserve to 'cheat'

2. Exercise has left me feeling crap and wanting to change that feeling by binge eating

The only point I ever saw in moving around on purpose was to aid weight loss. I had no experience of it being useful for much else. And certainly no experience of it ever being enjoyable in itself. The closest I'd ever got was on the rare occasions when I'd enjoy that euphoric (and smug) feeling afterwards.

Now, I know that I could have been easing myself in from day one by doing things like getting off the Tube one stop early on the way to work and walking the rest of the way, or trying out a gentle exercise class that wasn't created with weight loss in mind. I could have downloaded free five-minute guided workouts on my iPad and, just once a week, done a little routine.

But no. The way I thought before, if I was going to exercise, I needed to be training for a marathon or already slim and just trying to keep it up. The old 'just take the stairs instead of the escalator now and then' stuff didn't fit into my extreme, quick-fix, boredom-fearing kind of thinking. As far as I was concerned, taking the stairs twice in a week wasn't going to make me lose weight and so there was no point feeling out of breath. It didn't occur to me that the more frequently I did it, the less out of breath it would make me, and that the reverse was also true. It didn't occur to me either that every day doesn't exist in isolation when it comes to my choices. That they all add up, regardless.

I realised that I was in fact getting more unfit every year, despite increasing the number of fitness programmes I'd signed up to every year. Looking back now, I always knew deep down that my all-or-nothing logic when it came to being more active was flawed. I know that because if someone I loved had come to me fifteen years ago and asked whether small changes adding up is a better long-term strategy for their body than a series of extreme false starts, I would have given them the kind advice. I just wasn't applying the same wisdom and consideration when it came to how I thought about and treated my own body.

I am delighted to report that I eventually started becoming more active. I'd like to say that's because I wanted to be, but it's not. In fact, it was because my body just felt stronger, more capable and easier to move around. I naturally felt more connected with it and its needs because I was finally paying attention to what those needs actually were. For the first time it felt like we were a team and I started wanting to see what my body could do. Surprising myself with the new eating habits I was managing to keep up made me want to start surprising myself in every other way, not least in ways that might speed up my weight loss.

Perhaps it was because my body was unfamiliar with exercise, but it responded quite dramatically to making my day even just a little more active. The things I decided to do had to be really easy, so that I would want to keep them up and repeat them enough times for them to become habits. When I finally gave the 'quantity not quality' approach a go, the results were amazing. By choosing tiny little missions throughout the day, I was able to measure how quickly I could see progress. This progress in both my fitness levels and the amount of weight I was losing convinced me I needed to give more organised exercise a chance again.

Now, I can tell you, hand on heart, I truly love the feeling of being generally active in everyday life, as well the process of organised exercise and of course the feeling I get afterwards. I have found ways of exercising that suit me, and ruled out ones that don't. I would even say I look forward to exercise these days. I now know what people mean when they say they are going to 'blow off some steam' with exercise. In fact, I have pretty much disassociated exercise from being something I do to help me remain slim. First and foremost, it's become one of the most effective methods I've found to improve my mental health.

I'm telling you this because it's an example of how quickly you can undo years of presumptions about yourself and exercise. If, five years ago, you had asked anyone who had known me for any amount of time whether they considered me physically active in any way, other than when I was answering the door to the pizza delivery man, they'd have said, without any hesitation or doubt, 'No'. Now, if you ask those same people and the ones who've met me in the last couple of years whether they consider me to be a fit, active and, dare I say, sporty kind of person, they'd say, without any hesitation or doubt, 'Yes'.

You too can change any self-limiting beliefs and decide on purpose 'what kind of person' you want to be when it comes to your physical fitness. There are a few pieces of advice relating to exercise that I wish I had known or believed sooner. I have recorded them below in case they are useful for anyone else who wants exercise to be part of their lives but has no experience of sustaining that in the past:

- All physical discomfort isn't bad. Trust that your body will tell you if you're about to have a heart attack

- Feeling out of breath is normal and gets better much more quickly than you expect

- Doing exercise you don't like is a false economy

- How great you feel after exercise is often related to how much you invest during exercise

- When it comes to choosing an exercise you want to take up, make it something you like the idea of getting better at

- Don't feel guilty about caring how you look when you exercise. If fancy gyms and buying new gym gear help you exercise more, then do it. You're investing in your body

- Other people aren't judging you. And even if they are, you have a much more important thing to be focusing on – yourself

- Don't make presumptions about what benefits you should be gaining from exercise. Just go through the motions as best you can for as long as you can. Your body will start showing you benefits you never expected

- Exercise can be a form of meditation, and not just in the obvious way, as with practices such as yoga. If you happen to feel most present, connected with your body and free of thought when you're in a dark spin studio with disco lights, doing highly choreographed, high-intensity exercise with dance music and motivational speeches blaring, then do that

- This 'zone' people brag about getting into is real. And trust me, you want some of it. It's so effective at helping you stop thinking that you don't even realise you were in it until you've left it. Don't go looking for it though, it'll find you as soon as you've gone through the physical motions enough times

- You don't have to exercise early in the morning for it to be useful. If you don't want to have to blow dry your hair before work or miss out on sleep to be fit, you don't have to

- Don't overload yourself with other people's opinions about what exercise you should be doing. Stick to the basics at first and learn to be guided by what your body is telling you makes it feel good overall

- Don't pre-pay for unappealing exercise plans offering miracle results assuming you'll learn to love them. You won't want to go back enough times to learn anything, and you'll be out of pocket

- Allow yourself to keep trying out new things and expect to keep changing your mind about what you want to be a fixture in your routine. Explore and experiment with every new type of exercise you can, in as many different settings as you can, before signing up to anything long term

- If for some reason you do choose to wake up early to exercise in the early days when you're still finding it difficult, try going to bed in your gym gear the night before

- Don't use progress with exercise as a measure of how well your weight loss is going. Make weight loss and maintenance a bonus. Remember that if you focus on exercising to improve your mental fitness, your body will naturally start taking care of your physical fitness

I will now invite you to consider what physical activity you might like to include in your plan of change. If, like me, you would prefer to address food first and bring in 'organised' exercise later on in the process, that's fine. But please learn from my mistake of associating all physical activity with pre-planned exercise by identifying how you can be more active in even the smallest of ways throughout your day.

Adding exercise to your three-week plans

Feel free to simply include a commitment to exercise in each of your plans. Review how you found each experiment as you do with food, and, if you find it useful, give yourself some more prescriptive guidelines to stick to.

You can use these enquiry questions for some inspiration.

- In what simple ways could I be slightly more active in the mornings?

- In what simple ways could I be slightly more active during my working day?

- In what simple ways I could be slightly more active during the evenings?

- What types of exercise would I like to start doing right away?

- What type of exercise that I already do would I like to continue doing?

- What types of exercise would I like to take up at some point?

- What types of exercise could I be excited to get better at?

- What types of exercises could I do that are designed to target the body areas I most want to work on?

- What types of exercise do I think would leave me feeling most invigorated?

- What types of exercise do I think could benefit my mental health?

- What types of exercise could enable me to enjoy active time with my loved ones?

- What types of enjoyable exercise could I plan to do during the weekends?

- What kind of physical activity can I do regardless of weather conditions?

- What kind of physical activity can I do to increase how much fresh air I get?

- What types of organised exercise would realistically fit into my routine?

- What time of the day does it most suit my body to exercise?

- If I try to imagine the type of exercise routine that I could maybe be convinced I'd keep up long term, what habits would it need to include?

Note that, in keeping with the spirit of The Last Diet, creating actions to improve your physical wellbeing extends to all aspects of your body. As such, if completing exercises like these makes you realise, for example, that in order to take up tennis again you'll finally need to make that appointment to get your back pain sorted, then be sure to make that an action too.

When the three-week reviews end

Eventually, a shift will take place that enables you to avoid the chore of planning. Naturally, when this is will differ from person to person.

Even though it took me eighteen months to lose all the weight I wanted to, at around month fourteen I noticed that I could gradually do my check-ins less and less frequently. I had got the hang of balancing out my choices and the habits that caused me to lose the last couple of stone are pretty much the same habits that helped me maintain the weight I was ultimately happy with. Many people reading this book will feel they can reduce the frequency of their check-ins long before I could. Either because they have much less to lose, or because they don't have as much investigation and unlearning to do. I grew to love my check-ins, as they punctuated my progress and reminded me that I'm investing time in diversifying my list of enjoyable food options. Ten minutes every three weeks was totally doable and fun.

If you commit to your AM check-in exercise and focus on your overall personal development, you'll naturally find yourself needing to be far less prescriptive when it comes to ensuring you make sensible decisions about food quantities that work for you. Things will get easier – and stay easier – when you start realising that your goals are being achieved with the help of an eating plan, not because of one. You will start respecting your own intelligence when it comes to excuses you'll accept for going off track. You'll be able to acknowledge that you're having to make difficult decisions and already be in the habit of reminding yourself, first by glancing at a map and eventually by just knowing, that you're capable of overcoming much more difficult challenges. You'll be in the habit of catching any unkind, unhelpful messages you're giving yourself. You'll be practising your new impulse-control skills daily and collecting examples of moments when you've been able to treat an urge as an alert, instead of a command. You'll be in the habit of reminding yourself that you always have a choice of what action to take when you're triggered in any area of your life. You will have gathered evidence of being able to stop a lapse in its tracks and challenge flawed thinking patterns once and for all.

If you commit to backing yourself long term by developing these habits, and simply seeing food plans as an aid for moments when common sense and trusting yourself aren't enough, the results can be transformative. The Last Diet process believes that it doesn't matter how many delicious on-plan meal options you assign yourself, there will be moments when you'll want to go off track, and that ultimately, no book is going to stop you from doing whatever you want. There will be moments you hadn't planned for, when you have to make a call. In order to feel empowered in the actions you take in those moments (and the ones you take straight after them), you ultimately need to trust and believe in yourself more than you trust and believe in any plan.

This process is not about controlling what you eat. It's about believing in your ability to apply common sense principles and not treat urges as commands. It's about exploring what foods stop you losing weight and teaching you to think differently about them until you can meet them head on and still trust that you'll make the best decision for you. And more importantly perhaps, trust that when you don't make the ideal choice, you have the ability to immediately make the next choice the best, most kind, most logical one, however difficult it may be. Once you've mastered this, a shift will take place that can benefit you in every area of your life. You'll then feel less need to keep planning.

Again, it will happen at different times for different people, depending on how things looked for them when they started this process. But when it happens, when you truly start believing in your ability to treat an urge as an alert instead of a command and become prepared to call yourself out on the spot, you won't need a plan to write down how many cashew nuts you're allowed to eat in order to still feel you're on track with weight loss or management.

Plan and review guidance

Now it's time for you to start working through your own plan using the guidance throughout this chapter and the maps you've created along the way. To recap, first you'll recreate a table like this one for yourself, either in a notebook or on a computer.

OFF TRACK	GATEWAY	ON TRACK	[OPTIONAL] FREQUENCY/ QUANTITY GUIDELINES

Then, when it comes to your first check-in, you'll simply sit down for ten minutes (or more if you like) and reflect on this table as well as your AM check-in exercises and decide what the next three weeks of your plan are going to look like.

It might be helpful to consider incorporating the below prompts if you find that you need a little more structure in your observations. Again, these are just suggestions. Feel free to word this however suits you best and add anything you feel would be helpful to each plan.

- I will complete my check-in at __AM everyday

- I will put aside thirty minutes, every three months to reflect on my check-in exercises and update my 'My Body Can' and 'My Body Has' maps

- What elements of my plan aren't helpful/sustainable?

- What tweaks will help make my eating plan feel sustainable long term?

- What is the combination of food, exercise and check-in habit actions that make up my new and improved plan?

- What habit actions make up my new 'normal' way of eating?

- What habit actions make up my new 'normal' way of being physically active?

And there you have it. For now, it might be an idea to do something nice for yourself, however small. Whether this chapter took you two hours or two weeks to complete, you deserve serious acknowledgment for the time and energy that you've put into creating a plan that affects what you do all day every day.

bring it on

If life is going to be filled with challenges
that make us stronger, why not choose
what some of them are going to be?

Through my work in addiction, I have discovered that when it
comes to the question of how best to manage high-risk situations
when we're in the process of changing habits, there are two main
schools of thought:

1. Focus your planning on avoiding triggers, as decreasing the
   frequency of exposure to risk will logically decrease the
   likelihood of unwanted lapse

Or,

2. Assume you will be around triggers all the time, so be
   aware of them, but focus more of your energy on building
   your self-belief to deal with unexpected ones

The Last Diet approach very much supports accepting, expecting
and preparing for triggers. It's not that I don't think we should

always be on the lookout for ways to minimise our experiences of stress or upset. But the way I see it, learning to better manage our overall wellbeing should be a lifelong, ongoing process. So, if you've identified that the eating habits you want to change are currently helping you manage stress, and you want to start to lose weight before you've developed effective long-term coping strategies for stress, then you should accept that you will probably feel more stress during the first stages of changing what you eat. And you're going to need both short- and long-term strategies for dealing with it.

That's why I think that when you feel strong enough – and only then – you should start to reintroduce some situations and circumstances that you enjoy but find it difficult to keep up your weight-loss plans in. Later in this chapter, you will complete an exercise to help you identify and prepare for these situations.

We can decide to accept that our plan of change will initially involve unpleasant things like annoyance and hunger. We can choose to not only prepare for these things if and when they crop up, but also use them to our advantage. We can reframe them as opportunities to fast-track the resilience-building process.

When I took time to reflect on which weight-loss plans I'd tried weren't right for me, I noticed many shared the characteristic of requiring me to feel in control of both my internal and external environments at all times in order to see results. These plans helped me lose weight, but in order to keep it up and keep seeing results, I had to create a protective bubble around myself since I always felt so deprived and ready to pounce at the first sign of a trigger. In my case, this meant isolating myself and staying indoors with only my (often tasteless) designated 'meal' to entertain me.

It just goes to show how much less I liked myself back then, because it's difficult to even imagine putting myself through that now.

While I know that some people strongly believe in avoiding facing high-risk situations in habit-change at every cost, it personally doesn't work for me because:

- It makes me feel like I'm just holding old habits at bay, as opposed to shedding them entirely

- It makes me feel like I can't trust myself to make the right choices in challenging and unforeseen circumstances

- It stops me having fun that I'd rather have with a bit of compromise as opposed to not have at all

In this chapter, you're going to draw from your 'Testing Times' exercise to create a collection of high-risk situations you will not only overcome, but you will attempt to welcome when they inevitably arise as an opportunity to practise your new skills and strengthen your resilience and self-belief. Overcoming the high-risk situations you do have some control over helps you to believe in your ability to overcome the ones that pop up out of nowhere.

I've often noticed those who are in long-term abstinent recovery from alcohol addiction to have notably high levels of resilience against temptation to relapse. It appears, though, that it's not in spite of alcohol being everywhere, it's *because* alcohol is everywhere. When it comes to sustaining motivation, repeatedly exposing themselves to the substance they are desperately trying not to consume can actually make it easier. I've gathered through conversations with those in long-term abstinent recovery from alcohol addiction that it's because they grew so aware of why they shouldn't drink, and had to remind themselves of the preferred life they're moving towards so often, that they just cut to the end and stopped even seeing having a drink as an option, let alone a temptation. Because alcohol is everywhere and associated with so many occasions, they had plenty of opportunities to practise showing themselves that they could be around it without consuming it. By committing to building their resilience, connection with their bodies, self-belief and self-awareness, over time they have desensitised themselves to it and made their peace with their default, automatic choices, safe in the knowledge that when they decided not to drink again, they had their own best interests at heart. This also meant that they felt they could still feel strong in situations where alcohol was around – or even appeared unexpectedly.

When I recently asked a client in long-term abstinent recovery from alcohol addiction how she managed to resist all the shelves of booze every single time she went grocery shopping, she told me:

> After hundreds of successful trips now I just instinctively
> know that some sections of the supermarket have things
> I don't need and that I know full well I will never need
> again. I was already used to thinking like this, not just
> because I've never needed nappies before, but because
> I'm lactose intolerant. I just told myself that another
> allergy I've discovered is the one I have to alcohol. It has
> side effects that are dangerous for my body and mind.
> So, the alcohol section is not for me and never will be.

No point debating about it, negotiating with myself is a waste of time. I just get on with the rest of my shopping and walk straight past it now.

This is how I'd like you to feel when it comes to how you approach weight management and unwanted food choices. Like you can cut to the end with your internal dialogue about why it's important for you to stay on track, and not feel like anywhere is out of bounds for you just because you could be exposed to triggers. I want you to feel like you're in control of how you behave regardless of where you are and what challenge you're faced with because you know yourself and you've laid strong internal foundations. Again, planning is of course important, and as I've mentioned before, just pre-empting triggers can be enough to make us change our response to them. But we can't always anticipate them and we will never be prepared for every possible risky scenario. We're better off doing what we can to make them less risky scenarios and eventually not risky at all scenarios. Plus, we don't want to spend our energy constantly trying not to ever become stressed or hungry or tired or in the company of someone irritating, or in the company of onion rings. This only reinforces the idea that our actions are at the mercy of these things, which they absolutely are not.

Coming back to alcohol, the focus of my work has more recently shifted to helping those who don't want to stop drinking, but who do feel they have a drinking problem and that they need a general plan to stick to. A 'way of drinking' that they'd never taken time to create on purpose. Those who succeed in doing this are extremely inspiring to me. That's because they're the ones I can relate to most when it comes to learning how to eat a human-sized portion of something I've only ever been able to eat a bear-sized portion of. I had to create my first 'way of eating' thirty-odd years after I began eating. I understand what it feels like to be around my substance of joy, comfort, protection, relief, distraction and despair all day, and constantly need to make new decisions about how you're going to behave around it. Abstinence from food is not an option (although at some points I've wished it was), so I have to see, smell and handle my substance all day every day for the rest of my life.

The clients who are successful in implementing alcohol-management plans long term seem to share something with those who are successful in implementing weight-loss plans long term: they frequently have to be in high-risk situations they can't avoid.

A common example of this is a parent whose weight-loss plan involves not eating the much more enticing food they have to pre-pare for their children. This gives them a number of opportunities to strengthen their resilience every day. Eventually when they push through it enough consecutive times, they stop associating the children's food preparation with their own and realise they've stopped feeling so powerless at these times.

During a period when I was receiving weekly counselling, I noticed that I came away feeling prouder of myself when I'd reported to the therapist that something negative had happened – and I had responded to it positively – than when I reported than nothing negative had happened at all. This happened enough times until the things I initially defined as negative events stopped coming up at all, because I hadn't even had to think about how I responded to them anymore. My new habits had become auto-matic ones, and so my triggers had become less triggering. That's what the exercise in this chapter will begin to help you to do for yourself.

It may sound silly, but these days when I'm met with internal or external challenge, I try to feel grateful for it. More and more every day, across every possible life area, I have committed to reframing challenge as an opportunity to practise my new strategies and have more say in what my soundtrack sounds like. I know that if I want to be 'the kind of person who can easily eat half a portion of popcorn and leave the rest', then I need to have shown myself that I can do that as many times as possible. If I want to be the kind of person who, when anxious, exercises instead of reaching for chocolate, then I need examples of having done that over and over again. Of course, I am presuming common sense tells you here that I don't recommend you intentionally making yourself feel anxious to practise easing it with exercise – you can wait for that trigger to find you. But becoming a slightly more frequent cinema-goer in order to collect more examples of when you managed to eat half of the popcorn isn't such a bad idea.

Written Exercise: Bring It On: Part 1

When it comes to keeping up your new eating plan for weight loss, what current high-risk situations for lapse would you like to eventually become low-risk situations?

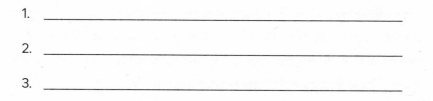

1. _____

2. _____

3. _____

4. _____

5. _____

6. _____

E.g. When I'm hungover, when I'm stressed at work, on Friday night, in a restaurant, after a row with my partner, when celebrating my success, when I've got my period

Map: Bring It On: Part 2

Now let's use this information to create a map. First write 'Bring it on' in the centre of a blank page, with a circle drawn around it. Then, use each item in your list above as further headings and circle those too, being sure to leave space under them for more notes.

Now, for each scenario, try to guess how many times you'd need to have responded to this situation in the way you want to in order to truly believe it's not a high-risk situation for going off track with a weight-loss plan anymore. Essentially, to genuinely believe you've changed. Then draw empty tick boxes under each heading, one for each occurrence. (Though if it's something like 100 times then you may want to just write 100 and commit to drawing yourself seven new empty tick boxes a week until you hit 100.)

The idea is not only that you boost your self-belief by recording your progress and achievement, but also that you start to get excited about practising your new responses – whether that's responses to challenges you put yourself in front of on purpose or those that present themselves out of nowhere.

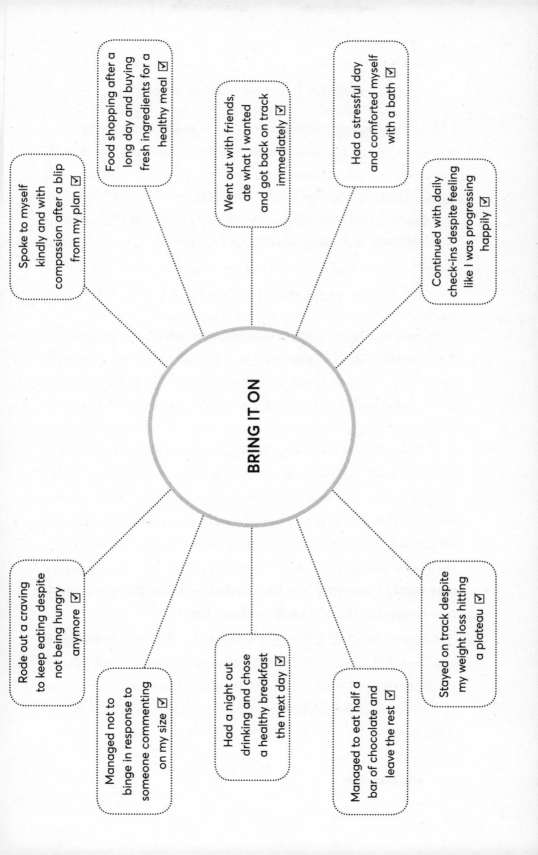

BRING IT ON

Spoke to myself kindly and with compassion after a blip from my plan ☑

Food shopping after a long day and buying fresh ingredients for a healthy meal ☑

Went out with friends, ate what I wanted and got back on track immediately ☑

Had a stressful day and comforted myself with a bath ☑

Continued with daily check-ins despite feeling like I was progressing happily ☑

Rode out a craving to keep eating despite not being hungry anymore ☑

Managed not to binge in response to someone commenting on my size ☑

Had a night out drinking and chose a healthy breakfast the next day ☑

Managed to eat half a bar of chocolate and leave the rest ☑

Stayed on track despite my weight loss hitting a plateau ☑

Written Exercise: Celebrations

I found it incredibly motivating to reward and celebrate myself for having ticked off a certain number of high-risk situations that I'd overcome in a row. Sometimes I felt I deserved a reward because I'd got through just one (usually this was a time when a number of triggers seemed to pile on top of each other and I handled it so well with my subsequent food choices I barely recognised myself). Either way, I started tuning in to what truly felt like an accomplishment to me and feeling prouder and worthier of acknowledgment and respect every day.

However, when it came to actually rewarding myself, I discovered, as many of my clients do, that I slipped back into old ways of thinking. The only rewards, celebrations and indeed punishments and commiserations I could think of involved eating. I do think rich, fattening, delicious food can be a great reward in the right circumstances, I just don't think it should be the only reward you have for managing not to eat rich, fattening, delicious foods. Not only are we worthy of more exciting and creative treats, this type of thinking makes us feel like the foods we have voluntarily chosen not to eat are forbidden and that the first chance we get we must consume them. You can eat whatever you want whenever you want – with The Last Diet you don't celebrate by letting yourself off the hook, because there is no hook.

Consider some of the ways you might be able to celebrate your personal milestones during this process (both to acknowledge yourself things for like pounds lost and to reward yourself for things like completing the written exercises for twenty-five consecutive days).

Write some suggestions of rewards and celebrations here:

1. _____

2. _____

3. _____

4. _____

5. _____

6. _____

E.g. Take a long candle lit bath, take myself to the theatre, treat myself to a massage, spend a Sunday in bed reading magazines, invite a friend out to raise a glass with me, buy myself some flowers

A final note on this chapter: even if you are quite far into your change process, if you don't feel comfortable with the 'putting yourself in front of stuff on purpose' idea, then just don't do it. Focus on building your resilience in preparation for the high-risk situations that come out of the blue. Then after you've dealt with them, log them on your 'Bring It On' map and/or your 'My Body Can' map.

damage control

It's not damage when you know
how to get back on track

This chapter will help you feel more equipped to get back on track from any blips as soon as possible. It builds on previous chapters which explain that there is a step we often overlook when it comes to how we behave towards ourselves when met with challenge.

To recap, in short, a 'lapse' is a planned or unplanned deviation from your 'on-track' general 'way of eating' that you can bounce back from quickly.

I would argue that if you adopt The Last Diet completely in the spirit it's intended, you will never consider anything a 'relapse' again, long term. That's because you won't see starting again practically as a false start anymore, rather as a signal that you need to review your plan more before it's perfect for you in the long term.

You know by now that eating and exercise make up just two of the many elements of The Last Diet. By the time you've attained your default way of eating, 'lapses' will just be the moments you choose to enjoy foods or ways of eating that you know aren't helpful for weight management before immediately going back to the ones that are. Provided you keep demonstrating to yourself that you can immediately bounce back to your default 'way of eating' without letting these lapses drag on, they will stop being lapses and start being your version of 'eating everything in moderation'.

Perhaps in the future, you'll realise that, for whatever reason, you've neglected your practical weight-management habits for a few weeks, perhaps because of a holiday. Maybe that's caused you to gain some weight. That's fine! If you still complete your AM check-ins, go back to your self-defined best 'way of eating' to manage your weight and how you're generally treating your body and mind with more kindness than you did before, then you're still on track with many of the important parts of The Last Diet.

One of the main challenges when changing habits around food is that we are exposed to food and food decisions all day every day in a range of different contexts which may well keep changing for the rest of our lives. Those of us who are highly skilled at negotiating with ourselves internally and finding reasons to go off track are simply given too many opportunities to make unkind decisions, full of technicalities and get-out clauses. That's why, when it comes to weight loss, we're better off trying to challenge flawed logic across all areas of our lives than focusing on food specifically. Even if you get a huge tattoo across your hand that says 'YOU KNOW THOUGHTS AND FEELINGS CAN'T FORCE ACTIONS', there will still be moments in the future when you choose to keep that hand in your pocket.

That's because before the bounce-back tools can work, you have to want to use them. You have to want to remind yourself that all-or-nothing thinking doesn't make sense, and that your plan is really important to you. You have to *want* to put steps between feeling an urge to do something you'll later regret and actually doing it. Sure, sometimes it feels as simple as:

High-risk situation = relapse

But in reality, it's:

High-risk situation + internal conversation = lapse
then
Lapse + internal conversation = relapse

There have been many occasions when my clients have pushed against The Last Diet's requirement to shine light on their excuses and question the validity of their internal justifications. As I often say, this is because they don't want to give up their 'fuck it'. They know deep down that their excuses and delay tactics make no logical sense. They know hunger pangs don't take the wheel and drive their body to KFC. But they don't want to give up that mindless but comforting option to escape from discomfort by allowing themselves to believe their own excuses. So they choose to keep their 'fuck it' as a security blanket.

Think back to one of those moments in the past when you've impulsively gone off track with a challenging diet plan. A time when you felt so desperate to give up that you threw in the towel and quickly binged on a vast buffet of foods you'd felt deprived of. You'd white-knuckled it through the tasteless meal choices but a bad day at work meant you finally just said, 'Fuck it'. Now you're slumped on the sofa post-major binge, feeling that horrible kind of full you'd forgotten about. The one that makes you feel physically sick and somehow still hungry at the same time. Would that moment have been the kind of time when you'd have wanted to go find a relapse management map to complete? Would it be a period of time when you'd be feeling really resilient against self-sabotaging thoughts?

Say you have plans to eat at a restaurant, and when you arrive you're starving and very angry at someone close to you. You already looked up the menu online beforehand and decided on what you'll order. It's a meal you're really looking forward to, as it's delicious but also keeps you on track and doesn't make you feel deprived or restricted. However, when you arrive at the restaurant, you're informed that the menu has changed. So much so in fact that now there isn't a single thing on the menu you can eat to keep you on-plan completely. Now you have to choose whether to remind yourself of what you know you should do, or simply revert easily into your old habit of using 'being caught out' as an opportunity to order yourself enough food for three people.

When thinking about what you'll do when faced with these sorts of dilemmas, even if 99 per cent of the time you made the kinder decision, the other 1 per cent can throw you off track. If that's combined with all-or-nothing thinking styles, then the 1 per cent can throw you off track for a while. You won't always *want* to tune in with your thoughts and bodily sensations enough for your excuses to become undeniably unconvincing.

So, what can we do to make it difficult for even that (very ambitious) 1 per cent of times to throw us off track for long? We can commit to designing the best possible environment in which mindful acts just make sense and mindless, unkind ones just don't. It's more obvious how to start creating these conditions externally.

Say, for example, you're months into your plan and you've developed a repertoire of recipes you're happy with and that align with your chosen 'way of eating' long term. You're weeks into an exercise routine and have friends who turn up every week to do that with you. Your check-ins have become part of your day-to-day routine. You've introduced kindness into your morning and your fridge is packed with healthy breakfast options. Everyone around you has grown used to seeing you take more pride in your appearance and care more about yourself in general. You're absolutely convinced now that self-sabotage only delays things and that you're in control of your actions.

But one evening, for a variety of different reasons, you decide to flick the 'fuck it' switch with your eating. However, you wake up in the morning and, whether or not you have the energy in that moment to challenge unhelpful thoughts, your entire life is already challenging unhelpful actions. You already have plans to meet your friends and exercise. You already have a new outfit you're looking forward to wearing. From the moment you get out of bed, you're performing kind actions for yourself. You have actually made it easier to carry out your plan than try to revert to old ways. In fact, going back to old ways requires much more effort on your part than getting back on track. There would be too much arduous and unwelcome undoing to be done.

As well as setting a more fitting scene in which to live, all those kinder habits dotted throughout your day are playing an important role in keeping planned and unplanned lapses from becoming relapses ever again: they are imposing friction. In that, they are creating as many speed bumps as possible between thinking about throwing in the towel and actually managing to do it.

Some speed bumps are of course choosing referring to your maps for the support and reassurance you need, or just opting for a short-term delaying tactic. But the real strength ultimately is in our default routine, which provides the infrastructure to get us back on track in those inevitable moments when we simply don't want to care, while our thoughts catch up.

We can use this 'speed bump' thinking in a range of ways when it comes to riding our short-term physical cravings during the initial stages of change. For example, if your plan includes not ordering take-aways from your phone anymore, don't just delete the app. Sign out of the app, after deleting your pre-filled payment and delivery details. Create more and more speed bumps; more effort required to follow through on your impulse to act; more steps to take between an idea and its execution. Even if you've logged back in and decided what to order, perhaps while you're looking for your credit card you'll catch sight of what you're doing and decide to stop that unwanted lapse in its tracks.

One great way of imposing a speed bump that requires no administration is simple delay tactics. Tell yourself that you have every intention on acting on whatever impulse that you want, but that you'll try to wait for thirty minutes before you do. When it comes to impulses to eat urgently in ways we quickly regret, imposing a delay can make all the difference. That's because very often when we've reassured ourselves that our guaranteed fix is available as if we need it, we feel more able to calm down, slow down and to try a new, healthier approach before we resort to it. Because of both the changing and usually fleeting nature of physical cravings, by the time it comes to allowing ourselves the fix we wanted, more often than not the urge has passed.

Removing speed bumps can then help us when trying to create new habits, especially in the early days of change. As soon as you think of a new kinder habit you'd like to make part of your routine, do everything you can to remove barriers between wanting to and doing it. I do this all the time and find every day that just a tiny bit of speed bump-flattening in advance can go a very long way.

For example, at one point I was struggling with a plan to do a very enjoyable thirty-minute online stretch routine every Sunday morning when I woke up. I knew this habit was one I wanted to adopt, since it was one where I could wake up whenever I wanted and do something that made my body feel good during and after. But despite this, I hadn't been able to keep it up. I knew there wasn't anything deeper to it than just forgetting about it as an action. So, I decided to transfer some speed bumps from Sunday morning to Saturday to create a plan of less resistance. I put an alarm on my phone that reminded me to do two things on Saturday in preparation for Sunday:

1. Charge my iPad and load up the guided stretching video

2. Put my yoga mat somewhere visible ready for the morning

Then, when I woke up on Sunday, I had to walk over a giant yellow mat to get from bed to coffee in the morning, which I absolutely noticed and remembered why it was there.

Sweet spots

When helping clients to reintroduce foods that they initially choose to cut out because they feel out of control around them, I encourage them to adopt what I call 'sweet spot' thinking. It's aligned with previous themes around illogical reasoning when it comes to eating behaviours.

I learned, while identifying my ideal way of eating, that the foods I didn't seem to think I could eat in small amounts weren't actually most enjoyable to me the large amounts I thought I wanted to consume them in. I was going by the logic that if the first slice of cake is delicious and the second is also delicious, then the fifth must still be delicious. When in fact, after the first couple of slices, the rewards started diminishing in terms of how much I was enjoying the experience. Not only because of side effects like bloating or feeling hyper, but because the fifteenth bite is completely different to the first bite. This realisation helped me identify the distinction between using and abusing foods that I haven't previously been able to consume in reasonable amounts.

If you think you could do with developing more 'sweet spot' thinking, cast your mind back to the last moment you had during a meal when you thought, 'I am truly enjoying this eating experience. This food is genuinely delicious.' Then consider:

How much had you eaten?

At what stage of the meal was it that you were you most enjoying your food?

Then, try to be more mindful of this concept as you go about your daily life making choices about when to stop eating.

Post-binge reactivation plan

If like me, you've been known to suffer with seriously uncomfortable post-binge withdrawals, I have an extra tip I'd like to share with you. For me and many of my clients, the first couple of days into a healthier diet after a stretch of heavily bingeing on unhealthy food is incredibly difficult physically, and can involve anything from pounding headaches and acid reflux to skin outbreaks and anxiety.

If you find yourself in a situation where, for whatever reason, you feel that physical withdrawals are holding you back from pushing through the first few days of a new eating plan and coming out the other side, then I recommend creating a little pre-activation plan that involves committing to just three days of general physical preparation before focusing on weight management.

For me, this involves steadily decreasing my intake of the foods I want to cut out while creating comfortable conditions to ride out my withdrawals in. For example, I will decide that for three days I will only snack on unlimited amounts on fruit that I enjoy, make sure I drink three litres of water and, when it comes to meals, eat things that I know won't leave me craving more soon after. I won't focus on losing weight yet, just on feeling less unwell and less full of physical urges for starchy foods or those that are high in sugar. Then, when it gets to re-activation day, things don't seem nearly as difficult. Any further cravings and urges become considerably more tolerable because I am no longer swimming against the very strong current of physical withdrawal.

Now you know what you need to know about the lapsing process, I'd like to help you create a couple of extra tools that will help further minimise the likelihood of unwanted lapses.

Written Exercise: Early Warning Signs

First, think about subtle ways in which you might start neglecting your commitment to your plan and giving your goals less importance. These are things to be on alert for going forward. Sometimes one or two at a time can be fine but when a few are allowed to worsen gradually and continue to add up however subtly for too long, plans can start derailing without us noticing.

1. _____

2. _____

3. _____

4. _____

5. _____

6. _____

E.g. Not completing my AM check-in, justifying why a blip should drag on, not making sure I review my plan regularly, isolating and not connecting with friends and family who make me feel positive

Map: Emergency Plan

First, write 'Emergency Plan' in the middle of a blank page and draw a circle around it. Now think of someone who you'd happily take advice from because you know they have your best interests at heart. Someone who cares deeply about your happiness and really wants to help you achieve your goals. They know your history well and they know exactly what you need to hear to stay on track using the tools and exercises you've picked up. Imagine you have bumped into this person either during or en route to an unwanted lapse. You tell them what's going on, and the combination of guidance, advice and reminders they give you convinces you to get back on track immediately. On your map, write down what they said, drawing a circle around each response as you go.

When you're finished, what you have in front of you is a snapshot of bespoke take-aways from this process that you can glance at all at once. It will provide you with the bounce-back guidance that gives you the greatest chance of getting back on track with a challenging eating plan ASAP.

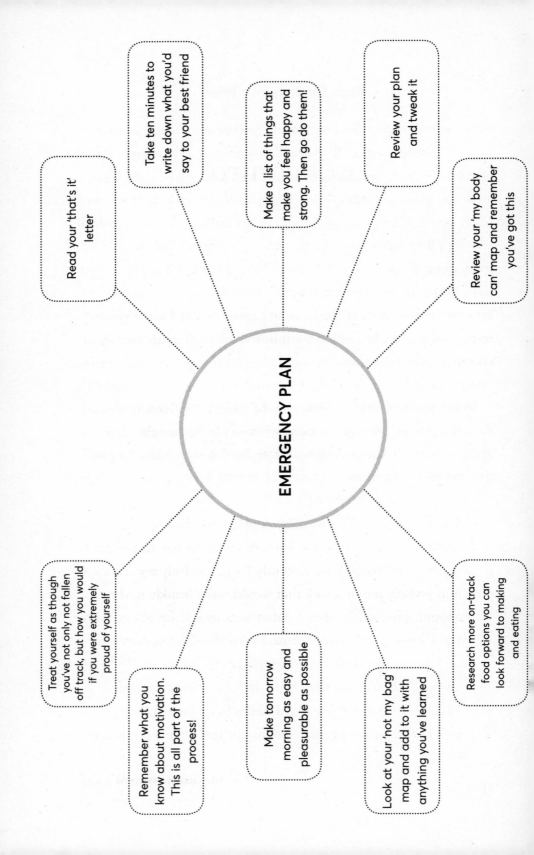

kind control

People often ask me how I can be so confident that I won't go back to my old ways. The simple truth is, I've made it unappealing for myself to do so, because:

- I've got a default 'healthy way of eating' I'm happy with that I now generally stick to without much thought. Any spontaneous decisions to deviate from it are conscious and I never regret them

- Since my body has always been prone to gaining weight quickly, I now accept that I will fluctuate in size throughout my life, and that's OK. Recently I went to Italy for ten days and joyfully ate in a way that would quite frankly make anyone gain weight. But I didn't beat myself up about this for a second. Not just because I recognised an opportunity to truly enjoy eating for the glorious experience that it is, or because I don't beat myself up about anything anymore. Mainly because I knew that I had a bespoke, effective weight-management plan waiting for me when I got home

- My response to even a tiny bit of weight gain is the opposite of what it was before. Now, I ramp up my self-care and ensure that I wear clothes that make me feel great and speak to myself in my most encouraging of voices. Before I know it I'm back at the weight I'm happy with

- When my body craves a behaviour pattern my mind knows I want to break in any area of my life, I observe it like a child who can't be blamed for wanting what it wants but whose demands simply won't be obeyed. I acknowledge it with compassion and understanding without feeling at the mercy of it. This has helped me feel incredibly capable of impulse control across a range of life areas

- I like how my body looks and feels, and that makes me feel strong and happy as a new baseline every day. I'm so aware of the habits that move me away from feeling like this that it's become a no-brainer not to engage in them

- If I wake up feeling bloated, I see it as just that. It's not a signal that I may as well keep eating bloating and fattening foods because I don't like how I look

- I place importance on how I see myself behaving when no one else is watching. If I don't feel happy with any behaviour I engage in, that's enough to make me want to change it. I don't need anyone else to witness my actions for me to want to change them

- I've done so many 'Gig's Up'-style maps that there are no more excuses or variations on excuses left to entertain, and now any new ones don't really stand a chance against my internal bullshit detector

- Whether it's a decision about what I'll eat or how I respond to an email that has angered me, I've taught myself through weight management to automatically project into the future and ask how I'll wish I behaved tomorrow and next week

- I am on a mission in every aspect of my life to reduce the time it takes to forgive myself for anything I didn't mean to do or later wish I hadn't done

- When I'm not sure whether an act towards my body is a kind one, I automatically consider what choice I'd want my mum to make for herself in that moment

- I have entirely new automatic self-care habits that were adopted not to remedy something, but purely to increase my enjoyment and wellbeing. They are absolutely a part of my daily routine and play an enormous part in me feeling happy with the day-to-day decisions I make across all areas of my life, including food. When I'm not behaving kindly towards myself in any way, I notice immediately

- I catch the moments when my first impulse to soothe or comfort myself is to eat food as opposed to trying a different coping strategy. If someone upsets me and I catch myself wanting to reach for something sugary, I can distinguish this from hunger. It's become such an obvious distinction now that I hear myself internally saying things like, 'I bet if you don't get the response you want to that text you'll immediately think you're hungry even though you just ate lunch.' It's become like an observation game of my thoughts and feelings, and I'm fully aware that they don't have to dictate my actions

- I genuinely enjoy keeping up my new kinder eating habits. These days, the fact they contribute to weight management is a bonus. I like striving every day to build a kinder, more positive internal and external world for myself, especially when it's challenging. One where acts and thoughts of unkindness are not welcome and stick out like a sore thumb. I'm finding it easier than I could ever have imagined to maintain my weight, because it makes me feel good to do so. After all, that's all The Last Diet was really ever about: finally learning to feel good in and about myself so I could make decisions on the spot about any part of my life that are in my best interests.

Now it's your turn.

NEW FRONTIERS OF SPACE, BODIES AND GENDER

Edited by
Rosa Ainley

London and New York

LEEDS METROPOLITAN
UNIVERSITY LIBRARY
7102365129x
HC BL
888653 19.1.99
305.42 NEW

LEEDS METROPOLITAN
UNIVERSITY LIBRARY
1702342361

First published 1998
by Routledge
11 New Fetter Lane, London EC4P 4EE

Simultaneously published in the USA and Canada
by Routledge
29 West 35th Street, New York, NY 10001

© 1998 Selection and editorial matter Rosa Ainley;
individual chapters © the contributors

The right of Rosa Ainley to be identified as the Editor of this Work has been
asserted by her in accordance with the Copyright, Designs and Patents Act 1988

Typeset in Sabon by Keystroke, Jacaranda Lodge, Wolverhampton
Printed and bound in Great Britain by
Biddles Ltd, Guildford and King's Lynn

All rights reserved. No part of this book may be reprinted or
reproduced or utilized in any form or by any electronic, mechanical, or
other means, now known or hereafter invented, including
photocopying and recording, or in any information storage or retrieval
system, without permission in writing from the publishers.

British Library Cataloguing in Publication Data
A catalogue record for this book is available from the British Library

Library of Congress Cataloguing in Publication Data
New frontiers of space, bodies and gender / edited by Rosa Ainley.
p.   cm.
Includes bibliographical references and index.
1. Urban women–Social conditions.   2. Urban women–Psychology.
3. Women–Identity.   4. Sex role.   5. Spatial behavior.   6. Personal
space.   7. Spatial ecology.   8. Feminist theory.   I. Ainley, Rosa.
HQ1154.S617   1998
305.4–dc21   97–33186

ISBN 0–415–15489–8 (hbk)
ISBN 0–415–15490–1 (pbk)

HARROGATE COLLEGE OF ARTS
AND TECHNOLOGY LIBRARY

CLASS   305.42
NEW

ACCESS No. 88342

DATE 2/3/99   LOCATION HP

Contents

Illustrations

Plates

Figures

Notes on contributors

Rosa Ainley is a writer and photographer. She is the author of *What Is She Like? Lesbian Identities from the 1950s to the 1990s* (London: Cassell, 1995) and editor of *Death of a Mother: Daughters' Stories* (London: Pandora, 1995). In 1997 she completed an MA in Photographic Studies at the University of Westminster. She lives in London.

Maher Anjum was brought up and educated in Bangladesh, Libya and Britain. At present she works as a lecturer in social policy and sociology with particular interest in issues of gender, race, class and regeneration. While completing her PhD from the University of Greenwich, London she is working as a consultant on organisational development within the public and voluntary sector service providers.

Jos Boys is a senior lecturer in architecture and urban studies at De Montfort University, Milton Keynes, UK. She was one of the founding members of the Matrix architectural practice and research group, and has written extensively on feminism and architecture. She is currently completing a PhD which explores the differences between professional architectural knowledges; development, design and building processes; popular and academic debates about buildings and cities; and the shape of the material landscape.

Jacquelin Burgess is a Reader in Geography at University College London. She believes passionately in the life-enhancing qualities of contact with nature and living landscapes. Through her work, she has raised awareness among environmental planners, landscape designers and local politicians about the importance of creating and managing green spaces for the many different groups who make up local communities.

Ali Grant is an independent researcher with interests in urban activism, gender and sexuality. She has recently completed a PhD at McMaster University, Hamilton, Canada on 'Geographies of oppression and resistance: contesting the reproduction of the heterosexual regime'.

Lesley Klein is a specialist in the urban regeneration field. She was director of the leading Technical Aid Centre, CLAWS, specialists in community participation, and then chief executive of Bethnal Green City Challenge. She currently works as a consultant, facilitating and developing partnerships on a wide range of projects.

Jacqueline Leavitt, Professor in the Department of Urban Planning at the University of California at Los Angeles's School of Public Policy and Social Welfare, co-authored *From Abandonment to Hope: Community Households in Harlem* (New York: 1990), coedited *The Hidden History of Low-Income Housing Cooperatives* (Davis, CA: 1995) and has written and lectured extensively on issues of housing, community development, and women.

Teresa Lingafelter is a graduate student in the Department of Urban Planning at the University of California at Los Angeles where her speciality is community development.

Robyn Longhurst is a lecturer in the Department of Geography at the University of Waikato, NZ/Aotearoa. Research interests include geographies of 'the body', critical social theory and urban cultural geographies of Aotearoa/New Zealand. She is a co-author of a forthcoming book entitled *Pleasure Zones: Sexualities, Cities and Space* (Syracuse University Press).

Doreen Massey is Professor of Geography at the Open University, Milton Keynes, UK. She is author of *Spatial Divisions of Labour* (London: Macmillan, 1995), *Space, Place and Gender* (Oxford: Polity Press, 1994) and, jointly with Paul Quintas and David Wield, *High-tech Fantasies* (London: Routledge, 1992). She is also co-founder and co-editor of *Soundings: A Journal of Politics and Culture*.

Claudia Morello is a graduate student in the Department of Urban Planning at the University of California at Los Angeles where she has combined her planning studies with a degree in architecture from UCLA's School of Art and Architecture.

Sally R. Munt is the author of *Heroic Desire: Lesbian Identity and Cultural Space* and the editor of *Butch/Femme: Inside Lesbian Gender* and (with Andy Medhurst) *Lesbian and Gay Studies: A Critical Introduction* (all London: Cassell, 1997).

Inga-Lisa Sangregorio is a freelance journalist and writer. She has written extensively on housing and planning and is a former editor of the feminist magazine *Kvinnobulletinen*. Her latest book is titled *Pä spaning efter ett bättre boende* ('On the lookout for better ways of housing ourselves') (Stockholm: 1994).

Tracey Skelton is a lecturer in geography and cultural studies at Nottingham Trent University. She has recently coedited two books, *Cool Places: Geographies of Youth Cultures* (London: 1997) and *Culture and Global Change* (London: forthcoming) and is currently working on a single-authored book about the Caribbean.

Affrica Taylor is a lecturer in the Centre for Indigenous Australian Cultural Studies at the University of Western Sydney–Macarthur, and a doctoral student in Women's Studies at the University of Sydney. She is currently working on the connections between identity, community and place across the relations of sexuality, gender and race.

Nina Wakeford is a lecturer in Sociology at the University of Sheffield. She is at work on a three-year project funded by the Economic and Social Research Council on 'Women's experiences in virtual communities' which forms the basis of the book *Networks of Desire*, to be published by Routledge. She is currently conducting fieldwork in Silicon Valley while a Visiting Scholar at the University of California at Berkeley.

Lynne Walker was formerly Senior Lecturer in Architecture and Design at the University of Northumbria and most recently a visiting lecturer at UEA and the University of Cambridge. Her latest publication on gender and space is *Drawing on Diversity: Women, Architecture and Practice* (London: RIBA Heinz Gallery, 1997).

Aylish Wood is a PhD student in Film Studies at the University of Nottingham. Her thesis topic is on representations of science and technology in contemporary film.

Acknowledgements

Mainly, a big thank you to all the contributors for their work in producing their chapters in the rather long and sometimes tortuous process of getting this book together.

Also thanks to everyone who said 'What do you mean, space?' and to the MAPS Ladies Team at Westminster who saw the pictures and then had to hear (I know it must have seemed endlessly) about the book.

And thank you to both Sarah Lloyd and Tristan Palmer for their enthusiasm and support.

I am grateful to John Wiley and Sons Limited for permission to publish Lynne Walker's work, a version of which appears in I. Borden, J. Kerr, A. Pivaro and J. Rendell (eds) (1997) *The Unknown City: Contesting Architecture and Social Space*, Chichester: Wiley.

Thanks to the following for permission to reproduce and describe their illustrative work:

Robyn Longhurst (Chapter 2)
John Sturrock/Network (Chapter 3)
Ebony, Jose, Melva, Leonel, Ashley, Star and Juana from the 4–H Program in LA (Chapter 6)
Baltimore Museum of Art: Friends of Photography Fund, BMA 1986.9, *Court of the First Model Tenement in New York City* (1936) by Berenice Abbott (Chapter 7)
Laura Barnes, for extracts from *Cruising* (1996) (Chapter 7)
Anna Sjödahl, for *Spring in the suburb of Hallonbergen* (property of the Museum of Boras) (Chapter 8)
Jacquelin Burgess (Chapter 9)
Lesbians on the Loose, 'Opera House Concert' advertisement, July 1991 (Chapter 10)
Linda Dawes, Department of International Studies at Nottingham Trent University (Chapter 11)
Section openers, Rosa Ainley

Every effort has been made to trace copyright holders. Any omissions brought to our attention will be remedied in future editions.

Introduction

'This is not star wars' says Affrica Taylor talking about the Sydney Lesbian Space Project in her chapter 'More than one imagined territory'. And it's not *Star Trek* either, which is what seemed to catch the imagination of those around me when I said I was working on a book about space. Intergalactic it isn't. That's a space both actual and imagined/dramatised, with a sense of boundlessness, 'in which all objects exist and move' (*Oxford Popular Dictionary* 1993). The dictionary definition there has a suggestion of a neutrality (which is generally absent from the discussions of space in this book) without restriction or border (which are very much present). The Oxford definition goes on to mention 'empty area' and 'interval' which again have interesting trajectories in relation to the conceptualisations of space presented here.

So, what it *is*.

New Frontiers of Space, Bodies and Gender presents a series of essays on gender and spaces: bodily, built, community, cultural, cyberspace and imagined environments. As it brings together contributions, some localised studies and others of a broader canvas, exploring (some very different) strands of feminist theory and practice, cultural and social geography and architecture, it also links across and interweaves analysis to activism, theory to practice, or conception to execution, as Doreen Massey calls it. This book does not seek to provide a definitive overview or a set of positions about space and gender but it presents instead a series of takes on the workings and interventions (and dysfunctions?) of the interrelationship between spaces and gender. 'The Space Book', as it became known, was always meant to be a diversity of positions (or lack of them) from a clutch of contributors in the fields of geography, urban regeneration, journalism, cultural studies, lesbian and gay studies, architecture, planning, film, music, social policy, activism, community development, housing, architectural history and photography.

With a scope of this kind a book needs a signage system. It also means that this is not going to be the kind of introduction which locates each piece within its broader discipline, because that would be another book. An introduction can work as a kind of explanatory note, a map even, to finding a way around the book. The pieces which follow will I hope make their own space – I long ago gave myself up to the inevitability of the spatial metaphor – within the interstices and overlaps between their subjects and disciplines. But they are not necessarily trying to plug the gaps, rather to flag them – or even to contribute to the recognition and establishment of newer ones.

The structure and content of *New Frontiers of Space, Bodies and Gender* are, in a sense, a response to nearly a decade spent working in the 'built environment' area, in institutions which included the whole gamut from the esoteric architectural to the more conventionally organised planning-related. While some of these were firmly and apparently securely positioned in their own space/culture, others both suffered and developed through an almost inbuilt tension between the need to work in 'practical' ways for improvements in real lived lives and the desire to move beyond the concrete, into the realm of the potential. Caught between the actual and the possible. It hardly needs saying that both approaches – the practical and the theoretical – have their own particular validity. Both are important and necessary, even perhaps simultaneously. Neither has primacy, each can inform and enrich the other. As organisations and individuals were forced into justifying their own positions, with the attendant exigencies of finance and funding, it seemed counterproductive that the two were often sited as oppositional. Without rehashing those debates here, *New Frontiers of Space, Bodies and Gender* attempts a *rapprochement*, a bringing together.

During the same ten-year period my own photographic work has moved from an early fixation on photographing buildings to making photographs about buildings and spaces. More recently, still using an architectural language, the work has concentrated on notions of 'home' and 'feeling at home' and, latterly, on pieces that use architectural glimpses to explore the production of social, cultural and personal memory. So I have been surrounded by and have engaged with work about lived experience and hard space as well as the imagined and discursive, and been involved in the creation of visual spaces that speak about the nature of all those kinds of space, to a point where they become much less separate, as Jacquelin Burgess says: 'what is perceived to be real, is real in its consequences' (see Chapter 9); and in a sense this book seems like an extension of all this or a culmination – although that suggests finality and it's really more of a marker.

Nowhere was this polarity more evident, and occasionally heated, than in the discussions around safety, and the book includes several pieces which explore different aspects of safety: Jacquelin Burgess's piece focusing on the lived experience of women using urban green spaces; Ali Grant's writing on the changes within organisations doing feminist anti-violence work; as well as the pieces by Sally R. Munt; Jacqueline Leavitt, Teresa Lingafelter and Claudia Morello; Maher Anjum and Lesley Klein; Affrica Taylor; and myself, looking at, in a sense, the security of having your own space.

The city isn't only about danger and fear (woman as perpetual victim), or boredom and limitation (woman as housewife), it is also a site of possibility, pleasure, excitement. A Women's Design Service *Broadsheet* puts it like this:

'Cities can represent great economic, social, political and cultural opportunities, if these are made accessible to all. . . . But cities are regarded by
many as being dangerous, unhealthy, or simply intrinsically hostile.' The
work of Elizabeth Wilson, in particular, on the city brings together the
danger and pleasures of the city for women. Which is one set of reasons
why people choose to live in them. A reconsideration of surveillance, often
implemented as a response to feelings of unsafety and also perhaps for more
pernicious and unsavoury reasons, is offered in Laura Barnes's work
Cruising (see Chapter 7, Plates 1 and 2) which explores a more pleasurable
side of surveillance, so often categorised as intrusive and malign, as well as
sometimes useless in effecting that for which it is installed.

Elizabeth Wilson has also pointed out the link between the growth of
urbanism and the emergence of 'the modern homosexual' into a space – the
city – that can bring both anonymity and visibility. Several pieces look at
the performance of the lesbian identities in space and in place: Sally R. Munt
on the discursive space of the lesbian nation; Nina Wakeford on the workings of community and identity of Bay Area dykes in cyberspaces; Ali Grant
on the importance of place in the formation of activist identities; Affrica
Taylor on the vulnerability/expansiveness of the ideas 'lesbian' and 'space'
that erupted with the attempt to create an entity that brought the two
together, coupled with the idea of 'safety'.

Long ago we moved on from the perennial questions of 'If there were
more women architects would buildings be different and if so how?'
(although on a strictly numerical basis this is hardly a resolved question)
and 'Is a feminist architecture possible?' and from the idea of consultation
consisting of asking women about kitchen layouts (although we have
not always moved as far as we might like to assume). We have needed to
find new ways to discuss built environment issues around race and gender
without falling into dead-end essentialisms, and assumptions of homogeneity within classes, races and genders are less prevalent. We have moved
on also from the traps of identity politics-as-straitjacket that so-called
'second wave' feminism fell into in the early 1980s (and so much of the
writing about built environment issues at the time – see Jos Boys's piece,
Chapter 15, which unpicks the architectural and theoretical implications of
a position that takes the built environment as reflecting received wisdom
about gender roles, and, through its construction and design, influencing
perceptions of them and how they are lived, seeing it as ultimately
reproducing an unhelpful fixed binary structure), and away from a simple
focus on woman-as-victim in the public arena, but no closer to 'post-
feminist ideology'.

New Frontiers of Space, Bodies and Gender looks at what we have
moved on to and, maybe, where next. If we have unravelled many of the
stereotypical ideas that have been seen as made solid in our cities, and in
gender-based assumptions therein, and if we see beyond this mapping/
reading-off approach (see Jos Boys, Chapter 15), *New Frontiers* offers
glimpses of how some of these ideas look in a more fluid or multi-faceted

state. Hopefully it also offers the possibility of shifting the parameters in the debates around issues of space and gender.

In the 1980s we witnessed a certain dissolution and reworking of spatial meaning when supermarkets were built to look like temples (of consumption), and now cyberspace and virtual reality have become, amongst many other possibilities, a new marketable commodity. Mass communication technologies (and multinational marketing strategies) have redefined, but *not* shrunk, global space and cyberspace has opened up new levels/worlds/forms of communication, which have also been recognised as marketable commodities, all of which adds to the debates about how space and gender work. At the same time, we acknowledge the shifting of the 'certainties' of gendered realities – taking gender as something that we *do* rather than something that we *are* (as Shere Hite says about sexuality: ' "lesbian", "homosexual" and "heterosexual" should be used as adjectives, not nouns' [1993: 85] – and of the distinctions between biology and culture, and sex and gender. Kate Bornstein says: 'Most of the behavioural clues [to gender] boil down to how we occupy space, both alone and with others' (Bornstein 1994: 27).

Gender then as how we do space, in addition to, rather than instead of, how space does us, which I write advisedly, if ungrammatically. The writings in this book examine, from a myriad of perspectives and disciplines, how such ideas are influenced by, and in turn influence, spaces and their construction. It looks from many angles at Shirley Ardener's comment that 'behaviour and space are mutually dependent' (Ardener 1993: 3). But as well as the question of feeling at home within the spaces built for us, or even by us, there are other spaces to consider: the bodies we inhabit; the interrelations between birth and reassigned genders and sexuality; cultural space; spaces created by specific communities – whether organised by location, race, sexuality, age, religion or whatever. Hence the scope of *New Frontiers of Space, Bodies and Gender*. A consideration of space, then, which looks beyond bricks and mortar.

Working out sections of the book then became crucial to understanding its purpose, and drawing diagrams became my preferred method of making decisions on organising the sections. The groupings under different section headings exist as a response to the nature of the collection, a reining-in against the possibility of fragmentation. If this introduction looks at the 'why' of the book, the sections suggest an answer to the 'how' of approaching it. That said, there are, of course, many overlaps and many absences. It is perhaps indicative of the kind of book *New Frontiers* is that many of the pieces could have sat happily in sections other than where they now are – an interconnected filing system, if you like.

The book is divided into four sections, each focusing on a different type or aspect of space: Bodies; Spaces; Cultural Planning; and Futures. The sections offer collections of pieces about the organisation and negotiating around, representation and theorisation of, and strategies of resistance to, that particular area. The purpose is to raise interesting questions and illuminate aspects of the section's theme: how the body functions in the public sphere; the reinscription of the built on the perception of the body; the influence architecture and planned spaces can have on behaviour and the possibilities of everyday life; the establishment and ramifications of cultural space; the construction and performance of gender and sexuality; the place of urban regeneration in the shifting of public gender roles; historical and contemporary uses of domestic space and the implications thereof; the creation of alternative spaces of the imagination or cyberspace; and the use and implications of technology in gendering or gendered identities.

Two last, topical and unashamedly local notes: first, it seems a touch ironic that finishing this book coincided with the publication of research about 'why little girls are sugar and spice' – it's genetic, apparently. This research, actually based on parents' assessments of their children's behaviour, was reported in *The Guardian* (12 June 1997) under the (front page) headline 'Genes say boys will be boys and girls will be sensitive'. No uncertainty there then. Second, with the Labour Party in Britain newly installed in government with a large majority, and a new socialist government in France, a pervasive euphoria envelops this land, or this writer at least, and it remains to be seen how both policy and culture changes will be made to the fabric of the environment of the country and the ways in which we perceive and make spaces within it.

Rosa Ainley
June 1997

I

COMING FROM THE SAME PLACE? BODIES

De La Warr Pavilion, Bexhill-on-Sea, Sussex: Rosa Ainley

Taking the body as the corporeal and the group, the corpus and the mass, this section explores questions of biology and place; 'unwomanly' activism in feminist anti-violence work; the lesbian nation; and the operations of regeneration initiatives in partnership. The different pieces are talking about various 'communities' and the nature of community itself, and a sense of home and belonging.

Community has become a word overburdened with meaning, often euphemised almost out of existence, and often used to suggest its opposite. And yet without falling into assumptions of homogeneity, there are common concerns, resulting in the establishment of common, shared spaces – organised along ethnic, cultural, racial, or sexual practice lines. How are they constructed, realised, experienced and talked about?

What do 'partnership' and 'participation', buzz words of regeneration culture, mean in practice? Partnership arrangements demand that 'the community' is consulted and involved, not only to fulfil grant-releasing conditions but also because the community is now seen as the key to getting it 'right'. Maher Anjum and Lesley Klein's close examination of several interrelated projects run as part of Bethnal Green City Challenge provides a detailed account of why participation by the public in regeneration initiatives is paramount to sustainable development, and demonstrates the need for adequate resourcing for participants to take a full role in it.

Ali Grant's piece looks at lesbian identity and place, through critiquing feminist anti-violence work in Hamilton, Canada, and its unwillingness to deal with heterosexuality. Taking lesbians as runaways from their class, not women (*à la* Wittig), in different locations and involved in 'unwomanly' practices that contest the 'heterosexual regime', e.g. activism, use of space, she raises questions about the nature of feminist activism and the importance of location in the development of political identities.

Moving on to lesbian nationalism, 'the counterpoint to years of felt exclusion and invisibility', Sally R. Munt offers an exploration of a virtual nation, one without land or state, a discursive space rather than a geographical one. Looking at the idea of the exclusivity of lesbian nation from the early 1970s onwards, often presented as a separatist state, contrasted with Queer Nation in the 1990s, intended, though not always experienced, as one of inclusiveness, she lights on the operation of a shame/pride binary. With a thorough examination of lesbian utopics this chapter exposes a battery of responses to the need for the chimerical social belonging.

Returning to the sexed body in space – in this case the pregnant woman's experience of a particular shopping centre – to the frame of feminist geography, reappraising the 'pitfalls' of biological essentialism, chapter 2 challenges the mind/body dualism encountered in some geographical knowledges. Robyn Longhurst unwraps the 'complex feedback relation' (Grosz 1992: 242) between the production and influence of bodies and environments.

1

Sisters in exile

The Lesbian Nation

Sally R. Munt

'So, that was my role in the growth of Queer Nation,' Troy Ruby told me, chomping on a cigarette. 'One minor character in a minor movement. *Queer* did get old very fast, nowadays only academics take it seriously. But *Nation* managed to live on in many fond conversations. Transgender Nation, Alien Nation, Reincar Nation. And all along the line no one noticed how much that word echoed with the secret store of nostalgic desire for normalcy, normalcy, normalcy. Those apple pies, warm kitchens and American flags that are trapped somewhere back there between the hypothalmus and the frontal lobe. Someplace in the Central Drawer where *One Nation Under God, Indivisible, With Liberty and Justice For All* resonates eternally. And that is why *Nation* is ultimately such a comforting word. And that is how I became an American poet.'

(Schulman 1995: 111)

Lesbian citizenship is located in space and time and self-consciously lived as a form of process, of relational movement. Like other oppressed cultures, lesbians hold fast to a dream of commonality and unification. An ethic of solidarity and commitment informs many liberation movements, and the drive for the 'rightful' colonisation of 'their' space – the desire to occupy their perceived constituency – fuels the imagination, and the movement, of radical struggles.

The idea of the Lesbian Nation developed from the lesbian feminisms formed in the USA during the 1970s, its most famous encapsulation appearing in Jill Johnston's eponymous *Lesbian Nation: The Feminist Solution*, published in 1973. The idea of Lesbian Nation as I intend to examine it here is of a utopic community and a fantasy of autonomy, which offered a kind of heroic narrative for the lesbian feminists of the 1970s. The idea of a Lesbian Nation provided a rhetoric of empowerment, and most significantly a cognitive space, for women experiencing *dis*placement from American culture. Further, as an imagined community, it was a metaphor of movement, of aggregation, of transit and progress to a *state* of belonging. It provided the sense of a bounded, shared identity of resistance which was conceptualised in relation to other political protest movements of the 1960s, notably the Black Civil Rights Movement, drawing from the longing of other excluded identities for their place in American society.

Several writers have explored spatial metaphors as a way of articulating lesbian occupation.[1] Some have written about the lesbian presence in the city as a localisation which makes lesbian identification possible. Jill Johnston's polemical project, in *Lesbian Nation* (1973), was to assemble the sentiment of radical and lesbian feminism into one metaphor, and then to claim the inauguration of a radical state, as a form of political mobilisation. Her brief introduction, 'Remarks', indicates her affiliation with nationalist ideology. It purports to be a 'true explanation' of 'collective memories' of an archetypal past; finally Johnston invokes 'the return to the harmony of statehood and biology through the remembered majesty of women' (Johnston 1973: 11). Homogeneity through nostalgia, naturalised truth-claims, and a heroic utopianism – these precepts are not unique to lesbian radicalism.

The liberal academic consensus on nationalisms is to bipolarise movements into 'good nationalisms' and 'bad nationalisms', depending on the perceived relative social power of disenfranchised/dominant minority groups.[2] A certain romanticisation of oppression is evident in the knee-jerk tendency to laud any territorial claim arising from marginalised groups, which often masks dominant historical discourses of regulation and displacement hovering in the wings, such as in the connotative Native American 'reservations'. Ideologies of race or ethnicity often compound the nationalist controversy, as they provoke the question of how that identity is being defined, specifically who is to be included and who is to be excluded, and who will be displaced. Any nationalism has a historical and ideological complexity which needs to be examined separately for just cause and expression (but by whom?). Lesbian nationalism became a mobilising force; the impetus for its ideology can be understood as the counterpoint to years of felt exclusion and invisibility. But we may also wish to consider who was excluded, what were the limits of its historical roots and ideological liaisons, what were its inadvertently destructive effects, and whether its agenda can ultimately be read simply as either radical or reactionary.

Nations and nationalism

Nations as a natural God-given way of classifying men, as an inherent . . . political destiny, are a myth; nationalism, which sometimes takes pre-existing cultures and turns them into nations, sometimes invents them, and often obliterates pre-existing cultures.

(Gellner 1983: 48)

Nations as we know them are social artefacts, belonging to a particular period of recent history. Nations appear under certain technological and linguistic conditions and are inherently unstable, due to the contingency of those conditions. Nationalism is defined by Ernest Gellner as primarily to mean 'a principle which holds that the political and national unit should be congruent' (Gellner 1983: 1). There are fissures within nationalism, as Eric Hobsbawm points out:

> First, official ideologies of states and movements are not guides to what is in the minds of even the most loyal citizens or supporters. Second, and more specifically, we cannot assume that for most people national identification – when it exists – excludes, or is always or ever superior to, the remainder of the set of identifications which constitute the social being. In fact it is always combined with identifications of another kind, even when it is felt to be superior to them. Thirdly, national identification and what it is believed to imply, can change and shift in time, even in the course of quite short periods.
>
> (Hobsbawm 1990: 11)

Already the idea of nationalism becomes complex.

For a nationalist ideology to form there must be some general functional prerequisites: first, there must be an emergent 'specialised clerical class', as Gellner called it, forming an intellectual culture which somewhat perversely, proselytised by the middle class, is one appropriated in the name of the 'folk'. Its symbolism draws heavily from a selective representation of the working class, repackaged and delivered back to 'the people' in a stylised, romanticised 'authenticity'. Second, despite the fact that nationalism preaches a historical continuity, paying homage to the 'folk culture' it has bowdlerised, it operates using a form of nostalgia which is intrinsically new and commensurate with the demands to amalgamate and reformulate 'the nation' according to contemporary criteria. Third, Gellner defines nationalism as a *sentiment* produced when the political and national unit is incongruent: 'the feeling of anger aroused by the violation of the principle, or the feeling of satisfaction aroused by its fulfilment. A nationalist *movement* is one actuated by a sentiment of this kind' (Gellner 1983: 11). If we understand nationalism as a sentiment, a feeling of exclusion which is articulated as a protest for inclusion, we must necessarily examine that feeling and the ways in which it is echoed and reproduced as an act of language, becoming in Foucault's words a 'discursive formation', a political structure, inventing the 'nation' where one previously did not exist.

Crucially we also need to conceive of how nationalism appears as a narrative, which inscribes its readers through a mechanism of identification. Nations are imaginary constructs that depend on a range of cultural fictions to maintain their mythic existence. Geoffrey Bennington highlights this connection: 'we undoubtedly find narration at the centre of nation: stories of national origins, myths of founding fathers, genealogies of heroes. At the origin of the nation, we find a story of the nation's origin. Which should be enough to inspire suspicion' (1994: 121).

Thus we need to approach any examination of nationalist sentiment with the tools of narrative analysis, to see how nations, as fictions, involve the curiosity and evoke the commitment of a reader, and ask why this particular story captures her/his intricate social imagination, at this specific fork in history.

Nation space

It seems axiomatic to claim that 'nation' is a spatial metaphor. Any thought of nationhood implies the construction of a bounded space, a place with borders and frontiers to enclose and, of course, exclude, containing a centre and margins. These borders are better perceived as permeable boundaries which permit communication with, and sometimes infusion by, the Other. The nation must have something to delineate itself against: meaning is created by a process of differentiation, and 'nation' as a concept contains its own deconstruction, as those boundaries bleed.

In considering the nation as a space from the point of view of the Other, the most cogent theorisation appears in Homi Bhabha's work, specifically in his essay 'Dissemination: time, narrative, and the margins of the modern nation' (Bhabha 1994), from which I wish to procure some significant premises. Bhabha speaks movingly of the gathering of scattered peoples: 'The nation fills the void left in the uprooting of communities and kin, and turns that loss into the language of metaphor' (Bhabha 1994: 139). Interestingly, the nation is for Bhabha what heterosexuality is for Judith Butler – the site of loss and melancholia.[3] The nation from this perspective is not 'here', but 'there', a desired object, representing a projected yearning for a perfectly consolidated self, paradoxically beyond the self. We might think of this nation as externalising the dream of integration. Interestingly, the profundity of this yearning can be revealed only metaphorically; in that sense linguistic expression is itself displaced, in a 'figure of speech'. So, the grief of unbelonging, of migrancy, is fixated by its own antithesis, a fantasy of transcendence, and immanence.

Bhabha also poses the question of representing the nation as a temporal process, a 'national time-space'. The people are not simply a series of historical events, an origin, or a national past, they also exist contemporaneously as signs of the present: 'The scraps, patches and rags of daily life must be repeatedly turned into the signs of a coherent national culture, while the very act of narrative performance interpellates a growing circle of national subjects. In the production of nation-as-narration there is a split between the continuist, accumulative temporality of the pedagogical, and the repetitious, recursive strategy of the performative' (Bhabha 1994: 45). In writing of the nation there is a temporal tear between the need to marshal the present and to perform the past. According to Bhabha this results in the splitting of the national subject, hence:

> the problem is not simply the 'selfhood' of the nation as opposed to the otherness of other nations. We are confronted with the nation split within itself. . . . The barred Nation It/Self, alienated from its eternal self-regeneration, becomes a liminal signifying space that is *internally* marked by the discourses of minorities, the heterogeneous histories of contending peoples, antagonistic authorities and tense locations of cultural difference.
> (Bhabha 1994: 148)

Bhabha is drawing attention to the instability of the nation, arguing that any notion of the people will emerge in narrative ambivalence, fluctuation and disjunction, in the 'abyss of enunciation' (Bhabha 1994: 154) produced by this rupture. He then argues that 'from the liminal movement of the culture of the nation . . . minority discourse emerges. . . . minority discourses that speak betwixt and between times and places' (Bhabha 1994: 155). The imagined nation of nationalism is fantasised as intact, impregnable, unitary, constant and monolithic; as a material entity the nation space is ruptured, it is mutable, temporal, limited and precarious, haunted by its own division.

Nationalism and sexuality

Corporeal metaphors are unavoidable as the nation is often depicted as a vital body with organs, mind and extremities. Nations/bodies have lives – they are born, get old and die; they are also sexed. Metaphors of contagion assail the nation/body. 'Nationalisms', as Anne McClintock underscores, 'are from the outset constituted in gender power' (McClintock 1995: 17). Despite the fact that citizenship has historically been denied to women, who have paradoxically been rendered stateless, in the rhetoric of war there is a deeply ingrained 'depiction of the homeland as the female body whose violation by foreigners requires its citizens and allies to rush to her defence' (Parker et al. 1992: 6). This rape analogy depends on the trope of nation-as-woman, but more specifically the patriarchal construction of the nation as Mother, nurturer and protector of the propagation of the national culture. In this heterosexist construct, the men impregnate the nation's 'soil' with their potent seed. Critics have observed how often liberation movements also employ this same predicate. In the erotic fervour of nationalism, heterosexual desire foments the ardour of the activist. Geraldine Heng and Janadas Devan have this to say regarding the nationalist politics which led to the Republic of Singapore:

> as patriotic duty for men grew out of the barrel of a gun (phallic nationalism, the wielding of a surrogate technology of the body in national defense), so would it grow, for women, out of the recesses of the womb (uterine nationalism, the body *as* a technology of defense wielded by the nation).
> (Heng and Devan 1992: 348)

In mapping out the field of nationalism it is essential to refer to the research that posits the homoerotic, rather than heterosexual, affiliations of nationhood. George Mosse's history of sexual norms in modern Europe, *Nationalism and Sexuality*, argues that our present notions of middle-class morality and 'respectability' are rooted in nineteenth- and twentieth-century ideologies of nation. He argues that nineteenth-century bourgeois ideal-isations of virility came to be sublimated as nationalist virtue, manliness and male beauty symbolising the nation's spiritual and material vitality. The 'back-to-nature' movement in England and Germany depended on the neo-classicist romantic revival of Greek models of (male) citizenship and the naturalisation of nudity. The covert homoeroticism abeyant in this cult of the body was made explicit by figures such as Edward Carpenter in England and the poet Stefan George in Germany. A reformist homosexual and a utopian socialist, Carpenter believed that nudity, 'the gospel of individual regeneration' (Mosse 1985: 63), would abolish discrimination. Carpenter was particularly interesting for his romanticisation of land and working-class labour, both factors that reoccurred in lesbian nationalism.

Nazi Germany provides Mosse with an example of established homo-erotic nationalism. The naked Greek youth distilled the aspirant imagery of the Third Reich, clearly a raced, as well as sexed, symbol. As Mosse comments: 'a beautiful Jew was a contradiction in terms' (Mosse 1985: 139). The Nazis built upon the nineteenth-century concept of the *Männerbund*, a passionate brotherhood formed primarily among elite youth, emphasising nature and physical strength. According to the historian Hans Blüher, homosexuality in the *Männerbund* represented spiritual principles – heroism, leadership and communality. Returning to Nazi Germany, however, within George's circle, homoeroticism was seen as the principal agent of national renewal. Mosse comments on how the distinction between homoeroticism and homosexuality became blurred:

> The rediscovery of the human body combined with the exclusively male nature of the early youth movement did raise the spectre of homoeroticism, even homosexuality. Those who tried to recapture their own bodies as well as nature from the hypocrisy as well as artificiality of bourgeois life, as they saw it, also wanted to find refuge in a true community of affinity. They began to perceive the nation as such a community. Moreover the nation helped spiritualise their new sensuality.
>
> (Mosse 1985: 57)

This middle-class rebellion also has parallels with sexual liberation, the (white) student resistance cultures of the 1960s and 1970s, and lesbian life in the 1970s and 1980s. Mosse concludes: 'As a living organism, filled with energy, nationalism tended to encourage male bonding, the *Männerbund*, which by its very nature presented a danger to that respectability the nation was supposed to preserve.'

Other critics locate homosexuality as proximate, even central to western culture – Eve Kosofsky Sedgwick (1991) Jonathan Dollimore (1991) and Terri Castle (1993). I am not proposing that homosexuality is the 'closet' secret of nationalism, but indeed, because the homoeroticism of the *Männerbund* led eventually to Hitler's *Reichszentrale* police,[4] the purging of homosexuals during *Kristallnacht*, Paragraph 175 and the pink triangle, I am obliged to Sedgwick's claim that gay proximity leads to gay panic:

> Because the paths of male entitlement, especially in the nineteenth century, required certain intense male bonds that were not readily distinguishable from the most reprobated bonds, an endemic and ineradicable state of what I am calling male homosexual panic became the normal condition of male heterosexual entitlement.
>
> (Sedgwick 1991: 185)

If we take this model in relation to nationalism, it is feasible to argue that the pervasive heterosexuality of most nationalisms is the manifestation of a kind of panicked response to the elemental structure of homoeroticism towards which it is compelled and which it is concomitantly desperate to repudiate. It is with these contradictory characteristics of nationalism in mind, that we turn again to lesbian nationalism.

Johnston argues in *Lesbian Nation* that prior to the Radicalesbians 'There was no lesbian identity. There was [only] lesbian activity' (Johnston 1973: 58). The narrative is a treatise of the move from personal experience to structural analysis, in line with the rhetoric of various liberation movements of the 1960s. Centrally, the political collectivity is formed around the expressive practices of identity, distinguished by the culmination of experience. The first shift is to claim an identity (lesbian), the second is to form an affinity group based on that identity ('the community') and the third is to define an enemy ('man as my natural enemy' (Johnston 1973: 92)); the fourth is to declare secession: 'to buy up a lot of space and establish a chain of lesbos on the mainland and invite the lesbian population and . . . just forget about the men' (Johnston 1973: 76). The fifth is to begin to colonise: 'All women are lesbians' (Johnston 1973: 90), and finally to reproduce: 'The order for the day for all women immediately is *psychic parthenogenesis*' (Johnston 1973: 258).

A call to parthenogenesis makes sense if we understand the psychic project of the book as an attempt to interrupt the real and metaphorical invasion of female body space, in a rejection of the permeated and 'besieged female' (Johnston 1973: 254) of heterosexist culture, and fulminate expansion instead of contraction. Its call to separatism can be read as an attempt to seal the boundaries of her imagined body. In particular the last chapter is awash with dualistic imagery of the 'intact' or 'violated' female, where the most articulated argument for the lesbian nation occurs. There is a metonymic replacement of the female body for the lesbian nation. In contrast to conventional nationalist ideology, here the female nation body prefigures Wittig's *Lesbian Body* in an intense eulogy to the actively desiring woman, an attempt to destroy the binary grammar of (male) subject/ (female) object (Wittig 1986). Johnston, like Wittig, recovers the Amazons as contemporary models of agency and autonomy, recalling the recourse to classical myths evident in other nationalisms. The active principle of the warrior woman does not merely replace soldiers with female counterparts – the female agent acting on the feminine groundspace of nature creates a lesbian text able to expose the erotics of nationalism and transform the linear antipathy of the traditional (heterosexist) configuration. Hence Amazon society's circular mantra:

> I am a woman who is a lesbian because I am a woman and a woman who loves herself naturally who is other women is a lesbian a woman who loves women loves herself naturally this is the case that is herself is all woman is a natural born lesbian.
>
> (Wittig 1986: 266)

The textual solipsism posits Woman as an exclusionary category. Johnston's model is further circumscribed by its class- and race-specific denotation. It is clear from the text's dismissal of existing 'old gay' cultures that, using Gellner's formulation, this nationalism is addressed to a clerisy: white, middle-class and educated. The 'temporal tear' that Homi Bhabha speaks of is here evident in the tendency to create 'Year Zero' in lesbian political identity, oblivious to the history of pre-Stonewall lesbians. The nationalism being espoused here is open only to the youth, or those wishing for a selective memory. Integral to this lesbian nation is the propensity to fracture, and forget, along the lines of its incompatible discourses. By mimicking nationalism, Johnston has pre-ordained the split of Woman into the competing identity groups, the split which characterised the feminist movement from 1973 to 1983. The centre could not hold.

The utopian rights movement of lesbian feminism both mimicked and subverted nationalism. The cultural feminist[5] nationalism of the 1970s was predicated on an ideological and material separatism which led to the creation of 'Wimmin's Land' throughout the USA, its existence in the real a shadow of its symbolic effect. By positing the category of Woman as individuated, no longer dependent on the qualifier 'Not-Man', the conceptual space of Woman as autonomous was squeezed open. The ideology of separatism, lived as an incarnation of the idea of the lesbian nation, dominated lesbian culture in the 1970s. It is to the lived experience of the lesbian nation that we now turn.

Utopianism and separatism in the 1970s

The lesbian nation of the 1970s constituted discursive rather than geographical space. There was no land to reclaim, and a predominantly anarchic movement meant there was no state to make. Lesbian nation was an imagined space, envisioned as the symbolic rupture of women from men. As Mary Daly put it: 'Patriarchy is the homeland of males; it is the Fatherland; and men are its agents' (Daly 1978: 28). Even if the impetus for separatism was contained within a binary, the establishment of lesbian space did create more freedom to centre the category Lesbian/Woman, providing manoeuvrability within that cipher to align an identity.

It has become formulaic to patronise the 'excesses' of 1970s lesbian feminism and I hope to avoid that in my appraisal of one of its most structuring totems. Even in the 1990s we can appreciate the legacy of lesbian activism in the feminist social infrastructure it produced: rape crisis helplines, battered women's shelters, women's centres, well-woman clinics, retreat centres, all these and more, staffed mainly by lesbians, are the material result of the vision for a safe, utopic space for women to affirm their separate identity. To be a separatist lesbian was endowed with the kudos of having made the total commitment to feminism, and separatist communities became the elected conscience of the (lesbian) nation. Dana R. Shugar makes the point that separatist groups were the first amongst White feminists to tackle 'competing' oppressions, even if they did often attribute them to a common cause (sexism) (Shugar 1995). Shugar has analysed the political outcomes of separatism:

> Creating a binary other in the figure of men compelled separatists to place all their collective conflicts outside the practice of women themselves. And while some of the opposition women faced did indeed come from external sources, much more of it came from conflicts among collective members themselves. . . . Construction of a demonic, binary other thus ironically provided the impetus toward female community and made the success of that community impossible.
>
> (Shugar 1995: 181)

Shugar observes that despite the numbers of black women living in separatist communities, in the period 1960–90 not one fictional utopia was written by a woman of colour, nor was there envisioned a utopia for women of colour. Clearly, black feminism was unmoved by the kind of binary reductionism at the centre of the utopian project.

Blame/victim culture was not left behind with the men, it osmosed through into the heart of the collectives themselves. Shugar again: 'women's conceptions of an always-oppressive patriarchy took away any effective method through which they could claim responsibility for their own destructive behaviours' (Shugar 1995: 89). Similarly, despite the romanticisation of poverty and of manual labour and trades, and the fashionability of ethnic working-class style (the infamous 'downward mobility'), the practices of separatist collectives remained securely middle-class, not least in the way that they were highly literate and mannered. With the appropriation of working-class skills came middle-class attitudes to work, with the expectation of recognition, reward and professionalisation. Significantly, cleaning, that staple of women's employment, never attracted the same cachet.

Still, the utopian discourse of lesbian nationalism in the 1970s can be seen to have resulted in utopian *practices* that had some positive effect on women's everyday lives. The first phase of lesbian separatism can be read as an anticipatory consciousness of hope which produced a range of utopian practices. The most crucial of these was the movement to form an identity not dependent on men, an attempt to break down the binary. The second phase, the reconstruction of Lesbian/Woman, floundered. Lesbian nationalism became a discourse of exclusion; in a desire to place and fix the meaning of this identity, the hope died.

Borderlands/La Frontera: Gloria Anzaldúa

The configuration of bounded categories such as race, nation, sexuality and even identity, is an inheritance of nineteenth-century imperial obsessions with naming, containing and blaming. The scurry to secure ambiguity and fix contradiction can also be read as expressive of a fear of the unknown and different, which can conversely be banished to the non-discursive or extra-symbolic. There is a contrary semiotic action evident here: difference is positioned as either supra- or under-representable, a slippery character indeed. We have seen Mosse's attempt to locate a nexus of sexuality, race and gender concerns in the nineteenth century. Judith Raiskin has drawn attention to the twin Victorian doctrines of evolution and degeneration, reminding us that 'hybrids' who crossed boundaries of race or sex were classified as deviant and regressive. Raiskin points out that even in the nineteenth century homosexual rights activists such as Edward Carpenter were advocating 'intermediacy' as 'a revolutionary step forward, not a degenerate state' (Raiskin 1994: 156). Raiskin locates the contemporary work of Gloria Anzaldúa within a tradition of radicalism which has transformed this conflation of racial/homosexual degeneracy, reworking it into the language of a strategically essentialist reverse discourse. Anzaldúa calls this emerging space the 'mestiza consciousness'.

Borderlands/La Frontera: The New Mestiza (1987) has functioned as a crossover text in the Anglophile academy, occupying the borderlands of canonised, yet 'racially marked', feminist theory. Earlier critics have already remarked on the implications of appropriating work by women of colour for predominantly white lesbian theory, but as Shane Phelan argues, the analogy of the mestiza is transferable *providing* the specificity of its origin in Chicana politics and Aztlàn history is remembered, and 'race' issues are not conveniently buried by the (white lesbian) privileging of the sexual (Phelan 1994: 68). As Raiskin identifies, Anzaldúa's model for the 'New Mestiza' draws on the work of Mexican nationalist writer José Vasconcelos, who in 1925 proposed that the ideal nation should be based on 'constructive miscegenation' or 'hybrid progeny', inverting nineteenth-century fears of degeneration. Anzaldúa rewrites his model of a unified Mexican nationhood based on heterosexual reproduction, as a queer consciousness 'experienced through the body' (Raiskin 1994: 162) – in Anzaldúa's case, a lesbian body predicated on active, plural ambiguity, not the passive, prescribed female body of conventional nationalism.

Anzaldúa, in tandem with the postmodern destruction of secure 'truth' categories, sees the mestiza consciousness as potentially deconstructive. Destabilising the givens of national belonging, she envisions a new space, a national consciousness that frees the self to wander, secure in spiritual belonging. The dispossessed, no longer confined to the binaries of inside/ outside, transcend the material altogether. She describes the Borderlands as a state of psychic unrest, which, like a cactus needle in the flesh, has to be excised by the process of writing. 'Nudge a Mexican and she or he will break out with a story'(Anzaldúa 1987: 65) she announces at the start of one chapter, and proceeds to explain the necessity of performative narrative in the making of tribal cultures. However, this myth-making is not so much nostalgic as an intentional and recognised evolvement based on experience:

When I write it feels like I'm carving bone. It feels like I'm creating my own face, my own heart – a Nahuatl concept. My soul makes itself through the creative act. It is constantly remaking and giving birth to itself through my body. It is this learning to live with this *la Coatlicue* that transforms living in the Borderlands from a nightmare into a numinous experience. It is always a path/state to something else.

(Anzaldúa 1987: 73)

The body is then as much a metaphor as anything else; she stresses that the mestiza consciousness is not literal, but a transformative affect which permeates all spatial relations. Thus 'home' is loosened from place, to become a state of mind.

By replacing 'truth' with 'fiction', by superseding 'place' with 'motion', and by disposing of the fixed body and in its place putting 'queer consciousness', Anzaldúa deconstructs the old ideal of identity as a totalising essence. In another essay she writes: ' "lesbian" is a cerebral word, white and middle-class, representing an English-only dominant culture, derived from the Greek word *lesbos* . . . "Lesbian" doesn't name anything in my homeland' (Anzaldúa 1987: 249). Lesbian nation, in her formulation, becomes redundant too:

As a *mestiza* I have no country, my homeland cast me out; yet all countries are mine because I am every woman's sister or potential lover. (As a lesbian I have no race, my own people disclaim me; but I am all races because there is the queer of me in all races.)

(Anzaldúa 1987: 80)

Anzaldúa rejects the confrontational stance intrinsic to 1970s lesbian nationalism as limited by its reactive status to the definitive manoeuvres of the oppressor, and repudiates anger and rage – the emotions that fuelled and then splintered much of lesbian feminism – on similar grounds. She sees separatism as one transitory potential among many, preferring a 'continual creative motion that keeps breaking down the unitary aspect of each new paradigm' (Anzaldúa 1987: 80):

La mestiza constantly has to shift out of habitual formations; from convergent thinking, analytic reasoning that tends to use rationality to move toward a single goal (a Western mode), to divergent thinking, characterised by movement away from set patterns and goals and toward a more whole perspective, one that includes rather than excludes.

(Anzaldúa 1987: 79)

Rather than fragment down into another enclosed identity position, she chooses to read her multiple and *simultaneous* identities as bridges (like Audre Lorde), within herself and connecting others. As Phelan points out, she emphatically rejects ontological separatism, which reifies absolute incompatibilities. This is not postmodern voluntarism, but an attempt to integrate (not merge) lived aspects of the self already present. It is an indictment of the postmodern equivocation that prevents political engagement and challenges the postmodern trivialising of the fractured self.

Drawing upon the black feminist critiques of the preceding decade, which refused single issue identity politics, Anzaldúa presents a new utopia based upon process, positive engagement, fluidity, ambiguity and, above all, inclusivity. Her desert 'mestiza consciousness' flowered into Queer Nation.

Queer Nation

Queer Nation was first started in New York in April 1990 primarily by people involved in AIDS activism who also wanted to respond politically to a number of lesbian- and gay-bashings in the East Village. So its origin in part was a desire to defend space. Queer Nation coalesced around a new generation which was both angry and ironic. Queer Nation assembled around an anarchist aesthetic which mobilised a 'cultural happening', a momentary incursion into the domain of representation. They wanted to create actions for maximum media effect, and their main target was heterosexuality. They aimed to challenge the public discourse of sexuality. Their anthem was 'We're here! We're Queer! Get used to it!' Anti-assimilationist in intent, their exhibitionist agenda was self-consciously to shove the homosexual into America's face.

The divide between them and the older Lesbian and Gay Liberation Movement seemed profound. Queer Nation saw older lesbians and gays (as one critic put it, the over-35s) as capitulating to capitalism and defeated by their own rigid identity politics; and they, in turn, patronised Queer Nation and accused it of risking the civil rights gained since the 1960s by alienating a largely liberal public, and of glossing over material inequalities in people's experience of queerness. At issue was the deconstruction of identity *per se*: Queer Nation celebrated liminality, alternative practices, sexual freedom, subversion and ambiguity. It opened the doors to the marginalised and excluded, especially those who were transgendered, bisexual, and/or sadomasochist who had borne the brunt of the exclusionary practices of the 'mainstream' movement during the sex wars of the 1970s and 1980s. Queers did not share an identity, only an opposition to the discipline of normalisation; pleasure and individual desire were their celebratory incentive. Queer Nation reversed the nationalist parameters of exclusion and focused on the inclusion of anyone who felt 'different', although, crucially, sexually different.

Queer Nation placed a postmodern emphasis on signification – it practised a form of cultural terrorism by incursions into the public realm of sexuality. This had the effect of disclosing the hetero-normative hegemony at the same time as camping it up. Its intent was to make the nation a space safe for queers, not just in the sense of being tolerated, 'but safe *for* demonstration, in the mode of patriotic ritual' (Berlant and Freeman 1993: 198). Queer Nation was a spatial politics of queer embodiment, as Lauren Berlant and Elizabeth Freeman argued: 'being queer is not about the right to privacy: it is about the freedom to be public' (Berlant and Freeman 1993: 201). Queer Nation inverted the liberal division of society into public/

private space to which lesbians in particular had been confined. The public spectacle of queer sexualities being performed was intended to displace heterosexuality to the margins and centre the queer. As a strategy of inversion it was risky – a reverse colonisation and a felt response to a hundred years of restraint: 'queers are thus using exhibitionism to make public space psychically unsafe for unexamined heterosexuality' (Berlant and Freeman 1993: 207). Its assertiveness in taking up public space gave Queer Nation an incipient masculinity it was never able to shake.

Despite the attempt to welcome social diversity into the Queer Nation, the phenomenon remains perceived as a white, middle-class eruption of *sexual* discontent. The quintessential protagonist is still the muscular white boy in a 'Queer as Fuck' t-shirt. In its rush to affirm a new political moment Queer Nation, like many nationalisms, refused and 'forgot' the complex lessons of history, and broke apart over the same social divisions evident in Lesbian Nation and other single-issue projects. Steven Seidman makes a hypothetical remark which I think bears further attention:

> Queer Nationals hope to avoid the self-limiting, fracturing dynamics of identification by an insistent disruptive subversion of identity. Yet . . . their subversive politics presupposes those very identifications and social anchorings. *Is it possible that underlying the refusal to name the subject (of knowledge and politics) is a utopian wish for a full, intact, organic experience of self and other?*
>
> (1993: 105; italics added)

By consolidating around the rubric of 'queer', young activists were organising around what they perceived to be the end of shame. But the renunciation of shame involves its invocation: secession was necessary in order to break the (Gay) Pride/Shame binary, but this was predetermined on a loss. That grief of denunciation persisted in resurfacing as the utopian desire for an anchored identity. Queer identity was fixed in romantic undifferentiation, but the present reality of inequality and regret kept breaking through. In a piece on 'Women as queer nationals' in *Out/Look* Maria Maggenti makes a similar point, bemoaning the loss of the agency of the Lesbian Nation of the 1970s she attends a Queer Nation meeting sensing 'an underlying desire, an unspoken yearning it seems, to be accepted instead of liberated. I go home that night worried' (Maggenti 1991: 23). Bemoaning the need for a young lesbian participant to find her home, she concludes with a fantasy refrain for the new nation:

> And I want to tell her to grab her female friends and run, run out into the rainy street shouting with power and anger and glee, shouting and dancing her way to some unknown place, some undiscovered continent, some still-unnamed territory.
>
> (Maggenti 1991: 23)

American lesbians are still 'lighting out for the territory'.

Imagined communities and
lesbian citizenship

Despite a powerful revolutionary optimism, both Lesbian Nation and Queer Nation were caught by the very political embeddedness they were trying to escape, by a syntax of forgetting which returned as the race and class politics they were attempting to repress, in the hierarchical name of a sexual 'greater good'. Nationalism was an understandable temptation to lesbians and queers, apparently offering them a place of belonging, but as a result of the tendencies of the discourse of nationalism both Lesbian Nation and Queer Nation were undone by a historical past which refused to be subsumed by homogenisation. American lesbians seized the imagery of nationalism only to discover that the implicit 'nostalgic desire for normalcy, normalcy, normalcy' (Schulman 1995: 111) unravelled the radical impetus for future structural change. Lesbian Nation and Queer Nation were specifically American nationalist formulations, their allure particular to the ideologies of the land of mixture, polyglot opportunity, individual freedom and ethnic rights.[6]

Benedict Anderson observes how nations, nationality and nationalisms are notoriously difficult to define. The wish for them originates from a fear of meaninglessness and death – in the lesbian context we can interpret nationalist desire as arising from a historical invisibility contingent on a dea(r)th of signification. Conversely, the separatist impulse involved wanting to remove lesbians from the cartography of heteropatriarchy. The seduction of nationalism lies in its promise of an 'imagined community', a mental image of communion powerful in evoking 'love, and often [a] profoundly self-sacrificing love' (Schulman 1995: 141). Anderson explains how nationalisms arise from the 'outsider within', and we have seen how the Lesbian Nation contrarily constituted a similar toehold in dominant culture, whose unacknowledged complicity fuelled a divisive exclusion of 'other others'. Thus nationalisms reproduce a cyclical inclusion and expulsion based on a need to fix identity in place – literally and metaphorically.

Shane Phelan's book *Identity Politics: Lesbian Feminism and the Limits of Community* (1989) elucidates the difficulties that lesbian feminism had in constituting a categorical identity – the lesbian – and explains how that identity operated to exclude difference:

> As they began, lesbian feminists fought to wrest the understandings and construction of lesbian identity from the grip of those who denied the self-understandings of lesbian women. In the process, however, they fell into the trap awaiting all moderns, all subjects of the regime of truth: the trap of counterreification, of justifying their existence by reference to transcendental standards of what a lesbian 'is'.
>
> (Phelan 1989: 156)

Phelan analyses the extent to which the construction of lesbian identity in the USA was predicated on an ontological liberal individualism, with its fantasy of autonomy. Nationalisms, like individualisms, are the inventions of modernity. An essentially Marxist model of revolution is a macro-narrative promising to seek total social change. Ironically, class undermined the lesbian feminist revolution by marking it as an activity affordable only by the middle-class women desirous of, and able to afford, the totalising gesture of separatism. As Phelan says, the problem is with the terms of the separatist identity, based as it is on a metaphysical and essential gender incompatibility. Separatism also imposes a categorical unity from within, twinned with a paranoid fear of deviation.

Phelan develops the renunciation of the single coherent lesbian identity in *Getting Specific: Postmodern Lesbian Politics* (1994). Having pointed out the confluence of US interest group politics with the imposition of a homogeneous identity, she reiterates how middle-class academic feminist theory often forecloses and subjugates real differences between women by invoking unified differences in deference to a hardly disguised transcendent lesbian or feminist subject. She is unequivocal on queer nationalism, which she says 'reanimates the problems of lesbian feminism in its cultural feminist versions without resolving them' (Phelan 1994: 153):

> To the extent that queers become nationalist, they will ignore or lose patience with those among them who do not fit their idea of the nation. This dynamic in nationalism will always limit its political usefulness. The only fruitful nationalism is one that has at its heart the idea of the nonnation – the nation of nonidentity, formed not by any shared attribute, but by a conscious weaving of threads between tattered fabrics. And at that point, why speak of nations?
>
> (Phelan 1994: 154)

Why speak? Perhaps because 'nation' carries the romantic rhetorical appeal that 'community', in its nebulousness, has lost. But even 'community' according to Phelan is a dangerous idea in modernity, despite its reading as antithetical to the state (and therefore potentially anti-nationalist). Community has been 'firmly entrenched within the logic of the same' (Phelan 1994: 82), a victim of identitarian politics which presumes that common action must be based in a shared identity.

Instead of deploying the nationalist metaphor of liberation, Phelan argues that lesbians must self-consciously work for power. In prioritising the local struggle above the national or global, the author clearly invokes a postmodern model of social change, built not upon identities but on the specificity of diverse oppressive experiences. Phelan is about fashioning a new morality, an active creation of values which seeks out alliances expressed as a form of love:

> It is a love of the world, a love of democracy, a love of others as inseparably part of the community within which we live. As an activity based on conscious commitment rather than a feeling, love can be chosen and it can be refused. Love need not entail self-negation, but it does entail a willingness to 'go under', to suffer the small deaths of humility and pain and self-examination. Just as love does not come from others unless we offer it to them, so allies will develop as we ally ourselves with their causes. And as we

increasingly open our eyes and hearts, we will help to create those fences against oppression by modelling decency. Without decency and love, bringing us toward one another without requiring sameness, our rhetorical and heartfelt commitments to others will continually be frustrated in the face of ineluctable difference.

(Phelan 1994: 158)

But, as Jeffrey Weeks asks, 'what do we mean by love? It is difficult to "love" humankind, except as a metaphysical flight' (Weeks 1995: 173). Certainly the love generated by nationalism is at least in part a response to the experience of aggression, in a desire to foreclose it, but as we know from Lacan, wherever love is, there also dwells aggression. Even so, in an historical moment characterised by the homophobia produced by AIDS, and in the general misogynistic milieu, a call to love is a heroic narrative invoked to sustain our spiritual survival, it is a working mestiza consciousness, inflected by the *utopian* hope that we will be able to create bonds across differences.

Whereas nationalism can foster the love of the same it also provokes a movement against others – it is insufficient for recognising our interdependence and need for others. We need a heroic desire that acknowledges and includes our commonalities and our differences without homogenising conflict, that eschews nations and embraces the specifics of people's real material needs. We must supersede the increasingly vacuous term 'community' with a concept that will invigorate people temporarily and contingently to vitalise the radical process and create safe spaces for lesbians to live in. Love is a contentious term to invoke, a discomforting concept within an academic work, as it is associated with unanalysed feeling, and imaginary enchantment. We need to deromanticise love and begin to openly acknowledge its presence, for lesbians and gays do love each other, practically and emotively, in the weaving interstices of our daily lives together. We have constructed an elaborate ethics of care that we check and refine and reference, that we measure ourselves and others against. Many lesbians now spend inordinate amounts of time in therapy learning to love, and yet we scorn this intimacy amongst those to whom we belong. I cannot help but suspect that shame is a negative player in this, an effect of melancholic displacement and repudiation, and that it is conceivable that the pride/shame dichotomy can be commuted into love. A call to love is not an invitation to easy sentiment, it is to arouse that most arduous and perceptible of practices.

In Edward Said's essay 'Reflections on Exile' he describes the heroic literature of exile as merely an effort to overcome the crippling sorrow of estrangement, and loss – the conditions of nationalism. But exile is a solitary experience, a sense of being outside a group: 'Exiles feel, therefore, an urgent need to reconstitute their broken lives, usually by choosing to see themselves as part of a triumphant ideology or a restored people' (Said 1990: 360). Clearly, the pride/shame dichotomy is in evidence here.[7] Conditions of exile create envy and destructiveness, and a defensive retrenchment. Elements of the Lesbian Nation can be seen to have perpetuated this and caused its implosion. But exile, like shame, can also fracture the self and permit new formations to erupt, and new connections to configure. As we understand from molecular science, it is the moment of separation that allows new elements to appear. Love can arise out of this conjunction only if first we are able to recognise the emotional profundity of our loss of that chimera: social belonging.

Notes

1 See Anzaldúa (1987), Pratt (1984: 9–64), Moraga (1983); on the city see Wilson (1991).
2 During the 1990s, with the growth of nationalisms and the resurgence in fascism in Europe, there is even more of a wish to try to distinguish between the radical, and the oppressive, discourses of nationalism.
3 Thank you to Sarah Chinn for this connection. See Butler (1990).
4 Formed in 1934 for the state persecution of homosexuals.
5 Cultural feminism was predicated on the opposition 'Man equals Culture' (negative) versus 'Woman equals Nature' (positive) – early indications of this position are evident in Johnston's *The Lesbian Nation*.
6 By comparison, Lesbian Nation and Queer Nation had no political currency in the UK, a country largely cynical towards nationalist movements and still bitterly reminiscent about the National Socialism of the Second World War.
7 On the mechanism of pride/shame see my *Heroic Desire: Lesbian Identity and Cultural Space* (London: Cassell, 1997 and New York: New York University Press, 1997). This chapter is an abridged version of 'The Lesbian Nation', which was published in that volume.

2

(Re)presenting shopping centres and bodies

Questions of pregnancy

Robyn Longhurst

Many geographical knowledges tend to be premised on a dualism between mind and body (Longhurst 1995). What is more, the divisions between mind and body are gendered/sexed. The mind (reason and rationality) has long been associated with masculinity while the body (emotion and irrationality) has long been associated with femininity (Lloyd 1993). The discourses of geography in various and complex ways assert a division between abstract, rational Man and embodied, emotional Woman (see Rose 1993). Of course, in 'reality', both men and women 'have bodies' but the difference lies in that men are thought to be able to pursue and speak universal knowledge, unencumbered by the limitations of a body placed in a particular time and place, whereas women are thought to be closely bound to the particular instincts, rhythms and desires of their fleshly, located bodies (Longhurst 1997: 491).

In this chapter I put bodies (bodies that are inseparable from minds – see Johnson 1989) centre-stage. Louise Johnson (1990: 18) argues that feminist geographers have tended to employ a dichotomy between gender and sex and that there are a number of implications of employing this distinction. One of these is 'the omission of the body as a vital element in the consti-tution of masculine and feminine identity and the consignment of those who argue for a "corporeal feminism" . . . into the nether world of biological essentialism'. Johnson (1990: 18) goes on to explain that geographers, 'in their zeal to avoid the accusation of biologism and by embracing the logics of historical materialism and liberalism, have ignored the possibilities of examining the sexed body in space'. Yet, as Johnson (1989) argues, there are rich possibilities for feminist geographers in examining biology as a social construct rather than treating it as a natural given and/or ignoring it (Longhurst 1995, 1997).

One possibility for studying embodiment more closely in geography is to examine the relations between bodies and cities as constitutive and mutually defining. Feminist geographers to date have carried out substantial work on how (male) bodies make or create ('man-made') cities (see Matrix 1984; Spain 1992; Weisman 1992) but have focused little attention on how cities make or create bodies with certain desires and capacities. By that I mean, there is a 'complex feedback relation' between bodies and environments in which each produces the other (Grosz 1992: 242). Elizabeth Grosz (1992: 242) argues: 'the city is one of the crucial factors in the social production of (sexed) corporeality'. Examining the ways in which bodies are 'psychically, socially, sexually and discursively or representationally produced, and the ways, in turn, that bodies reinscribe and project themselves onto their sociocultural environment so that this environment both produces and reflects the form and interests of the body' (Grosz 1992: 242), is a potentially rich area of research for geographers (Longhurst 1997: 496).

I begin to examine some of the ways in which a specific space within a city might produce or create bodies with certain desires and capacities. This does not mean that essentialist accounts of the body have to give way to social constructionist accounts but rather that geographers and others could develop further some of the strategic possibilities for reconceptualising studies of people/environment relations by using a range of approaches in innovative ways. I focus on one distinctive mode of corporeality within a specific historical and geographical context. I examine some of the ways in which the corporeal can condition and mediate pregnant women's experiences of a specific place.

Studying pregnant women offers possibilities for disrupting masculinism in geography (see Rose 1993) in that pregnant women effectively illustrate the notion of Other being Self or Same. Pregnant women undergo a bodily process that transgresses the boundary between inside and outside, self and other, subject and object (Young 1990). This serves to problematise the framework of binary opposition through which the authority of key concepts is established in geography. I focus on pregnant women's relationship not with cities *per se* but with one shopping centre – Centre Place – in Hamilton, Aotearoa/New Zealand.[1] More specifically, I examine how the discursive and material fields of Centre Place reinforce a notion of feminine beauty as slim and of pregnant women as unattractive and no longer sexually desirable.

This chapter is based on stories collected from thirty-one pregnant women, all of whom were pregnant for the first time and living in Hamilton. Sometimes I also spoke with pregnant women's husbands or partners. The data were collected over a period of approximately two years – May 1992 through to July 1994. I conducted focus groups with sixteen women, individual one-off interviews with eleven women and a series of in-depth interviews and ethnographic work (which included visiting Centre Place) with four women for the duration of their pregnancy.

All of the women involved in the interviews and focus groups were near the end of their pregnancies. There was a large variation in the participants' personal and household income. Many had stopped full-time and part-time work. Over half the participants, that is, 61 per cent, were aged between 24 and 29 years old. Only one participant was aged over 35. There were no participants under the age of 15 years but five were aged under 19 years. In terms of ethnicity, twenty-seven participants defined themselves as Pakeha,[2] while four defined themselves as Maori.[3] The conversations with these women were not solely about Centre Place. Usually we talked more generally about their experiences of a variety of public places and activities. The agenda of questions that I used was as follows:

- What activities have you continued to carry out during pregnancy and what activities have you reduced or stopped carrying out during pregnancy?
- Which places have you continued to visit during pregnancy and which places have you reduced or stopped visiting during pregnancy?
- In what ways, if any, have your relationships with family, friends, colleagues and so on changed since you have been pregnant?
- Are there any activities that you have been advised (by family, friends, colleagues, strangers, doctor, midwife and so on) not to engage in during pregnancy?
- What could be done to help improve the quality of life (in terms of both the physical and social environment) for pregnant women who live in Hamilton?

In the course of addressing these questions many of the women discussed Centre Place maybe because it is one of Hamilton's most central shopping malls. I offer the stories in this chapter not as a way of securing 'true knowledge' but as a way of beginning to unravel some of the ways in which bodies are socially, sexually and discursively produced through inhabiting particular sociocultural environments.

Centre Place

Centre Place is situated in down-town Hamilton. Hamilton is a city of 102,000 people (Census of Population and Dwellings 1991) located to the west in the northern half of the North Island of Aotearoa/New Zealand. The city grew as a service centre for the outlying rural Waikato dairy industry and has a reputation for being rather 'conservative'. Centre Place covers approximately five acres, contains large skylight windows in the roof and comprises two levels (see Plate 2/1). Development of the centre started in 1984. When it opened in 1985, and for the next decade, it was heavily marketed as the 'Heart of the City' (a heart motif was used in its advertising) in an attempt to restore profitability to the city centre. Recently 'Heart of the City' was replaced with the slogan 'Your Complete Shopping and Entertainment Centre'. This coincided with a number of other changes. A second cinema complex – Village Showcase – opened in the Centre. The outside walls of the Centre were repainted pale mustard, trimmed with forest green. Yet another change was that the previous name, 'Centreplace', was broken into two – 'Centre Place' – presumably in an attempt to emphasise its (physical and symbolic) central location. The heart motif was replaced with a spiral.

Plate 2.1 Centre Place Shopping and Entertainment Centre:
Robyn Longhurst

Facilities at Centre Place currently include a multi-storey car park, toilets, a 'lotto' (New Zealand Lotteries Commission) outlet, and a security and information centre. The major attractions include a Food Court, the Fox and Hounds English Tavern, the Village 7 Cinema, the newly opened Village Showcase which contains three cinemas, and a range of shops (about ninety-five in total). These include boutiques, a fashion accessory shop, a swim and surf shop, a perfumery, a jeweller's, a florist, an art gallery, two appliance stores and a gift shop. Unlike most shopping centres Centre Place is not anchored by a supermarket or large department store. It is comprised solely of speciality shops many of which target their goods at (mainly Pakeha) women with access to middle/high incomes (Fergusson 1991: 23).

Sexy bodies

In the 'culture' of Centre Place women are frequently positioned as objects/subjects of (a presumed male) sexual desire. In the window of Christies Chemist a large poster advertising 'Piz Buin Suncare Products' shows a 'beautiful', slim, sun-tanned woman wearing a white bikini. She is reclining, partly supported by the arm of a 'handsome', sun-tanned, muscled man. Her eyes are shut as he gazes upon her (see Plate 2/2). Slim, white mannequins clad in black lacy underwear occupy the window of a lingerie shop called 'Hot Gossip' (see Plate 2/3). Advertising in Bennett & Bain's lingerie shop claims their collection is 'gorgeously romantic for Christmas'. These are but a few examples of representations of a shopping centre culture that portrays women as normatively glamorous, erotic, alluring and seductive. A culture that encourages women to display their bodies but only so long as their bodies are slim, sexy and attractive in ways that befit the dominant culture.

Representations of pregnant bodies are largely absent in this highly charged, sexualised environment. This is in one sense absurd since pregnant bodies are clearly marked as having been sexually active. Although not all women have heterosexual intercourse in order to conceive (some choose different methods such as inserting a donation of sperm from a friend into their own vagina with a syringe), pregnant bodies tend to be read as material manifestations of sexual intercourse. Yet pregnant bodies are not the kind of markers of sexuality that the mall managers and retailers promote. Instead there exists an uneasiness about the public exposure of pregnant bodies. This uneasiness is not simply the prerogative of retailers who sell goods in Centre Place, rather it is part of a wider discourse shared by pregnant women themselves as well as those who view pregnant women. Howard (Christine's husband)[4] claims:

> I've seen pregnant women in all sorts of states of dress and undress and it seems quite a normal, ordinary course of events. Yet it is different . . . I guess something in me tells me that a pregnant woman is somehow in a different status to a non-pregnant woman, in a way a pregnant woman is sort of non-sexual, outside of courtship rules.
>
> (Individual interview)

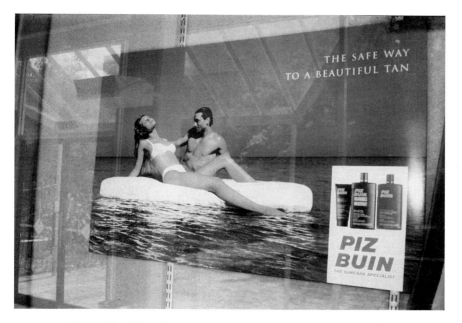

Plate 2.2 Advertisement in the window of Christies Chemist:
Robyn Longhurst

Howard raises an important point. Pregnant women are often perceived as being 'outside of courtship rules' – they are (ironically) constructed as 'non-sexual'. Once a woman is pregnant she is often considered to be no longer sexually available, active or desirable, even though her own desires may have increased. Young (1990: 166) argues that the pregnant woman's

> male partner, if she has one, may decline to share in her sexuality, and her physician may advise her to restrict sexual activity. To the degree that a woman derives a sense of self-worth from looking 'sexy' in the manner promoted by dominant cultural images she may experience her pregnant body as being ugly, and alien.

Many pregnant women with whom I spoke claimed that they tend to dress in baggy garments that act to disguise their swelling stomach especially if going out to places such as shopping centres, 'you do cover up your pregnancy. You always wear big clothes that are bigger than your tummy' says Jude, a university student who was 33 weeks pregnant (individual interview). This 'covering up' is not surprising since images of fatness, disability, incapacitation, uncomfortableness and ugliness were abundant in the research participants' accounts of their pregnancies. Paula recounts a story of a friend visiting her at home.

> At about 22 weeks pregnant, a friend, whom I see probably at least once per fortnight, came to dinner. As I opened the door to her, her first exclamation was 'Gosh, you get worse every time I see you.'
>
> (In-depth case study)

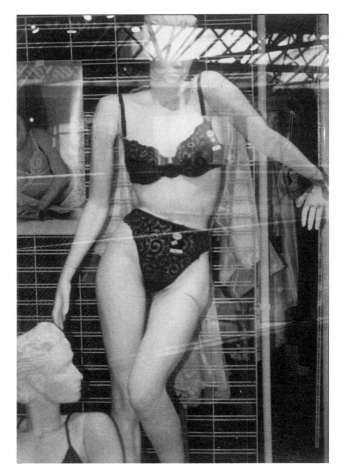

Plate 2.3 Mannequin in a lingerie shop – 'Hot Gossip':
Robyn Longhurst

Paula explained that in this instance, 'get worse' was equated with looking larger. Paula's pregnant stomach had become more evident since she last saw her friend. Kerry recounts a conversation that she had with a 14-year-old boy. The boy's feelings of abjection, and his representation of the pregnant body as ugly, are clearly revealed in the conversation.

> I was reading out the um week by week thing [a summary calendar of the various developmental stages of the fetus] to this fourteen year old that comes and milks with us – Mark. And um [laughter] I read out week twenty . . . and it said somethin' about um 'in week twenty your navel should pop out at any stage from now on'. . . . He's going, 'O o o *yuck*', he said, 'Oh you're going through a real ugly stage now Ker', and I said, 'Bloody hell' [laughter] and then I was in the shower this morning and I've got all these veins comin' up

on my legs and I'm thinking 'Gees, I'm going to the pack, I'm going [laughter] Oh Gees' and 'Oh I'm horrible'. And he said, 'Oh my aunty . . . I saw her just about two days before she went in' and he said, 'It's so ugly' [laughter].

(Joint in-depth case study)

One of Kerry's male colleagues described the ultrasound scan to her in the following way: 'For fifteen to twenty minutes you lie there with all this gel all over you with your *guts sticking out*' (emphasis added). Clearly his use of the phrase 'guts sticking out' to describe Kerry's pregnant stomach is interesting in that it does nothing to indicate the attractiveness of her stomach, rather to the contrary.

In relation to pregnant embodiment, it is useful to examine the words and phrases used not only by others, but also by pregnant women them-selves, to discuss their own embodiment and the bodies of other pregnant women. 'We were gonna park in the disabled car park,' says Denise. Denise's statement draws a correlation between being pregnant and being disabled. Christine claims: 'People sometimes treat you like you're just about handicapped when you're pregnant.' Ngahuia, although much less directly, also draws a correlation between being pregnant and disabled. 'I use the paraplegic toilets,' she says.

Pregnant women often discussed their perceptions of their bodies when I asked whether they had any photographs of themselves pregnant. When I asked Mary Anne, who was 36 weeks pregnant at the time of the interview, this question, she replied:

No and I don't intend to have any . . . I don't want anyone to look at my big bum. I don't mind my body shape of the baby, it's my hips and thighs that I don't like the thought of looking at.

(Individual interview)

Denise was concerned that her breasts had become larger during pregnancy and that people would see her 'boobs' bouncing up and down when she ran. She is of slim build and was 27 weeks pregnant at the time of this interview.

I was running across the street today in the rain 'cause it was raining and we had to run across the pedestrian crossing and I was running along and your boobs bounce up and down . . . I was concerned 'cause I thought there were people parked in cars waiting for the lights and I was running along. I knew they'd bounce up and down.

(In-depth case study)

Only two of the thrity-one respondents claimed that they liked their new body shape. Michelle, a dance teacher, says:

A pregnant body is really quite beautiful, it is just the feeling of, I don't know, it's like I feel good about being pregnant. One of the really nice things is I've got breasts. I was always one of these flat-chested people and so I feel so voluptuous during pregnancy.

(Individual interview)

In response to the question 'How do you feel about your pregnant body?' Ngahuia, the university lecturer, replied:

> I love it. I think it's good to have a positive attitude about it because so many women get put off by the fact that being pregnant means your body changes and you look awful, but let's face it, it is natural to look like that when you are pregnant and it's good to have a positive attitude and to set positive examples to other women to encourage them.
>
> (Individual interview)

By and large though, the pregnant women with whom I spoke did not like their new shape. These constructions of the pregnant body as ugly, alien and not sexy or sexual help to explain why it is so often considered to be private and in need of concealment. It is a body that is marked by a sexual act and sexual acts (although not the fantasy or anticipation of sexual acts) are usually confined to the private realm.

Yet a contradiction exists here. When pregnant women do enter public space their foetus is often treated as though it were a public concern. Pregnant women's rights to bodily autonomy are considered to be questionable (see Chavkin 1992: 193). This leads to pregnant women's stomachs being subject to public gaze and often touch. Their 'bodily space' is frequently invaded. Paula sums this up:

> Sometimes I feel as though being pregnant automatically deprives me of any individual identity and personal space. People seem to have a fascination with pregnant women's stomachs and want to pat them. It's not something they would normally do, but because I've got a bump it seems that I've become public property.
>
> (In-depth case study)

Although pregnant women sometimes feel as though they have 'become public property', images of the pregnant body are certainly not publicly displayed in shopping centres such as Centre Place. In the culture of Centre Place the discourse of pregnant women as having bodies that do not conform to the idealised norm of slim beauty positions pregnant women in ambiguous ways.

Many of the pregnant women whom I interviewed stopped visiting Centre Place. This is perhaps not surprising given that most of the shops that occupy prime sites in Centre Place and that focus on women's fashion and clothing (for example, Max, Denim and Blues, Underground Fashions, Esprit, Sportsgirl, Young World Fashion, Sussan and Stax) do not stock clothing above size 16. Several of the pregnant women claimed that prior to pregnancy they had enjoyed browsing and occasionally purchasing items of clothing in these shops but as they grew increasingly large they lost interest in browsing and felt less welcome there. This loss of interest in browsing and purchasing clothes could in part be attributed to a decline in income for most of the pregnant women as they gave up full-time employment, but I suggest much more is at stake. For example, one respondent said that she received a 'frosty' response from the shop attendant when she entered a lingerie shop not to buy a feeding or maternity bra but to outfit herself in some of the latest sexy underwear. This is despite the fact that the shop advertises that it sells 'Nitewear, Underwear, Bodywear, Maternity'.

When pregnant women disobey the unwritten cultural rules of pregnancy (for example, buying sexy underwear, engaging in 'extreme' sport or drinking alcohol) they risk disapproval by medical and health professionals, acquaintances, peers, friends, 'loved ones' and sometimes even strangers. It is not surprising, therefore, that during pregnancy in some places women find that their usual behaviours in public become increasingly socially unacceptable the more visibly pregnant they become. The familiar, the 'everyday' of some places through the medium/experience/physicality of their pregnant corporeality can become unfamiliar zones in which they at times feel uncomfortable and unwelcome. For example, during my first pregnancy I learned that in terms of dress codes, comportment and movement in public space, there are norms to which pregnant bodies are expected to adhere. For many complex reasons I became increasingly uncomfortable occupying public spaces such as pubs, nightclubs, beaches, public swimming pools, inner city business areas and ski-fields (ski-fields were places of both recreation and of employment for me).

Being visibly pregnant can also initiate access into specific environments. Many of the places into which I was suddenly welcomed and to which I felt a sense of belonging were places associated with the realms of domesticity – antenatal classes, maternity facilities at the hospital, doctors' surgeries, crèches, children's birthday parties and the homes of previously unknown neighbours and acquaintances (all of whom had children). However, one space where an atmosphere of belonging and approval did not prevail was 'pubs' or bars.

One of the respondents, Mary Anne, an international travel consultant who was 36 weeks pregnant at the time of interview, claimed that she became increasingly uncomfortable occupying Centre Place's tavern – Fox and Hounds. This pub is used mainly by inner city business men and women in their twenties. Not only did the atmosphere of the pub lose its appeal for Mary Anne (a place for 'single' people to meet?) but also the physical environment no longer met her needs.

Built environment of Centre Place

Patrons at the Fox and Hounds tavern are supplied with high, backless bar stools rather than chairs. There are only eight chairs in the entire tavern. These stools were described by Mary Anne as: 'impossible – I was sitting there thinking "where's a proper seat?" I was getting sore and so I'd rather not go any more' (individual interview).

It is perhaps no surprise that pregnant women's specific corporeal needs have not been considered by those who designed the tavern since such environments (long associated with alcohol and smoke) are not usually considered by society to be particularly 'appropriate' for pregnant women.

It is widely believed that a pregnant woman's primary concern ought to be for her unborn child. The pregnancy in many ways does not belong to the woman herself. Rather, the 'mother' is simply thought to be 'the site of her proceedings' (Kristeva 1980: 237).

Many of the pregnant women reported feeling discomfort in relation to the design and construction of Centre Place. To begin, the toilet facilities were reported as somewhat inadequate for pregnant women on two accounts: first, there are not enough toilets, leading to frequent queuing; and second, the cubicles themselves are small with one of them being positioned very close to a large structural pillar which makes it almost impossible for a visibly pregnant woman to enter. Given that the need to urinate with increased frequency is commonly met at the beginning and especially the end of pregnancy this is problematic.

Another point noted by pregnant women in regard to Centre Place was having to rely largely on stairs or escalators for access to the various levels. Climbing stairs can be tiring for pregnant women and mounting escalators can be problematic due to a change in their centre of balance. Although there are elevators in Centre Place these are small and there are often many people waiting to use them. Obviously there are many people who experience problems using stairs and/or escalators – people with strollers and prams, people with physical disabilities, elderly people, young children and so on.

Yet another problem identified by pregnant women who use Centre Place is that on wet days the flooring becomes slippery as water is tramped inside by users of the centre. Mats are laid out in some areas identified as particularly slippery (such as on ramps) in an attempt to improve the surface. For the pregnant women I spoke to, however, this did little to ease their worries about the possibility of falling and harming their unborn child.

Another problem that was identified for women in the advanced stages of pregnancy was 'fitting' into rows of seats in the Village 7 Cinema in Centre Place. Not only can it be difficult for pregnant women to sit comfortably for any period of time (there is no interval during movies screened at Village 7) in theatre seats but also it is often difficult for them to get to their seats. In the Village 7 Cinema complex four of the theatres have a reasonable amount of room between rows but the other three are cramped. Michelle, who was 33 weeks pregnant, commented: 'Trying to squeeze past people in the row in an attempt to get to your seat is difficult.' Joanne commented: 'People actually got up and moved into the aisle for me – it was really embarrassing.' Some pregnant women also mentioned these problems of uncomfortable seats and access to seats in relation to university lecture theatres and theatres used for live performance. For others, however, these were not considered problems.

Escaping the 'slim culture'

I am not proposing that the experiences of all the participants in this study were uniform: pregnant women and their experiences of Centre Place do not constitute a unified essential corporeality which effects solidarity between them. Not all of the women found the physical environment difficult to negotiate and not all of the women derived self-worth from looking sexy in the manner represented by the retailers in the shopping centre. Therefore. they did not all feel a sense of exclusion when their bodies no longer conformed to these representations. For many of the women their bodies did not conform to the dominant image prior to pregnancy.

In fact, rather than feeling excluded some of the pregnant women found it empowering to be temporarily located outside of the dominant cultural images of attractiveness, sexiness and slimness. For example, Jude, a university student aged between 25 and 29 years, and 33 weeks pregnant, claims that pregnancy can be a way of escaping some of the dietary constraints frequently placed on women such as the need to eat non-fattening foods in order to appear slim. Jude explains:

> It's nice to escape into pregnancy too, to get away from a slim culture. As a person who has never been particularly pencil thin it is really nice to eat lots of chocolate biscuits and not worry – to be able to hide it with pregnancy. To say 'I'm pregnant, of course I'm big. What do you expect? There's a baby in there.'
>
> (Individual interview)

Being able to walk around Centre Place and feel exempt from the 'slim culture' can be enormously empowering. For some women pregnancy offers an escape from feeling that they need to appear extraordinarily fit, trim, cheerful, playful, exciting, sexy and youthful. Becoming a mother can offer new and different roles for women.

Domesticity and motherhood

Hilary Winchester (1992: 148) notes in her study of Wollongong Mall in Australia: 'Women in their roles as wives and mothers are often the people who spend most time and money shopping and are therefore the main target for marketing.' Yet, interestingly, there are few spaces in Centre Place that promote (stereotypical notions of) domesticity and motherhood. As stated earlier Centre Place is not anchored by a department store or supermarket – it is comprised of speciality stores. In the early 1990s there were some spaces that reinforced traditional notions of women's domesticity, for example, Pumpkin Patch (a shop selling children's clothes and toys) and a crèche for shoppers' children. Some of the pregnant women whom I interviewed reported feeling initiated and welcomed into these places (the participants were pregnant for the first time). For some of the pregnant women their new body shape in the mall made them feel like they were somehow approved of and accepted for fulfilling that role that women have always fulfilled – the carrying and bearing of children. They were met with affirmation and their reproductive capacity was accorded social significance and value by other shoppers and workers in Centre Place.

More recently Pumpkin Patch and the crèche have closed. There are now even fewer representations of traditional domesticity and motherhood in Centre Place. The few that do exist are Hallensteins Kids (a shop selling children's clothing), Bye Gones (a shop selling ornaments/crafts), Heathcote Appliances (which sells some 'whitewear' but mainly television and stereo equipment) and Sussan (this shop sells trendy clothes for a young, slim clientele but currently has a large poster of a 'handsome', white man, woman and baby in the window).

There is also a clothes shop that caters specifically for women who are pregnant or have a 'fuller figure'. The (rather expensive) clothes in this shop, ironically, are displayed not on fuller figured, or even slim, mannequins but on coat hangers. The clothes hang, disembodied. The shop used to be called 'Preggy Gear', but in the early 1990s, in an attempt to increase their market share, the name changed to 'Kooky Fashions' (see Plate 2/4). 'Kooky' do not 'sell sex', rather, they sell the idea of being a little crazy, eccentric, foolish and/or hysterical. It is, I suspect, no coincidence that these 'attributes' are commonly associated with pregnant women. The *Collins English Dictionary* (1979: 724) states that the word hysteric is derived from seventeenth-century Latin *hystericus* literally meaning 'of the womb' and that there was a belief that hysteria in women originated in disorders of the womb (see Morgan and Scott 1993: 7). The one shop in Centre Place, therefore, that caters specifically for the clothing needs of pregnant women reinforces through its name the discourse and material construction of pregnant women not as sexy but as irrational, hysterical and 'kooky'.

Robbie Davis-Floyd (1986), in relation to the United States, argues that pregnancy has come out of the closet. We see pregnant women everywhere, from the night club to the formal dinner, and it is only a few old die-hards who mutter under their breath about unseemly display' (Davis-Floyd 1986: 47). Nowadays it is supposedly possible to be pregnant, attractive and sexy yet this research indicates that Centre Place opens up little discursive or material space for expectant mothers to be 'style-conscious', instead pregnant women's bodies are reinscripted as 'kooky'.

There is little doubt that changes have begun to occur in the discursive constructions of pregnancy: consider, for example, the appearance of actor and model Demi Moore on the cover of the glossy magazine *Vanity Fair* naked and eight months pregnant (see Jackson 1993: 220–1) and Joanna Paul (a New Zealand current affairs television reporter) on the cover of a magazine *New Spirit* 'heavily' pregnant. But such representations are yet to enter the realm of Centre Place. The circulation of these counter-discourses could potentially work to reinscript the bodies of pregnant women who use the shopping centre in 'new' ways. The formation of a new urban landscape could facilitate the formation of new identities for pregnant women in Hamilton, Aotearoa/New Zealand.

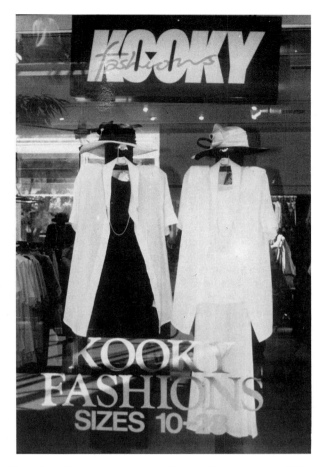

Plate 2.4 Formerly known as 'Preggy Gear', renamed 'Kooky':
Robyn Longhurst

The final, and more general, point that I want to make is that geography and geographers have a great deal to gain from current feminist scholarship, especially work on the body. Anglo-American feminist geography has, until recently, focused almost exclusively on gendered social relations in the 'real' material world rather than on questions of discourse, culture, power, representations and knowledge. This is not meant to imply that there exists a definitive split between the discursive and the material (rather it seems more likely that the material world is known through representational fields) but simply that the geographers' emphasis must not fall solely on the material world or on social relationships and activities as they vary across space.

Notes

Some sections of this chapter have been published in Longhurst, R. (1994) 'The geography closest in – the body . . . the politics of pregnability', *Australian Geographical Studies* 32(2): 214–23.

1 Aotearoa is the Maori term for what is commonly known as New Zealand. Over the last decade, especially since 1987 when the Maori Language Act was passed making Maori an official language, the term Aotearoa has been used increasingly by various individuals and groups. For example, all government ministries and departments now have Maori names which are used, in conjunction with their English names, on all documents. Despite these moves, however, the naming of place is a contestatory process (see Berg and Kearns 1996) and I use the term Aotearoa/New Zealand in an attempt to highlight this.

2 'Pakeha' here refers to Aotearoa/New Zealand-born people of 'European' descent. Although the term 'Pakeha' has been (and at times still is) highly contested in Aotearoa/New Zealand (see Spoonley 1995) it is now used as a standard term of classification of ethnicity in the New Zealand Census.

3 'Maori' is the term commonly used to refer to the *tangata whenua* (literally 'people of the land') or indigenous peoples of Aotearoa/New Zealand. I use this term here, but wish to problematise such use. As Spoonley (1995) points out, the word 'Maori' is really a convenience for Pakeha/European to lump together divergent groups. The inverse of this, however, does not apply since Pakeha/ European do not tend to identify themselves in terms of tribal affiliations.

4 The names of all participants, including the partners/husbands of pregnant women, have been changed. I attempted to retain some of the integrity of people's names by replacing Maori names with Maori pseudonyms and English names with English pseudonyms.

3

Involving black and minority women in regeneration initiatives

A case study of Bethnal Green City Challenge

Maher Anjum and Lesley Klein

'Redevelopment', 'regeneration', 'partnership', 'participation': these were some of the key buzz words being used in City Challenge and the Single Regeneration Budget (SRB), the latest in a long line of major urban renewal initiatives by the Department of Environment (DoE), to describe the culture of funding schemes for inner cities of England and Wales. These terms are designed to take away the negative images and connotations related to deprived inner city areas and instead instil feelings of 'hope, possibilities and new beginnings'. They also mark out new ideologies and approaches to old problems.

Assessing the Impact of Urban Policy (Robson *et al.* 1996), an evaluation of the earlier Action for Cities Programme, had in fact set the groundwork for the introduction of some of this new terminology through its recommendations. These recommendations highlighted certain areas of concern, including the need for more effective coalitions of local actors; for local authorities to play a significant part in such coalitions as enablers and facilitators; for local communities to play a part and for capacity-building (DoE 1996: 2).

> City Challenge was intended to be different from earlier initiatives in terms of its values, organisation and priorities. The diversity of local circumstances, needs and opportunities was recognised. Priorities were to be determined, not by central government, but by local partners defining an end-state vision, and linking specific programmes, projects and resources to that vision in a strategic way.
>
> (Department of the Environment 1996: 3)

In this way City Challenge, and the SRB which was to follow, was held up as the initiative that would address many of the needs identified, and unfulfilled, in previous regeneration programmes.

The summer of 1991 saw the launch of the first of two rounds of a competition in which local authorities could bid for money worth up to £37.5 million over five years. This new experimental programme was called

City Challenge; its initiatives were to be area-focused, delivered by independent bodies (i.e. independent from local authorities) and representing all local interests and 'players', and would be measured by a series of contractual outputs, particularly the leverage of private investment. By 1993, at the end of the second and final round, a total of thirty-one previous Urban Programme authorities across the country had qualified for these bids. All these programmes will have finished by 1998 having spawned the Single Regeneration Budget (SRB) as a follow-on initiative which has already started to provide major regeneration funding.

Regeneration programmes in the competition model like City Challenge and the SRB replaced all previous sources of money given out by the then government for the development of urban areas. So, in the absence of any other sources of finance to rebuild and regenerate inner city areas, and due to their very emphasis on identifying and meeting local needs, working in partnership with the public, private and voluntary sectors, encouraging real participation with service users, and addressing (locally) issues of poverty, unemployment, poor housing and crime, it becomes essential to assess whether or not such regeneration programmes have truly addressed the needs of the whole population.

This case study focuses on black and minority women as groups within the population whose needs are, as is well documented, too often sidelined. Women make up 52 per cent of the population but are also one of the largest groups to be socially and economically disadvantaged. A large proportion of the very old in Britain are women; most carers, single parents and disabled people are women; women are employed mainly in part-time, poorly paid, unsafe jobs with no security; women are most dependent on public sector housing and rented accommodation which are often of poor quality; women make up a substantial proportion of the homeless, although this often remains undocumented; women face violence both within the home and outside it (Women's Design Service 1992). Women not only predominate in most of the indices of 'deprived' groups but they are also the ones who often face and experience problems within their neighbourhoods.

The 1991 census identified that though there are great geographical variations within Great Britain itself in its ethnic composition, the majority of ethnic groups are concentrated in England. The south-east has the highest concentration of ethnic minority people followed by the West Midlands. Greater London itself has 44.6 per cent of the entire ethnic minority population of Great Britain (Butt and Kurshida 1996). The significance of these statistics for the purposes of this chapter is that women from minority groups live mostly in urban areas and therefore in some of the most socially and economically deprived areas of the country. So when regeneration programmes like City Challenge and the SRB are looking to address the needs of the whole community this must include the particular needs of women, and among them, of black and minority women, if they are to succeed in the long term within their own terms of reference.

With the emphasis on 'participation and partnership' between the private, statutory, voluntary and community sectors to formulate programmes to deliver services and meet the particular needs of the area, it is vital to assess how politically, socially and economically under-represented groups have become partners in the City Challenge and SRB process and participated in such programmes. This chapter then intends to examine the impact and involvement of women, particularly black and other ethnic minority women, in a major regeneration programme, Bethnal Green City Challenge (BGCC), in the London Borough of Tower Hamlets.

The Bethnal Green City Challenge Area

Prior to being awarded the City Challenge in the first round of bidding in 1992, the Tower Hamlets Bethnal Green area was very much like most other inner city areas in its economic make-up, if not socially or culturally.

> An area with a history and cultural diversity like nowhere else, Spitalfields, in particular, has been the focus of successive waves of immigration from Huguenots, to the Jews at the turn of the century and the Bangladeshis from the 1960s onwards. These immigrant communities have come to an area with its own rich traditions built up through hundreds of years of struggle and survival by the working-class communities of London's East End.
>
> (Bethnal Green City Challenge 1994: 11)

Among the key characteristics of this area is that it has one of the youngest and fastest-growing populations in England and Wales with 33 per cent of the local population under the age of 16 compared with 20 per cent nationally. Of the population 60 per cent are from ethnic minority groups, the vast majority being from Bangladesh. The level of poverty, if measured by statistics of unemployment and housing, is again significantly high in the area: 32 per cent for men and 19 per cent for women. However, if the figures are examined further, the rates of unemployment amongst the black and ethnic minority community are 44 per cent for Asian and black men, and 41 per cent and 27 per cent for Asian and black women respectively. The majority of households live in public housing: 59 per cent compared with 20 per cent nationally, and the levels of overcrowding are 22 per cent compared with 2 per cent nationally (Census for Ethnic Groups in Tower Hamlets 1991).

As one of the main sources, if not the only source, of major funding available from the DoE, City Challenge, SRB and their predecessors have tried to address the issues of urban decline. The more recent initiatives have been designed to put in an intensive amount of funding for regeneration schemes contained in the area programme over a relatively short period of time. This source of money was not tied to local authority budgets and other restraints; therefore it was possible – uniquely for the time – to have major housing refurbishment programmes along with newbuilds. The programmes have also been involved in extensive measures to set up employment training schemes, assist local small businesses and help voluntary sector organisations to provide services not, or no longer, covered by the statutory agencies, which are more needs-led, as well as establishing courses to create employment opportunities for its participants with local partners. However, at the end of such initiatives (it was April 1997 in the case of BGCC) there is the danger that, unless the specific projects have been picked up by the local authority or some other source of funding has been established for them, or the City Challenge company has reconstituted itself in order to sustain the work and the gains and carry through the 'end vision', they will all disappear. Sustainability of regeneration measures is then a crucial issue as it is at the point of the programme's closure that we will be able to assess and evaluate the true success of such initiatives.

Bethnal Green City Challenge was set up as a limited company to deliver the objectives detailed in the original action plan (the document put together as the competition bid). It aimed to

> make a significant, sustainable impact through a practical partnership of private, public and community based bodies which will deliver an imaginative, integrated programme that will change the economic and social fabric of the area, change local people's lives through providing access to new opportunities, and confer important benefits on London as a whole.
>
> (Bethnal Green City Challenge 1994: 6)

Ambitious plans included: providing a ladder of opportunity to equip the people of the Challenge area and surrounding neighbourhoods with the confidence and skills to take part in the mainstream economy; releasing and supporting local development potential in a way that maximises access to opportunities for local people to ensure they share fully in the jobs and wealth created; building a stronger, more vibrant local economy that offers a diverse range of employment opportunities at reasonable rates of pay; and enabling local people to live in harmony, take control of their lives, and choose their own futures in an attractive environment with a mix of quality housing and with good public transport.

The starting-point for achieving this vision was to improve the language and literacy skills of local residents. Without this, other planned developments and opportunities were in danger of simply passing local people by. Vitally, City Challenge could unlock opportunities by providing residents with access to English language skills as the front end of a set of linked language skills training and employment programmes. The success of the initiative would be measured, according to the action plan, by the extent of this integration; by lasting improvements in the levels of literacy, employment, skills and business activity in the area; and by sustained reduction in the levels of unemployment, dereliction and overcrowding, relative to the averages for London and the borough as a whole (Bethnal Green City Challenge 1994). BGCC set up a structure of programmes with scores of projects relating to education and training, enterprise support, community development, housing and environmental development to tackle the area's problems during its five-year life.

As a means of assessing and evaluating the process of consultation, role and purpose of involvement of women in this programme, four projects and organisations, partly or wholly funded for either or both specific and general work, have been selected for closer analysis. The four projects are Language 2000, Heba Women's Project, Women's Youth Work Training Course and Jagonari Women's Centre.

Language 2000

Language 2000 was seen as a 'flagship' project of BGCC – another term which formed part of 'CC-speak', meaning that the project exemplified the BGCC philosophy of regeneration. Its stated aim was to ensure that 'every resident of the BGCC area [will] have access to English Language classes or ESOL (English for speakers of other languages)'. This was directly based on the original action plan: '[the] starting point for achieving this vision is improving the language and literacy skills of local residents' (Bethnal Green City Challenge 1994). The concentration of the local population consisted mainly of Bangladeshi people followed by a growing Somali community along with the existing white residents. The needs of the different communities while diverse were similar in some areas: poor housing, high unemployment, crime levels, lack of facilities, to name but a few.

Prior to the City Challenge proposal a language audit of the local population had been carried out by Tower Hamlets College. It was this audit which had established that local people felt language or, to be more specific, fluency and literacy in the English language, was a major barrier

Plate 3.1 Language 2000 crèche: John Sturrock/Network

to accessing employment or even training in some cases. Existing provisions did not, it was clear, cater for the needs of the local population. The audit exposed barriers – the location of venues, the teachers, the curriculum, the timing of classes, the lack of child-care facilities and, often, insensitivity to cultural issues – to both men and women accessing the available resources.

Language 2000, however, consciously set out to provide services to the local community including women from all cultural groups. Its aims were to provide language training and parent education to increase independence and raise aspirations; to link language provision to customised training and to access to higher education; and to promote nationally significant pilot schemes which explored the new National Language Standards and the Post-16 Qualifications Framework. Courses were set up at different times, in various venues, with both women-only and mixed options, with same-language teachers and teachers speaking only English. Basically a wide range of options was provided so that people could readily access the service that best suited their situation.

Although the services and provisions were based on the original language audit document, direct community involvement, particularly with women, did not take place at the initial stage, primarily because the period of submission of a bid for the City Challenge competition was very short. But later on, the curriculum was used to work with women attending Heba Women's Project's ESOL and craft sessions, so the feedback from the audit was incorporated directly into the actual curriculum that Language 2000 introduced.

In the first year of the project local women and men were recruited to become trained as ESOL tutors. (Interestingly some of the male tutors recruited already had qualifications from their country of origin.) They then went on to become qualified with RSA/TESOL diplomas in teaching English. This approach was successful in recruiting local Bangladeshi women in particular, who were out of full-time education or who had been looking after children. It was considered very important that the prospective students could identify with their tutors and vice versa. This also meant that as the curriculum developed it further reflected and included cultural norms and practices within its exercises and examples. Furthermore, the venues for the classes were all easily accessible as most of them were based in local primary schools as well as in community centres or tenants' halls, all with child-care facilities.

Though the project was intended to appeal to the whole community, women and particularly Bangladeshi women made up the majority of the service users. It was due to this that in the second year of the project, more mixed provisions were introduced on to the programme and more computer-related and information technology courses (IT) were set up. Most of the women who attended the courses started off on the 'Basic Skills' units and, as they progressed, were able to take up sessions in computer skills, word-processing and other IT-related subjects.

Plate 3.2 IT Training: John Sturrock/Network

The project's ability to respond to 'local need' through service delivery and not just through its provisions was identified as vital for its success. At the end of all courses students filled out evaluation and monitoring forms, and any student who had dropped out was contacted either by the course tutor or through a questionnaire. It was generally considered that part of the success of this project was due directly to its local connections – that the tutors were mostly local women, who having themselves become qualified, and so able to act as role models, were also well placed to contact and recruit other local women to enrol on the courses. This type of informal outreach development work was assisted by the appointment of an outreach coordinator. Besides the tutors being locals themselves, these additional posts were created to work with local groups and organisations to promote the project but also to get feedback on what people wanted. This gave the project a high profile in the area. Estimates suggest that during its life-span Language 2000 provided adult education to over 3,000 people. There was a general feeling of 'upskilling' within the community, especially amongst women, higher levels of parental participation within schools, particularly at primary level, and increased confidence amongst women. A number of spin-off projects were created, mainly in the fields of parent education and involvement in schools.

Heba women's project

This project was launched in 1990 as a number of small-scale training sessions set up by Spitalfields Small Business Association (SSBA) for the

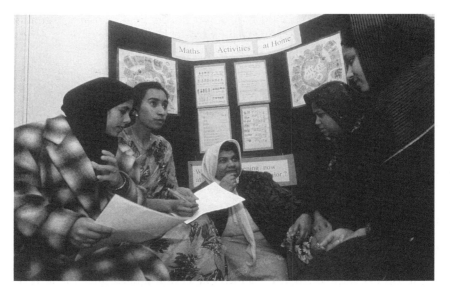

Plate 3.3 Parents and tutor at Parents' Centre:
John Sturrock/Network

LEEDS METROPOLITAN
UNIVERSITY LIBRARY

wives of the men working in the sweatshops in the area. Initially at least, this mainly involved Bangladeshi women, who had been identified as a group which was not being catered for by any existing provisions and therefore left marginalised and isolated. The aims of the programme were outlined as follows:

> [To] build up confidence, extending knowledge and improving literacy and numeracy skills . . . to equip the women so that they can take advantage of further training opportunities in this or other programmes in the area.
>
> The training will be based around three ideas of co-operative working, childcare, horticulture and interior decoration. Included in these will be an integrated programme of literacy, numeracy and language training. Set along-side them will be a parallel programme of confidence and assertiveness training.
>
> As a foundation and/or access course it will concentrate on developing these essential basic components within a programme of skill based training centred around the co-operative work ideas. The skills training will have both theoretical and practical elements located in Princelet St. [the main venue of the project] but linked, where appropriate, to other projects and training schemes in the area.
>
> All training will be delivered by women and where possible these will be bilingual. It is recognised that in most areas of the training this will be difficult and it is therefore envisaged that throughout the duration of the course a translator will be needed to work alongside the trainers in an active way.
>
> (Spitalfields Small Business Association 1991)

By the time Language 2000 had started on its first-year programme in 1994–5, SSBA was already running its own ESOL and craft sessions. From their own experience of working with local women, SSBA had suggested that there existed a need to put on English-language classes for local women in community settings. As mentioned above, Language 2000's initial curriculum was tried and tested on the women's sessions run by SSBA. Some of the SSBA's own tutors were recruited and trained as ESOL tutors by Language 2000. Women who attended the sessions were eager for them to continue and, at the end of the trial period, petitioned to have further English-language classes. The sessions ran both during the week and at weekends, and during the day and in the evening.

The sessions run initially were all based on crafts and language. This was partially due to the fact that some of the SSBA's small business tenants were skilled craftspeople who became directly involved with the delivery of the sessions. European Social Fund money was obtained eventually to fund the sessions but also to provide training allowances for women attending the sessions. This was fundamental; though the amount was very little, it was an incentive for the women to come and, importantly, represented a 'value' attached to the individual's attending. It helped to portray the sessions as more than just language classes. Though the majority of the women wanted to learn English in order to be able to access resources and provisions or become less dependent on their husbands or children, they also wanted to learn English to access training courses and employment. Hence the teaching of English occurred hand in hand with crafts, horticulture and sewing sessions. The products from these sessions were then sold in the open market. This then gave the project a further sense of being more than a language session. As translators were provided where possible, women attending a crafts session, for example, would also learn the necessary language and gain self-confidence as they improved their skills.

The SSBA worked together with Heba Women's Project, Language 2000 and other funding sources from BGCC, which enabled them to establish the project to a high status. As a project it definitely benefited from the regeneration programme. It now has its own shopfront premises from which it sells, jointly with another SSBA project, crafts, headscarves and other items of clothing made by women in various sessions. The project was very much user-led in its expansion even if in its conception the 'need' was identified by professionals at SSBA and BGCC, in a similar fashion to the development of Language 2000 during the City Challenge programme. The project, as it is today, has grown to reflect demand and the needs of its users.

Mohila/Hawan course for working with young people: women in youth work training

'Mohila/Hawan' means 'woman' in Bengali and Somali. This was a specially designed course to deliver the main elements of the Stage 1

Introductory Course of the Certificate in Basic Youth Work for Bengali and Somali women to become part-time youth workers in the BGCC area. The course was funded by BGCC and run by Goldsmiths' College, University of London. The steering group consisted of representatives from Avenues Unlimited, a local youth work organisation, and Jagonari Women's Centre, the local women's centre (Salvat 1996).

The first stage of the course began in April 1996, though initial planning had started in Spring 1995 and the funding was approved by BGCC by November 1995. The need for such a course had been identified earlier through the Youth Consultation programme carried out by BGCC. The consultation established that there were very few trained Bengali or Somali women youth workers and that there was a definite need to recruit and train within this group. A youth work training course had been implemented in conjunction with Goldsmiths' College but very few women participated and even fewer completed the course. It was evident that this course had failed to address certain needs which would have enabled and encouraged more women to attend. Some of these were to do with the actual course structure, and so the Mohila/Hawan course had these provisions built into it: close supervision and monitoring in placements by a tutor, support for carrying out written course work and ongoing individual supervision. This provided essential support to the students who came from varied backgrounds. Some of the women had postgraduate qualifications from their country of origin while others had no academic qualifications; some were born and brought up in the UK and others in Bangladesh and Somalia; some had in-depth knowledge and experience of youth and community work while others were just starting out. There was also a wide age-difference among the students.

The Women's Community Development worker at BGCC, a Bangladeshi herself, was instrumental in identifying the gaps in the existing course, including the needs of the targeted women, and in the actual recruitment of women to the course. English-language support in the form of women interpreters, transport to take the women home at the end of each session, child-care, placement supervision, tutorials and women-only venues were put in place. Thirty women applied to go on the course – testimony to the success of her work, considering that the course had been planned originally for only ten students. This was a response so positive that BGCC agreed to provide extra funding for an additional ten places. At the end of the first stage sixteen women had completed the initial course and were able to progress to the second stage, which began in October 1996.

While Stages One and Two of the course were very much 'women only', Stage Three, run in conjunction with the local authority, required the women to gain specific knowledge and experience in one area of youth work. This specialist training is offered in a mixed setting to all youth workers across the board, but there were no objections voiced by the women to this part of the course.

The Mohila/Hawan Course is similar to the previous projects discussed, in that it was conceptualised and set up without participation or involvement from local women, although widespread consultation had taken place. Being able to take account of the local issues and to address them within the course through a tailor-made programme increased the rate of success and retention of the women who joined the course.

Jagonari Women's Centre

Jagonari Women's Centre, a purpose-built centre, was established in Whitechapel in 1987/8. It was set up following a long campaign, by Bangladeshi women in particular, to highlight the need for a focal point to raise issues of concern for all local women as neighbourhood agencies and services had failed to cater for the growing number of Bangladeshi residents. Over the years Jagonari has had a turbulent history and it has never received funding to realise its full capacity to function as a centre although it has provided services for young women, day-care in its purpose-built nursery and after-school homework sessions, and has run specific projects in conjunction with other organisations such as the Whitechapel Art Gallery.

Aside from insufficient finance the centre has suffered from low staffing levels and management problems and in April 1995 Jagonari was almost closed down due to lack of funding and questions raised by funders about its level of success in meeting the needs of local women. At this time there were in fact very few activities taking place at the centre and the number of women attending ranged from very few to none at all. This crisis brought together various sets of people from the voluntary and statutory agencies along with local trusts and charities who had been funding the organisation. It also involved local women who saw Jagonari as a potentially valuable asset in the neighbourhood and who did not want to lose it.

BGCC, one of the project's funders, suggested that a detailed review and redevelopment plan of the organisation should be carried out which would include consultation with local women and agencies. This consultation formed the basis of Jagonari's redevelopment plan, the idea being that this would then reflect what local women themselves wanted, what they felt the gaps in services were. Rather than starting from the position that Jagonari had outgrown its purpose, the consultation took as its baseline that the centre was failing to provide services required and that it needed to have an appropriate structure to support its work.

BGCC's input involved making finance available over a three-month period, initially for five consultants to carry out various aspects of the consultation exercise and redevelopment plan. Following this, two consultants provided ongoing support by working with an interim management committee, local women and interested organisations to develop the new structure, aims and objectives in line with the feedback from the consultation process. This work allowed Jagonari to remain open and become operative.

Plate 3.4 Training women lifesavers: John Sturrock/Network

The redevelopment programme gave the centre the opportunity to involve local women directly in all stages of its new structure rather than the more 'top-down' method of professionals deciding what should happen. This had definite impact: for example, the majority of the women interviewed in the consultation exercise wanted the centre to be a place where they could come in and relax without feeling pressurised to do anything or take part in activities and training. They wanted a space for themselves and this need had not been previously identified or acknowledged by any of the agencies or individuals involved. Further, activities offered at the centre were usually limited to sewing, child-care and ESOL classes, thus confirming perceived 'cultural norms'. Only very rarely were courses like the Youth Training Introductory course or Heba's crafts-based sessions offered. Without the redevelopment plan these important pointers to providing services that women actually wanted to use would have remained hidden.

Conclusions

We can draw a series of conclusions from these examples of black and ethnic minority women's involvement in the City Challenge regeneration process. First, three out of the four projects – Language 2000, Heba Women's Project and the Mohila/Hawan Course for Working with Young People – were set up in circumstances where the initial identification of a need or a gap in service delivery did not come from 'the women' themselves. Yet in the case of Jagonari the original campaign for a women's centre was run by local women and workers, and the consultation and redevelopment plan carried out in 1995/6 involved local women at every stage. It is then not possible to say conclusively that involvement of women from the initial stage – true partnership and full participation, to return to the buzz words of regeneration – will result in success.

The success of the other three projects underlines the importance of creating the right atmosphere or, rather, taking the specific needs of the target group as the starting-point, prior to the project opening. In other words, participation must begin at the point of conception if the project is to reflect anything more than the beliefs of interested professionals, community leaders and so on, about what women want to do. They may, as we have seen, be wrong. It is also clear that factors such as child-care, single-sex sessions, timing, transport, safety, language, acknowledgement of diverse cultures, racism, poverty, unemployment, lack of access to training, which may influence a woman's ability or desire to attend on a regular basis, need to be examined and responded to within the provisions offered.

The audit which formed the basis of Language 2000 and featured in the BGCC programme focused on the need to have English skills to access training and raise levels and opportunities for employment of the Bangladeshi, Somali and majority populations. These courses emphasised both directly and indirectly the importance of proficiency in English-language and literacy skills as a basic requirement for seeking employment or training. But they failed to acknowledge that the students already had skills in their own language and so missed the possibilities for building on that. The training courses that women have gone on to attend have generally been in the areas of child-minding and crèche support and, for some of the younger women born and brought up in Britain, office skills. Certainly there is a need for trained Bangladeshi women in these fields but these courses fail to provide the students with skills which would enable them to compete in the open market. For instance, in the child-care field only mainstream qualifications like that from the National Nursery Education Board are recognised and valid, and outside Tower Hamlets or other densely populated Bangladeshi localities, the demand for such bilingual skills is very low. So women are spending time studying to become fluent in English and then to gain qualifications with which they will still be unable to enter the mainstream job market.

Second, the importance of direct contact through outreach and development work, or whatever means, comes sharply into relief. Many other women were recruited on to the course through the women who became tutors for Language 2000. A similar situation was apparent in the SSBA crafts and language sessions with the outreach work undertaken by the BGCC women's development officer along with the course's support tutor enabling students to become more confident while on the course.

Without these methods of recruitment it is possible that courses and projects will continue to be set up which will never attract women, and especially black and ethnic minority women. This is amply portrayed in the case of Jagonari Women's Centre where although all members of staff were Bangladeshi and the centre was a women-only space, which celebrated the cultural and religious events of the community, it was barely used – so having the right environment, while necessary, is not enough.

A third point concerns the viability of the work done with the women involved and the way in which their needs are met. It is well documented that there is a high proportion of black and ethnic minority women employed in 'homeworking' and that far from this being about filling spare time it is about earning a wage for the household. Again, this explains the success of the Mohila/Hawan course and the Heba Project which both took a 'holistic' approach, that is, one that provided a transferrable skill at the end, rather than being an end in itself. This demonstrates that limiting the project to immediate concerns – for example, lack of proficiency in the majority language – or taking a 'cultural relativist' position which inevitably confirms and perpetuates assumed restrictions on Bangladeshi women, is not enough.

Inner city regeneration through City Challenge and SRB programmes has been able to help improve services and resources purely because they have the means to inject sums of money in more flexible ways. All the projects discussed here would have had extreme difficulty in securing funding and support for their work from sources other than a regeneration programme. Local authorities may be able to identify such needs but are usually tied to trying to keep essential public services running rather than funding 'untried' projects, perhaps with less conventional approaches. Lack of finance and the need to show 'results' quickly mean that a project has to show evidence of success early on in order to get renewed funding. Work with community groups can take more than a year to achieve results; organisations like City Challenge with their five-year time-span had the flexibility to wait for results in a way that the local authority does not.

Regeneration programmes are able to look at all aspects of a geographical area and work out a 'grand plan' for it. In other words strategic decisions can be made about all aspects of a particular area which will have long- and short-term effects, whereas local authorities are no longer in a position to take a holistic approach. They certainly would not be able to fund support services which were crucial to the success of the examples above, like safe transport, child-care, language support tutors, etc., for every project to enable the target groups to participate in different programmes and activities, or in consultation programmes about the needs for services and support.

As in other under-represented minority groups, the involvement of black and minority women in regeneration programmes is essential, as this is their only opportunity to set their own agenda and take a measure of control in the local sphere and so become a vocal part of the mainstream, participating in the planning of their own neighbourhood and their future. The benefits of regeneration projects can only be limited, and their success only partial, if they fail to address the needs of the whole population. In that case, phrases like 'redevelopment, regeneration, partnership and participation' will lose their meaning and become only another catchphrase to be supplanted by another equally empty terminology and ideology in the future as new initiatives replace those currently in force, unless long-term plans for the projects' futures become part of the regeneration packages from the start.

4

UnWomanly acts

Struggling over sites of resistance

Ali Grant

Introduction: losing site(s)

In communities all across Canada, political activists of many stripes have been feeling the chilling effects of a general swing to the right and a conservative backlash against all and any progressive social movements. Feminist anti-violence activists have found themselves in a particularly difficult situation: while the issue of violence against women has been enjoying a high political and public profile, anti-feminist sentiment has become a frequent, and largely acceptable, component of contemporary public discourse and practices throughout the nation.[1] Feminist analysts and activists[2] have argued that 'the movement' has been institutionalised and that in the process, many shelters and rape crisis centres have become little more than traditional social service agencies with a twist[3] (Dobash and Dobash 1992; Timmins 1995; Walker 1990).

Feminist anti-violence activism can usefully be thought of as 'UnWomanly acts'. That is, understanding violence against women as one process in the manufacture of women (and maintenance of gender hierarchy) and feminist activism as resistance to this process can help make better sense of the ways in which certain spaces of organised feminist activism have become 'de-radicalised'. Funding and regulatory bodies, as well as 'the public', often condemn those activities that appear to challenge the heterosexual regime[4] (Wittig 1992). To avoid this, and to maintain legitimacy, many shelters and rape crisis centres have been forced to illustrate that they are neither disloyal to men ('anti-men', 'man-hating', 'anti-police') nor lesbian. Using the accusation of lesbianism as a slur is an old but still effective way of maintaining a strict gender hierarchy (Frye 1992; Grant forthcoming). The gravity of the sin of disloyalty to men is illustrated annually in the national furore over the exclusion of men from Take Back The Night[5] and in less public daily struggles over the rights of men to access services of sexual assault centres and to serve on boards and staff of these centres and shelters, and the provision of counselling programmes for abusive men.

Although much has been written about the implications of these changes for the struggle over how violence against women will be understood and how it will be tackled (and by whom), here I am interested in what these changes might mean for the development of political identities in place. In this chapter, I take a brief look at struggles over particular sites of political resistance and investigate the implications of these for the regeneration of local capacities for collective action. I draw on doctoral research[6] carried out in the city of Hamilton,[7] Canada during the first half of the 1990s to offer a concrete illustration of the importance of space in identity formation, political mobilisation and the performance of sex.

Contesting gender: unwomanly activism

The issue of violence against women has been an important one in Canadian feminist activism over the last three decades (Backhouse and Flaherty 1992; Carty 1993; Wine and Ristock 1991). Women have created a nation-wide network of shelters and rape crisis centres as well as contributing to a huge expansion in public consciousness of the issue. Analyses of the issue have of course developed and become more sophisticated over time. As members of the mental health and social services industries have come to view violence against women as squarely within their professional realm, the messages that we receive in the public domain about this violence have become a confusing and contradictory mix of competing concepts including power and control, the cycle of violence, learned behaviours, and dysfunctional families (Timmins 1995; Yllö and Bograd 1988).

Still, feminist anti-violence activism can usefully be viewed as most clearly contesting the oppressive system of gender, directly and openly challenging the rights of men in a sexist society. That is, as a set of counter-hegemonic practices and ideas, it shines a spotlight on the realities of men's violence; for example, that when it is used against their wives, lovers, daughters and so on, it is punished much less severely than when it is used against other men (and/or 'other men's women'). This type of feminist activism, then, contests the reproduction of the heterosexual regime.

Just as there have been struggles over how this violence should be understood and tackled, so there have been ongoing struggles over shelters and sexual assault centres – their funding, their control and their activities.[8] Activists and analysts alike note that organised anti-violence activism has lost its earlier radical political message and that traditional sites of resistance, such as shelters and rape crisis centres, have been institution-alised[9] (for example, see Findlay 1988; Gold 1991; Timmins 1995; Walker 1990). These processes have seen many go from grass-roots, informal, peer-counselling organisations to government-funded 'social service agencies' employing professionals.[10] Discussing the changes in the shelter movement in north-western Ontario, for example, Leni Untinen (1995: 175) notes, 'Workers have difficulty relating to this early period when shelters had little or no money for salaries, and activism translated directly into volunteer, front-line work. It wasn't unusual to reach into your own cupboard and bring back as much food as you could afford to give.'

It was also not unusual to find lesbians at the front and centre in the early days; however, few of the writings on the institutionalisation of anti-violence activism investigate the roles that normative gender scripts (Butler 1990) and the 'lesbian threat' have played in its de-radicalisation. Despite the recent surge in the critical analysis of sexuality as a vital component of subjectivity, there is still little recognition in social theory that hetero-sexuality constitutes a system of economic and political exploitation (as has happened with race and class and so on). Critical lesbian interventions have, however, illustrated that we are surrounded by heterosexuality as normative and regulatory; on television and radio, in films, in church, and in the assumptions of the health, legal and social services systems (Bell and Valentine 1995; Grant 1997; Valentine 1993a, 1993b and 1993c).

The practices and ideas, subtle and not so subtle, which work to order society as heterosexual are uncovered in investigations of various ways in which women challenge the boundaries of acceptable behaviours, desires, attitudes, activities and employment. The regulations of the heterosexual regime are often deployed in the punishment and disciplining of those acts which most obviously transgress the boundaries of what is acceptable in a society ordered on a strict gender hierarchy. In Canada, a country still dominated by the societal values of a white, male, heterosexual, non-disabled, middle-class culture, the contours of the acceptable Woman are very different from those which are constructed in other cultures and groups both within and outside of this particular location. The transgressable boundaries, then, are those of a culturally and otherwise contingent, politic-ally and socially constructed category. The dominant one in Canada is that of 'nice white girls'. What might these 'de- radicalising' processes mean for the development of counter-hegemonic political identities in different places?

Identity and the politics of location

Location matters for the development of political identities and for the possibilities, in place, for collective political action. This is not to suggest locations or identities that are given or stable. It is instead to invoke a politics of location which Adrienne Rich (1986) argued entails a recognition of where we are in the world, in relation to others, and of our location within certain webs of oppressive material and ideological relations. As a self-consciously politicised lesbian in a heterosexist society, for example, I recognise myself as never either completely inside or completely outside the heterosexual regime. I am, to an extent, always out of place, located, through a combination of choice and force, in the margins: in my pro-duction and consumption of culture; in my romantic, economic, political and sexual attachments; and in the temporary nature of my travel in mainstream institutions such as the academy. My identity is constructed and reconstructed in and through these particular locations. When feminist anti-violence activists talk of 'coming from the same place', they are invoking a locational politics, referring to their common locations in alliances against particular sets of power relations. In this way, the bases of 'community' may be a shared sense of political identity rather than a shared physical location or biology. By focusing on the different locations of political subjects and what this might mean for their subjection to heterosexual rule and the possibilities for collective struggles against it (and other systems of oppression), we can move away from an essentialist identity politics and all of its associated dangers towards a more self-conscious coalitional politics.

One of the factors involved in identity formation, in the process through which we come to see the world differently and act on it, is our interactions with others. Women who contest and transgress gender materially and symbolically expose the manufactured nature of the category 'women'. The possibility and existence of various locations beyond gender, such as lesbian, are made unintelligible, denied (Durocher 1990; Frye 1992; Wittig 1992). As mentioned above, transgressive females have tended to be marginalised, as spaces of resistance have been institutionalised. Removing these transgressive bodies and ideas not only affects the kinds of services offered, for example, but also reduces the possibilities in place for the continuation of the development of radical counter-hegemonic identities. As I illustrate below, the outcome of struggles over sites of resistance matters for identity formation in place, and for the regeneration of local capacities for collective political action. As William Carroll (1992: 10) notes, in his discussion of counter-hegemonic social movements:

> By contesting the discourses of capital, patriarchy, industrialism, racism and colonialism, and heterosexism, movements destabilize the identities of compliant worker, subservient wife, or closeted queer and create new ways of thinking about ourselves and the world around us.

The political identities of different activists are constituted in part through their subjection and resistance to heterosexual rule. These experiences affect the possibilities, in place, for organised challenges to the heterosexual regime. In suppressing the ideas, experiences and practices of those females who have self-consciously transgressed the boundaries of the heterosexual regime, who have most clearly challenged the 'doing' of gender (Butler 1990), mainstream feminism loses critical insights into the possibilities of undoing the system of gender (and the system of men's violence which is endemic to it). In the following sections I introduce local activists who were centrally involved in organised feminist anti-violence activism in Hamilton in the early 1990s, focusing on factors involved in the development, performance and regulation of their individual and collective political identities.

The importance of space: performing sex

What processes are involved in forcing us to take that crucial step out of our place in the world, to have a sense that it is not in fact immutable, nor is the 'natural' sex upon which it is supposedly based? Local activists pointed to the importance of particular spaces of resistance for the development of political identities, articulating the notion that identities are developed in and through space. This activist is worth quoting at length on the process of developing her lesbian and feminist identities:

> I can remember sitting on the floor at OISE [Ontario Institute for Studies in Education], at the break, not even at the conference, but at the break and all these women coming round and eating fruit and tofu and all that crap and yak yak yak, yak, and just sitting there and feeling like I was in a little oasis, and being aware that I'd never felt like this in my life. I'd never known such contentment. I couldn't even figure out what it was, just smiling a lot. I was so happy, you know. And everywhere I turned there were new things to learn, it was like, holy shit! It's a wonder my brain didn't get overloaded, I mean, I read everything. I listened to women's music, I'm sure I must have driven my friends nuts, it was all I listened to, all I talked about were women's issues . . . and then of course, it went from there to suddenly 'they are having a Take Back The Night march, do you want to go?' and me saying, 'what's that?' Imagine saying 'what's that'? Imagine not knowing!! [laughing]. So I said, 'oh that sounds like fun' . . . and off we go and it was like wow! This was Toronto, a thousand women on the street. There they are, standing up at a microphone, actually saying they're lesbians, and actually saying they're prostitutes and I'm thinking, holy shit! . . . Well then we just kept going to conferences and I don't know what happened but I just kept listening to all these things and looking at all these women and thinking 'wow, thank goodness, I have finally found where I belong. This is my place.'
>
> (Activist 23)[11]

The important spaces in and through which identities are developed include lesbian and feminist conferences, demonstrations, music and books. As one activist described her feminist politics, 'I caught it like a cold, this had to happen' (activist 8). Politics, however, has to be around to catch. In communities where there are no sexual assault centres, no women's centres, no lesbian organisations, or where these spaces have been so thoroughly incorporated as to be no different from more traditional social service organisations, there are fewer opportunities for the development of counter-hegemonic identities (and movements). Sites in Hamilton, such as the Sexual Assault Centre, Interval House (a women's shelter) and the Women's Centre have historically (and at different times, more or less so) played an important role in presenting these opportunities. These activists pointed to the importance of local spaces:

> When I came back to Hamilton I went around town looking for a women's organization . . . I went everywhere except the Sexual Assault Centre and everyone kept telling me to go there, right? 'That's where you go', 'You go talk to —— '. I thought, oh my god, this is like, unanimous, everywhere I go. So, I went.
>
> (Activist 15)

> To me, the only places in Hamilton to be in the women's movement was to be at the Sexual Assault Centre, or the Women's Centre.
>
> (Activist 13)

> I slowly decided that I wanted to become involved with some more radical politics and had heard that the Hamilton Rape Crisis Centre was an organization of women who were primarily lesbian radical feminists, and I found that really appealing. So I made contact with the women in Hamilton.
>
> (Activist 11)

More transient spaces of resistance are also created, outside of these more formalised sites; for example, in the development of local, independent activist groups such as the Justice For Women Coalition (discussed below), or in demonstrations such as Take Back The Night and the Montreal Memorial,[12] or through the repeated inscription of public spaces. In Hamilton in the early 1990s a downtown courthouse became the site of multiple demonstrations protesting violence against women (and the justice system's treatment of it). Activists effectively reinscribed that very public space from one of 'justice' to one of injustice. In explaining why the 1992 Take Back The Night rally was being held in front of that courthouse instead of in its traditional site in front of city hall, a committee spokeswoman stated, 'This is the place women go for justice, but they don't get any' (Todd 1992: B1).

Local activists also pointed to the importance of their interaction with other politicised subjects, for the development of their own identities; for example, these women argued:

> Look at the movement in terms of the second wave of feminism and the anti-violence against women movement, the establishment of shelters and rape crisis centres. There was a lot of consciousness-raising that preceded the establishment of those groups and I think that a lot of women who would identify themselves as political lesbians came out at a time when women were deconstructing the whole notion of sexuality.
>
> (Activist 11)

> If I think of myself personally, in some ways identifying as a lesbian was a natural outcome of that work. In some ways if you do that work for a long time, I don't know how you can stay involved with men. So that's part of it, I think. You just more and more see the limitations of having men be involved in your life in any central way. A number of lesbian women arrive at it [that identity] through the work.
>
> (Activist 19)

These comments point to the fact that it is not only the existence of spaces of resistance that is important in the development of counter-hegemonic identities, but also who is and is not involved in those spaces. The process of identity formation involves our interaction with others, and, as Adrienne Rich and other lesbian theorists have illustrated, this point is not lost on those who have power. Women are kept from knowing that lesbians exist or that lesbian existence is in fact a viable alternative to a regulatory heterosexuality.

The regulation of certain gendered and sexed identities in more formalised sites of resistance has increased over the years. The outlawing or demonisation of certain performances as, for example, 'lesbian', 'anti-male', 'angry', 'anti-police' and 'political' helps to regulate the kinds of activities which take place in and through these spaces of resistance. In the case of Hamilton, the naming and/or criticisms of particular local feminists and/or organisations as anti-men, anti-police and having a lesbian bias, reached a wide audience through being played out in the local media. The concrete consequences of UnWomanly acts, such as organisational reviews, threatened loss of funding, loss of employment, and public vilification, all send a message to other women's organisations and individual activists.

Below, I discuss several of the local events in Hamilton which most clearly illustrate the performance and regulation of sexed and gendered identities[13] in place.

Regulating identity: local struggles

Two of the most critical events[14] with respect to local activists' experiences of and interactions with 'justice' in the city of Hamilton in the early 1990s, concerned the police and the legal system's treatment of two violent men. The first was Guy Ellul who was acquitted (based on self-defence) by a jury of a charge of first-degree murder in the death of his estranged wife Debra. Ellul had stabbed Debra twenty-one times and left her to be found dead the following morning by her mother, Ruth Williams. A group made up of representatives from various women's groups was quickly formed to meet with the provincial Attorney-General to express their outrage and demand an appeal. Problems arose almost immediately over gendered identities and UnWomanly activism. This founding member noted:

> We got together initially as a group of social service agencies who were quite horrified at the acquittal . . . we began meeting with Howard Hampton [Attorney-General] and some of the members of that coalition felt that we were becoming too radical, or that they couldn't speak on behalf of their agencies so they had to withdraw.[15]

Out of that group an important local activist organisation was developed: the Justice For Women Coalition. A radical direct action and advocacy group with an individually based membership of women's advocates and survivors, it stated its purpose as:

> We are working to stop violence against women. This includes male violence against women, lesbian battering, rape etc. Violence happens whenever a person, group, institution or culture uses its power to control another person, group, institution or culture with lesser power.[16]

Over the next several years, the coalition was extremely vocal in its criticism of the legal and police systems. Both the group and individual members of it consistently engaged in UnWomanly activism, articulating a radical political identity which contested gender at every turn. Being an unaligned group without any kind of funding or ties to the state, the group placed itself relatively beyond the reaches of regulation (although individual members were reached through other sites, especially their workplaces). Justice For Women and Ruth Williams did not receive justice, however, in spite of years of letter-writing, petitions, demonstrations and actions, locally, provincially and nationally (Casella 1992; Davy 1992; Deverell 1992; Prokaska 1993a and 1993b).

The second case was that of Larry Fodor. Early in December 1991, Justice For Women was continuing its high profile with a four-part forum, 'Women Rights – Men's Responsibilities', which brought together shelter and other social service workers, abused women and other interested persons from across the province to discuss the contentious issue[17] of men's counselling groups. The forum, however, was overshadowed by events sparked by an investigative report by the city's newspaper, *The Hamilton Spectator*, on the Hamilton–Wentworth Police Department's treatment of an officer with a history of woman abuse (Holt 1991). Despite having broken his second wife's nose in a recent assault, Constable Larry Fodor had been able to plead guilty to a charge of common assault and receive counselling, probation and a suspended sentence. The article quoted the Chief of Police as saying, 'I have no qualms about putting him back on the street', and, using an analogy, 'Who better to send to talk to an alcoholic than another alcoholic?' (Holt 1991: A1). With support and representation from a multitude of local women's organisations, Justice For Women held a press conference and called for a review of the police department, criticising its and the court's handling of the case.

The Hamilton Spectator gave extensive coverage to the press conference the following day as well as publishing a photograph of a United Empire Loyalists statue in front of the county courthouse downtown, newly sprayed with graffiti. A workman could be seen removing the slogans 'Justice For Women Now!' and 'Police Protect Their Own!'

Over the next two days, the executive director of Hamilton's Sexual Assault Centre and a counsellor in the Family Violence Program of Family Services of Hamilton–Wentworth were arrested, charged with public mischief of under $1,000, and released in connection with the graffiti. Both were members of Justice For Women and the coalition subsequently organised several rallies in support of the charged women. One of them asked, 'How is it that police will act so quickly to charge someone with such a minor crime yet we are hearing from abused women that they can't get the police to come to their houses?'[18] And despite many years of involvement in community activism, paying for the cost of the clean-up, and having no prior criminal record, the women were found guilty as charged and ordered to pay a fine of $500 each or spend thirty days in jail (Lefaive 1992). Justice For Women was quick to highlight the disparity between the treatment of the spray-painters and abusive men. Outside the courthouse, a spokeswoman noted, 'The most common punishment for wife assault in this community is either a conditional discharge or a fine of $300' (Lefaive 1992: B1).

Both these local and non-local experiences of subjection to the state are important in understanding the development and regulation of activists' identities. Since political identities are developed, regulated and negotiated in and through space, a multitude of factors affects these processes in place, including experiences of local relations of power, regulation, contestation, and our interpretations and analyses of these. The Guy Ellul case had been regarded in the women's community as an 'open and shut case'. However, in court the defence portrayed Debra as a 'slut', and as a 'bad wife', calling on a local policeman to confirm this opinion. Ellul's behaviour prior to the murder was outlined in court; it included calling his estranged wife up to ten times a day and driving past her house. In his charge to the jury, however, Judge Walter Stayshyn asked:

> Does it [Ellul's behaviour] show a vindictive man or does it show one concerned with his children and wishing to have the wife and mother home with the children? I think it is clear that he was a loving and concerned father.
> (Davy 1994: D1)

The message taken from this case was that in Hamilton, abusive men were literally getting away with murder[19] and feminist activists were being punished, excessively, for acts of civil disobedience. Defying the sanctions against UnWomanly praxis, Justice For Women none the less continued to articulate its radical political identity. And late in 1992 regulation of particular identities was stepped up.

Two different women's organisations (one shelter, one sexual assault centre) ran employment ads a few months apart; both ads included 'lesbian' as one of the designated categories from which they especially wanted applications (a fairly standard employment equity statement in progressive organisations). Controversy erupted in both cases involving local councillors, media and community organisations. In the first case, members of Hamilton Rotary Clubs[20] threatened to withdraw a pledge for $500,000 (for a new twenty-bed shelter) and were quickly joined by regional councillors in demanding an explanation for the inclusion of the category 'lesbian'. A quick apology from the executive director and a promise that future ads would use the less controversial 'we are an equal opportunity employer' ensured that the organisation and the $500,000 pledge survived the controversy (Longbottom 1992; Tait 1992).

In the second case, Hamilton's Sexual Assault Centre would neither apologise nor back down. The debate about the legitimacy and intent of including 'lesbian' in the list of categories dragged on for several months before, under related accusations of being 'anti-men' and 'anti-police', the organisation asked its funders for an operational review.

Conclusions: the price of marginalisation

In this chapter I have provided a taste of local struggles over sites of resistance and what takes place in them. I have concentrated on a few of the processes which have worked to domesticate and de-radicalise UnWomanly praxis. Radical activists who most clearly unsettle the limits of Women's place(s) in this society, and/or their practices and ideas have been marginalised as 'the movement' has sought (and been forced) to become 'legitimate'. 'Lesbian' and 'anti-men', locations beyond the limits of the category Woman, have been effectively used in the regulation of particular sexed and gendered performances.

The processes which worked locally to contain anti-violence activism can be understood as being, in part, punitive consequences of activists not 'doing gender right', individually, collectively, and/or institutionally. In allowing rather than resisting the power of the term 'lesbian' and/or the term 'Woman' to regulate what will be accepted as legitimate action within shelters and rape crisis centres, anti-violence activists help to reproduce rather than contest the political regime of heterosexuality. That is, in not challenging the regulatory power of the fiction of gender (Butler 1990), we make it possible for these terms to continue to be used against females (and organisations) who transgress the limits of Woman's place(s) in society. The organisation which apologised for the 'lesbian ad' essentially agreed that women's shelters were in fact no place for the performance of trans-gressive female identities. The popular criticisms which were laid at the organisation which would not apologise – that it was too lesbian, too anti-men, too anti-police, too political – confirmed this view.

In Hamilton during a relatively short period, collective and institutional transgression of the boundaries of the category Woman were multiple, frequent and public, and more females were radicalised in the process. Local activists' identities were, in part, constituted through their experiences of local justice. The subsequent discipline and punishment (and the lack of sustained, organised resistance of any depth) partially depoliticised the community and this has reduced the possibilities for political development in place.

Effective regulation was certainly made easier because of the funding factor – funding bodies were able to exert considerable control over what identities could be performed in those sites. However, other regulatory bodies, social service agencies and 'the public' were also able to exert control by blurring the distinction between various sites of resistance. That is, although Justice For Women was a harbour from the storm for the performance of clearly counter-hegemonic identities, individual members could still be demonised in and through other sites. The women found that despite being performed outside more clearly regulated sites of resistance (most obviously their workplaces) their activities were regulated by control exerted in and through these.

What this raises then is the question of alternative sites of resistance which will have the ability to be spaces of regeneration for collective political action on this issue. As shelters and sexual assault centres become further institutionalised and their very existence comes into question (with the spread of neo-conservatism in Canada), what goes on in these becomes almost a moot point. What new sites will provide us with the all-critical collective space we need?

Notes

1 A defining moment in this developing discourse was 6 December 1989. At L'Ecole Polytechnique in Montreal, a heavily armed man targeted and murdered fourteen women (after shouting that he hated feminists). Most women in Canada remember where they were and what they were doing when they first heard about it.

2 Although the distinction between the two is not always clear (or even present) I make a distinction here to indicate that neither are the two always inter-changeable. For example, feminist analysts in academia are not always activists, although this depends on one's definition of activism.

3 Where shelters and rape crisis centres once rose up in opposition to traditional (and unsatisfactory) social services, many are now working in conjunction with them, as well as recruiting the same sorts of 'professionals'.

4 I am using this term rather than heterosexism and/or heterosexuality, and am using it after radical lesbians such as Monique Wittig and Louise Turcotte. It is used interchangeably with the political regime of heterosexuality throughout the chapter.

5 Take Back The Night marches and demonstrations take place annually in towns and cities across North America to protest against violence towards women and girls.

6 The research is based on local anti-violence struggles, my own involvement in those, and interviews with twenty-five 'white feminist anti-violence activists'. I wanted to critically explore this infrequently problematised group and investi-gate some of the differences found *within* categories. See Grant 1996 for a fuller discussion of these.

7 Steel City, as Hamilton is popularly known, is a municipality of over 300,000 which sits at the western edge of Lake Ontario, in the heart of southern Ontario's industrial region. It is also in the shadow of Toronto, located about 70 kilometres around the lake (Statistics Canada 1992).

8 For a more detailed discussion of this issue, see Grant 1996 and Timmins 1995.

9 This is discussed in detail in Grant 1996; many of these writers do of course recognise that state funding, for an example, was a 'necessary evil'. The history of feminism in relation to the state in Canada is an interesting one (see Wine and Ristock 1991).

10 The move towards professionalisation is complicated. Whilst for sexual assault centres and shelters, making sure that books are in order and that there are clear policies and procedures in place are good moves, the increasing distinction between 'provider' and 'user' and the increasing division of labour amongst workers (as, for example, administrators, executive directors and counsellors) are not.

11 Activists were numbered quite simply, that is, in the order of being interviewed. Although the lack of detail is problematic, the size of the 'community' made it impossible to use more satisfying descriptions such as 'shelter worker, lesbian, mid-40s'. The interviews were conducted during a very difficult time in Hamilton and the activists had been assured of confidentiality.

12 A memorial is held annually in Hamilton (and other towns and cities across the country) to remember the fourteen women massacred in Montreal on 6 December 1989, and to protest against violence against women.

13 This is discussed at length in Grant 1996: Chapter 4.

14 Many other critical issues and events, including counselling groups for abusive men and racism in women's organisations, are discussed in Grant 1996.

15 Interview with Vilma Rossi, 25 March 1993.

16 Justice for Women Coalition, information sheet (n.d.).

17 Contentious since many feminist activists and survivors argued publicly that men were being ordered into counselling groups in lieu of being incarcerated despite the fact that there was evidence of counselling groups being ineffective. Further it was argued that the groups were dangerous in that men involved in them were learning more sophisticated forms of abuse, and women were being put in danger with the false hope that counselling would ensure that their partners would change their ways.

18 The executive director of the Sexual Assault Centre quoted in *The Hamilton Spectator*, 5 December 1991.

19 As part of the Justice For Debra campaign, Justice For Women wrote to several current affairs programmes across Canada suggesting a storyline for their programmes, 'abusive men are literally getting away with murder'.

20 Local branches of Rotary International, a charitable society of 'businessmen'.

II

TAKING ANOTHER LOOK: SPACES

De La Warr Pavilion, Bexhill-on-Sea, Sussex:
Rosa Ainley

Architecture and design have been used as means to exert control, across lines of class, race, gender and nation, in a myriad of ways: the imposition of physical barriers; limiting access to public, shared spaces and facilities; restrictive and inappropriate models of housing organisation; even down to the right to change colour schemes. Restricting access to space has been, as Dolores Hayden says, 'one of the consistent ways to limit the economic and political rights of groups' (Hayden 1995: 22).

Clearly, the layout of cities, buildings, spaces in between, their services and how these things interrelate and function are factors that have immense impact on the quality of their citizens' lives. A chaotically woven set of assumptions is made about how society operates, who does what and who goes where. From the 'homes for heroes' postwar housing design based around the stringent gender-role stereotyping of woman as housewife and man as full-time wage earner, to recent examples such as the spate of car breakdown adverts that rely heavily on identification by women viewers who fear attack, the built environment has reflected received wisdom about gender roles.

Jacqueline Leavitt, Teresa Lingafelter and Claudia Morello's chapter gives visual and written documentation of a photographic project in LA. Children of colour from 7 to 13 years old living in public housing photographed their own neighbourhood – an environment often ignored or stereotyped – using disposable cameras. The results document their worlds and their resistance to the limits of their space, and offer a reinterpretation of stereotypes of public housing tenants.

'Having it all?' by Inga-Lisa Sangregorio offers a discussion about the design and actual negotiation of shared space in a Swedish housing initiative where residents have private apartments, share common space and equipment, and collaborate in various decisions about their housing. This piece provides a different (reclaimed?) view on 'multi-unit housing': domestic labour and spatial design, the possibilities of sharing and a reassessment of the separations of public/social, private/family.

Writing of a time when 'public woman' was a euphemism for prostitute, Lynne Walker escorts the reader on a tour of the West End of London in the late nineteenth century, in a consideration of the reworking of the private domain for more public uses. 'Home and away' is an A–Z of the use of domestic space for political organisation amongst middle-class feminists in Victorian London.

Rosa Ainley's piece on surveillance and representation combines a consideration of the panoptic structure – built or not – and more contemporary methods, both technological and 'architectural', with an examination of related photographic and filmic portrayals. As technology becomes a part of the spaces we move within, can we inhibit the assumptions that these developments are based upon, and subvert or even find enjoyment in what has been termed the carceral city?

5

Home and away

The feminist remapping of public and private space in Victorian London

Lynne Walker

The West End of Victorian London is normally understood as the centre of the world of work and of institutions of power, 'the masculine domain of modern, public, urban life' (Tickner 1987: 14) from which women were excluded.[1] But viewed in another way through the experience of the independent middle-class women who lived and worked there, this highly masculinised terrain can be remapped as a site of women's buildings and places within the urban centre, associated with the social networks, alliances and organisations of the nineteenth-century Women's Movement. This focus on a single strand is not intended to overshadow other readings of the sexed city, but adds another layer to the meanings of its diverse gendered spaces and their occupants.

Between 1850 and 1900, members of Victorian women's groups and circles experienced and reconceived 'London's heavily patriarchal public and private spheres' in new ways which offered women opportunities for 'control over their social actions and identity' (Borden *et al.* 1996: 12). Normally, the identity of Victorian women was closely bound up in the home and their removal from public life. The so-called 'ideal divide' (Pollock 1988: 68) which separated the legitimate spheres of men and women was deeply drawn between the public (masculine) world of remuneration, work and recognition and the private (feminine) domestic realm of home and family responsibilities which were undertaken for love rather than money. Ideologically, the stakes were high; social stability, the good order of society, and even human happiness were perceived to be dependent on woman's presence in the home.[2]

At mid-century, middle-class woman's place in the home distinguished respectable femininity in opposition to the prostitute, the fallen woman of the streets, whom Mayhew called the 'public woman' (Mayhew 1861: 218). But partly in response to changing connotations of public in relation to woman and partly constitutive of new definitions of public and woman, independent middle-class women in London were able to take up public roles without losing respectability and at the same time change the nature of home and domesticity to include their work. Leaders of the Women's Movement, such as Barbara Leigh Smith Bodichon, Dr Elizabeth Garrett

Anderson, Emily Davies, Emily Faithfull and Millicent Fawcett, who lived in London, were able to build identities as respectable public women with roles and activities linked to the public realm. Working from home or in premises nearby, philanthropists, reformers and professionals used their London homes as political bases from which to address the wider world of public affairs.

This juxtaposition of home and work made the home a political space in which social initiatives germinated and developed. As we shall see, feminists, such as Emmeline Pankhurst and Barbara Bodichon, adapted their family homes for meetings and other events associated with women's rights, while the offices of related projects for women's organisations, clubs and restaurants were located within walking distance of their homes in Marylebone and Bloomsbury. This 'neighbourliness', on the one hand, was the social glue of the Women's Movement in central London and, on the other, it generated sites for political activities as well as providing easy access to the public realm on their doorstep. The apparatus of their 'staged identities'[3] as white, middle-class, British women: the well-ordered home, the 'good' address at the heart of London and of the empire, the round of formal introductions, social calls and duties, as well as a sense of neighbourly connection for those who lived nearby, provided the private, social matrix for public, political action. In addition the presence and propinquity in the city of feminist activists, such as Dr Elizabeth Garrett Anderson, Barbara Bodichon and Emily Davies in Marylebone and Emily Faithfull, Rhoda Garrett and Millicent Fawcett in Bloomsbury facilitated building projects which developed from feminist concerns for women's education, employment, health and financial and personal independence. These independent middle-class women were well placed to cross and redraw the boundaries between public and private. As this chapter will explore, they devised tactics based on necessity and opportunity: working from home, gaining access to the professions, providing accommodation for their own needs (most notably in housing, health and women's clubs and organisations) and appropriating space for women on the less familiar ground of public institutions.

In the late nineteenth-century city, the implication of the intersection of gender, space and experience for these independent middle-class women was that control, or at least a sense of control, of social actions and identity was produced. The positions that they took up remained deeply contested and within certain boundaries, but opportunities for developing new identities which differed from the social norm were offered at various sites in the city, both public and private. Related to these concerns, I want to suggest not only that their groups and networks were critical to the successful struggle for women's rights, but that their socially lived identities were partly defined by the spaces they occupied – and that in turn their presence produced the social spaces and buildings which they occupied: a process which was cumulative and reflexive, taking place over time, producing, and being produced by and within, dynamic, gendered space. In this sense, late Victorian women were producers as well as consumers of the built environment, whose presence helped determine the spaces that were provided, the building types constructed, the needs represented and, most importantly, how it felt to be in public space: the ideas people received about themselves and the representations they were able to make when using architecture and the public realm.

Working from home

An important tactic that women adopted to negotiate a public presence was to work from home. In her many campaigns and projects, the artist and feminist Barbara Leigh Smith Bodichon operated from her house in Marylebone, which in the early years of the organised Women's Movement provided a meeting place for the group that petitioned in support of the Married Women's Property Bill in 1855 (Gandy *et al.* 1991: 3). From there, the first petition for female suffrage was assembled and dispatched to John Stuart Mill at the Houses of Parliament. It was delivered by Emily Davies and Elizabeth Garrett (Anderson) who had been recruited into the Women's Movement over tea at No. 5, Blandford Square (Manton 1987: 48).

Later, Emily Davies and Barbara Bodichon worked successfully for women's admission to university examinations and together produced one of the central achievements of nineteenth-century education, Girton College, Cambridge, which opened in 1873. For this venture, Bodichon's house was again called into action as an examination hall for the first candidates and later functioned as a place of entertainment and moral support for Girton students (Gandy *et al.* 1991: 5). Personally, Elizabeth Garrett (Anderson) gained support, introductions and encouragement at Bodichon's house for a career in medicine, which she achieved, becoming England's first female physician. After qualifying, she followed a similar pattern to Bodichon, setting up both her home and place of work over the years on various sites in the West End.

After their first meeting, Barbara Bodichon sent Emily Davies and Elizabeth Garrett (Anderson) round to the *English Woman's Journal*, the voice and centre of the Women's Movement, which then had an office in Prince's Street, Cavendish Square. Bodichon funded the journal and was a founder member of the Langham Place group, as the network of women who wrote for the journal and were associated with its related projects were known (after its most famous site). In three different locations in the Oxford Street area (Prince's Street, Langham Place and Berners Street) and in various combinations, a loose alliance of associated groups was accommodated with the *English Woman's Journal* (later the *English-woman's Review*), including the Society for Promoting the Employment of Women (SPEW), the Ladies Sanitary Association, the National Association for the Promotion of Social Science, and the Ladies' Institute.[4] That these organisations drew on the identity of the journal, and each other, as well as the advantages of a central site and the pull of a familiar place, is demonstrated by the way they either stayed with the journal over the years or spun off into nearby streets.

Like education and property rights, employment for women was a major theme of the movement which the Society for Promoting the Employment of Women approached by taking practical steps to help women gain marketable skills and find jobs. Like the National Association for the Promotion of Social Science, SPEW helped establish new work for women, such as the Ladies Tracing Society (established 1875), which provided training and employment for women to copy architectural plans from an office in Westminster (*Englishwoman's Review* 1876: 223).

Members of the Langham Place group collaborated on projects that were motivated by feminist politics, philanthropy and business necessity, and these mutually beneficial activities were developed and facilitated by the proximity of home and work. A resident of Bloomsbury (No. 10, Taviton Street), the printer and philanthropist Emily Faithfull served on the women's employment committee of the National Association for the Promotion of Social Science and established the Victoria Press in Bloomsbury (Great Coram Street), with the feminist and SPEW member Bessie Rayner Parkes, who edited the *English Woman's Journal*, which the Victoria Press published (Bloomfield 1993: 220).

Unlike Emily Faithfull who operated professionally on a number of sites a short walk from home, Emmeline Pankhurst, on moving to London in the 1880s, initially made arrangements similar to those of generations of women: putting home, work and family together by living over the shop. After three years selling arts and crafts products in the Hampstead Road, in the 1880s (Pankhurst 1979: 13), Emmeline Pankhurst and her family moved to Russell Square (No. 8, demolished, now the Russell Hotel). There, she again ellided public and private space but this time to political ends, adapting her house for meetings of the Women's Franchise League (an organisation which contrary to its title addressed a variety of social and political problems and was coeducational in its membership). In Russell Square, Mrs Pankhurst gave birth to her fifth child, directed the upbringing of two other leaders of the Edwardian suffrage movement (daughters Christabel and Sylvia Pankhurst) and received a stream of highly politicised visitors, 'Socialists, Anarchists, Radicals, Republicans, Nationalists, suffragists, free thinkers, agnostics, atheists and humanitarians of all kinds' from Louise Michel (La Petroleuse) to William Morris (Pankhurst 1979: 15).

A stone's throw from the Pankhursts' was No. 61, Russell Square (now the Imperial Hotel), the home (1881–91) of Mary Ward, the writer and philanthropist who founded and built the Passmore Edwards Settlement in nearby Tavistock Place. A great believer in higher education and a member of the council of Somerville Hall, Oxford's first college for women, from its opening in 1879, she nevertheless later became an active anti-suffrage campaigner and suffragists' bugbear (Sutherland n.d.).

Like her neighbour, Mrs Pankhurst, Mary Ward worked from home.

From a small study, she produced her best-selling book *Robert Elsmere* (1889), about a clergyman who refound his lost faith through social work with the London poor. This successful novel signalled the building of the Mary Ward settlement house, a local project which combined religious belief, philanthropy and public service. By 1914, there were two dozen settlement houses in London where middle-class young men lived and worked to help the poor. At the heart of the settlement movement was the idea that the bringing together of the classes would address the perceived social crisis in the cities and ultimately regenerate the nation. Having imbibed the settlement idea at Oxford, and following Keble College's Oxford House and Toynbee Hall in the East End, Mary Ward established her settlement house, after two earlier false starts also in Bloomsbury. A powerful committee, which included the feminists Frances Power Cobbe, a member of the Langham Place circle, and Beatrice Potter (Webb), helped to found the Mary Ward settlement. This provided new accommodation for an ambitious social programme to meet the needs of the local working-class community and provide living quarters for the young idealistic middle-class residents who had come to share their lives in a way which would, they believed, heal class divisions and create a better urban environment for all (Forty 1989: 28).

Access to the professions

The struggle for access to the professions for training and membership by women can be (re)mapped in the streets and buildings of the West End. University College London, the Architectural Association, Middlesex Hospital, the Royal Institute of British Architects and the University of London were all located in the West End of London and during the period in question were among the institutions that blocked or resisted women's medical or architectural education – and eventually responded to pressure from women to open their doors.

Among the many women seeking a route into professional training and practice were the cousins Agnes and Rhoda Garrett, who pioneered interior design from their studio/home in Gower Street (No. 2), Bloomsbury. The Garretts were members of the famous family which included Agnes's sisters, Dr Elizabeth Garrett Anderson and Millicent Garrett Fawcett, leaders of the nineteenth-century Women's Movement, and both clients of the design firm. For Agnes and Rhoda Garrett, like many women in 'the arena of high culture' (Cherry 1995: 49), design and the campaign for women's rights were a joint project. Their agenda included the entry of women into the professions, as well as full suffrage and the repeal of the Contagious Diseases Act. Rhoda Garrett published *The Electoral Disabilities of Women*, and according to Ray Strachey, was an effective, impressive speaker on behalf of women's rights (Strachey 1927: 12). At the same time, their design book, *Suggestions on House Decoration in Painting, Woodwork and Furniture* (1876), one of many advice and information books written by women for women in the late nineteenth century, claimed a substantial role for interior designers, and for themselves, in the design process.

Accommodating women

Among feminist priorities in the last quarter of the nineteenth century was the provision of respectable accommodation for single middle-class women working in the city. Agnes Garrett and her sister Dr Elizabeth Garrett Anderson were directors of the Ladies Dwellings Company (LDC) which built the Chenies Street Chambers, around the corner from Agnes's house in Gower Street. Aimed at accommodating professional women at a moderate cost, Chenies Street Chambers (1889) and York Street Chambers in Marylebone (1891) were the most successful and architecturally ambitious schemes of their kind in central London, while other similar residential projects developed by the LDC flourished in the affluent inner suburbs of Kensington, Chelsea and Earl's Court (*Queen* 1890: 507).

In Chenies Street, co-operative principles applied in which individual households retained their privacy but combined to pay the costs and share mutual facilities for cleaning, cooking and laundry. Individual flats were of two, three or four rooms, and although meals could be taken communally in the basement dining-room, accommodation was self-contained with either scullery or kitchen, and w.c., larder, cupboard, coal bunker and dust shoot. R. W. Hitchen's system of silicate cotton and plaster slabs was employed for sound-deadening and fireproofing. Rents were from ten to twenty-five shillings per week with ten shillings for dining-room and caretaker charges (*Builder* 1889: 332).

These arrangements suited such residents as Olive Schreiner, the South African feminist who wrote *The Story of an African Farm* and *Woman and Labour* and who lived in Chenies Street in 1899 (Davin 1978: 8[5]) and Ethel and Bessie Charles, the first women members of the Royal Institute of British Architects (RIBA), who ran their architectural practice from the York Street flats.

Feminist networks extended to male allies, such as the architect of Chenies Street Chambers, J. M. Brydon, who trained Agnes and Rhoda Garrett and supported Ethel and Bessie Charles for membership in the RIBA (Charles 1898). While the access of middle-class women to design was restricted, their participation was welcomed in the role of client and patron, which empowered many women in the public sphere. Through Dr Anderson, Brydon was employed again for two other important women's buildings: the Hospital for Women (opened 1890) in Euston Road, and the London School of Medicine for Women (opened 1898), in Hunter Street near Brunswick Square. These women also relied on networks of kinship and patronage. Commissions for interiors and furnishings were forthcoming from Agnes's sister and Rhoda's cousin Millicent Garrett Fawcett in Cambridge and in London, and from Dr Anderson for her own mansion flat in Upper Berkeley Street, and furniture was designed for their Beale cousins' new country house, Standen in Sussex. It was the intervention of Florence Nightingale, Barbara Bodichon's cousin, that ensured the funding and completion of Dr Anderson's hospital in the Euston Road (Manton 1987: 286). While as late as the 1920s the architect Ethel Charles was designing a decorative scheme for her soldier brother at Camberley.[6]

An effective practitioner of doorstep philanthropy and one of the key members of the campaign for a Married Woman's Property Act which sought to secure property rights for middle-class women was Octavia Hill. Unlike the comfortable backgrounds of many feminists, she had known financial insecurity personally and experienced first-hand the dire living conditions of the poor in the homes of toyworkers whom she had taught when earning her own living. Although her philanthropic schemes extended throughout London and her principles of housing management were widely influential, Octavia Hill's first experiment in architectural and social reform was undertaken about a hundred yards from her own house in Nottingham Place (No. 14), Marylebone, at the inappropriately named Paradise Place (Darley 1990: 91). By the early 1870s, her most ambitious programme to date was only a short walk away in St Christopher's Place, off Oxford Street, and involved the refurbishment and partial rebuilding of Barrett's Court, which was purchased with subventions from Lady Ducie and from Mrs Stopford Brooke (Darley 1990: 132).

Women's clubland in Mayfair

Women's place in the public sphere was supported and encouraged by clubs for women which became a prominent feature of the West End in the second half of the nineteenth century. Access to the city gave feminists a base from which to promote their agenda, while the poor provision of facilities directed their concerns to meeting women's basic needs. The Ladies' Institute was one of the first nineteenth-century clubs where women could eat, read and meet their friends when away from home.[7] Nevertheless, even in the early clubs, class lines were rarely crossed when it came to membership or location. Some clubs, such as the New Somerville, the Victoria and the Tea & Shopping, were located in Oxford Street and Regent Street, but in the main, women's clubs clustered off the main thoroughfares in the Mayfair streets associated with aristocratic shopping and elegant eighteenth-century mansions.[8]

Around 1900, the highest concentration of clubs was in Dover Street and its continuation, Grafton Street, the Pall Mall of women's clubland. As Erica Rappaport has pointed out, the trend was from earlier, consciously feminist, political clubs to later, more social, apolitical ones. The idea of private clubs for women was developed by female entrepreneurs, feminists and philanthropists, and more popularly at the beginning of the twentieth century, by the department stores, most notably, Debenham & Freebody, Harrod's, Selfridge's and Whiteley's. The feminist innovation of the Ladies'

Institute and its latter-day incarnation the Berners Club and, most prominently, the Pioneer Club were, however, models for dozens of clubs which were set up for middle- and upper-class women who were away from home working, shopping or enjoying other urban pleasures (Rappaport 1993: 170–98)

Located on various Mayfair sites over the years, the most long-lived of all the women's clubs is the University Club for Ladies (today the University Women's Club) with a membership profile in 1898 of 'graduates, undergraduates, students, fee lecturers, and medical practitioners' (*Queen* 1898). In addition to supplying facilities to meet the needs of women in the city, feminist clubs provided within the public sphere a private space which produced public women. Their identity was formed through shared social interactions in a supportive and stimulating network, and forged in debate and discussion on a wide range of subjects. At the feminist Pioneer Club, a public identity was negotiated across gender and class lines which drew on the status and respectability of their location in a grand townhouse in aristocratic Mayfair and on representations of femininity in architecture, design and fashion. The decorative language of the 'Queen Anne' style which was employed at the Pioneer Club was perceived as most appropriate for the modern independent woman and for her femininity. The decorated interiors and their generous spaces were considered by contemporary observers to be elegant, refined and suitably domestic for their female occupants. At the same time, other signifiers of class and rank, such as oriental carpets and old oak furniture, found in the houses of the rich in the West End, were used or referenced by the club and were valuable for creating a respectable (classed) identity.[9] The deeply contested position that these feminists took up in the late nineteenth century and the protection the new boundaries provided is represented in the motto inscribed on the drawing room walls: 'They Say – What Say They? Let Them Say!' (see Figure 5/1). This inscription expressed feminist defiance within the Pioneer's fashionable, decorative interior, which smacked of modernity but negotiated their radical, outspoken sentiments and position through traditional signifiers of the dominant class.

Often modelled on the club's founder Mrs Massingberd (*Queen* 1898: 1081), the identity of a feminist public woman was also produced and reproduced at the Pioneer Club through dress codes, demeanour and bodily presentation (Beckett and Cherry n.d.: 3): short hair, upright posture, tailored frocks and badges (inscribed with their membership numbers). The use of nicknames and abstinence from alcohol were the norm.

Familiar ground

Retracing the sites and spaces of Victorian London, new meanings can be read from familiar buildings and greater texture can be given to a new social mapping of the city. At the British Museum, for example, women readers were a feature both of the old library and of the domed Reading Room

Figure 5.1 The Pioneer Club, Cork Street: *Queen*, December 1893

which opened in 1857.[10] Many were involved in systematic programmes of self-education or in professional research and writing, such as Eleanor Marx, who lived across from the museum, and Clementina Black who campaigned for equal pay and improved living conditions for working women and supported herself through her research and writing at the museum, while sharing a bedsit with her sister across Tottenham Court Road in Fitzroy Street (Davin 1978: 7, 10). Two rows of ladies-only seating were provided in the Reading Room until 1907, but were treated as unnecessary and were generally unoccupied (Barker and Jackson 1985: 302). In the museum itself, the expertise and authority of women guides were exercised and accepted by visitors who were taken around the exhibits by peripatetic lecturers.[11]

Space for women

The buildings and places, both public and private, which were the arena of women's groups and networks and the sites and spaces of lived female identities in London constitute a different mapping of the city. However, drawing out a single narrative strand from the larger urban fabric is problematic, highlighting women's presence and achievement and perhaps thereby blunting the critique of sexual difference which accounts for their absence. Certainly, the focus on one group of women (i.e. those associated with the Women's Movement) does eradicate, if only temporarily, the representation of the experience of numerous and divergent other urban women, also users and producers of the spaces of the West End: working-class women, many of whom also lived there and toiled in their thousands as servants in the great houses of the West End; street sellers and entertainers; barmaids and female drinkers; prostitutes and performers; middle-class proprietors of shops – more than forty women shop-owners were listed in Regent Street alone in 1891;[12] lower middle-class and working-class shop assistants in the burgeoning department stores of Oxford Street and Regent Street; many kinds of students and lesson takers and teachers, and thousands of consuming visitors, both foreign and domestic.[13] Sheer numbers, or at least critical mass, were important to women's identity and experience of the city, and to their impact on spatial definitions and material culture – however, in late nineteenth-century London, class divisions remained as sizeable as gender bonds.

Unlike the usual architectural history of London, which focuses on architects and their monumental buildings, retracing and remapping the sites and spaces of the nineteenth-century Women's Movement has prompted narratives of women's lives and experience, taking us into the domestic sphere, to the gendered spaces of Victorian architecture; to sites of long-demolished buildings associated with the suffrage movement, philanthropy and women's education, employment and entry into the professions; and to a variety of architectural and social projects devised by women clients and patrons.

Although using the home for political ends was not new – it was familiar from anti-slavery campaigns (Walker and Ware forthcoming) – the politi-cised home was a powerful political space for women. By eliding public and private spheres through the conjunction of home and work, these women created new social spaces which challenged the traditional division between the public male institutions and the private female place of home.

While the home became both centre and origin of women's organisations and networks, the activities of these nineteenth-century feminists were not, as we have seen, restricted to domestic space or identities. Public space, such as the offices of the *English Woman's Journal* and its associated organ-isations, was claimed and utilised to promote feminist goals and projects, which, by extension, normalised women's presence in the city. This presence and proximity of women in the city, combined with their privileged backgrounds and positions, helped secure access to the public sphere and facilitated women's participation in public life and the development of a public ideology for women.

Notes

1 For the purposes of this chapter, the boundaries are Regent's Park (N), Haymarket/Piccadilly (S), Marble Arch (W) and Holborn (E). Cf., for instance, P. J. Atkins, 'The spatial configuration of class solidarity in London's West End

1792–1939', *Urban History Yearbook 1990*, ed. R. Rodger, Leicester: Leicester University Press, pp. 36–65.

2 Davidoff and Hall (1987); and, for example, Davidoff *et al.* (1976).

3 Jane Beckett's phrase.

4 Street addresses in this chapter were derived from and/or checked in the volumes of *Kelly's Post Office Directory*, 1850–1900.

5 I am grateful to Jane Beckett who recommended this publication and to its author who generously shared her copy with me.

6 Deposited in the British Architectural Library Drawings Collection.

7 *London Illustrated News*, 28 January 1860, clipping in Westminster Archives. Set up by Bessie Parkes in Prince's Street, the Ladies' Institute moved with the journal to Langham Place where it expanded with the addition of a luncheon room.

8 For street addresses and dates, see Walker (1996), notes for an architectural walk organised by the Victorian Society.

9 Rappaport, for example, refers to *Young Woman* (1895: 302); *Queen* (December 1898: 1081).

10 Engraving by H. Melville after T. H. Sheperd, illus. in Barker and Jackson (1974: 303, Figs 7 and 6 respectively).

11 *Graphic* (1881), illustrated in Bolt (1932: 155).

12 *Kelly's Post Office Directory*, entry for Regent Street 1891. These included a chiropodist, a decorative artist, a photographer, a restaurant owner, numerous milliners, court dress and glovemakers and makers of stays and mantles, as well as agencies owned by women for governesses, schools and domestic staff.

13 See Nava and O'Shea (1996: 38–76); Wilson (1985 and 1991); and Walkowitz (1992), Rappaport (1993), Walker (1995) and Campbell Orr (Cherry 1995). For theoretical reorientation, Vickery (1993).

6

Through their eyes

Young girls look at their Los Angeles neighbourhood

Jacqueline Leavitt, Teresa Lingafelter and Claudia Morello

A traffic island between an on-ramp to a major freeway and a row of southbound traffic lanes seems an unlikely place to locate a children's after-school centre. For freeway drivers the centre, with its two-storey high mural of the Virgin of Guadalupe, signals arrival in and departure from the Flats section of Boyle Heights in East Los Angeles. To neighbourhood residents, the mural is a reminder of the alternative high school that was once here. Although youths of high-school age still come to the centre, it is a destination now primarily for younger children, the supervisor of the 4-H after-school programme and his assistants.

Mention 4-H in the USA and gender-stereotyped images spring to mind of girls baking pies and boys milking cows. Long after participants reach adulthood, they are likely to recall the emblem of a four-leaf clover and the motto which they committed to memory: 'I pledge my *head* to clearer thinking, my *heart* to greater loyalty, my *hands* to larger service, and my *health* to better living, for my club, my community, my country, and my world' (author's emphases). The 4-H programme began when turn-of-the-century progressive educators thought nature study should be introduced into agricultural education for boys and girls. Farmers' institutes and school superintendents sponsored contests and projects on soil, plants and production. Parents in rural areas volunteered as leaders in after-school 4-H clubs and received support from county extension agents affiliated to the Department of Agriculture and state land-grant universities that were built on federal land after 1862. Thus the clubs became part of the educational infrastructure that supported rural settlement. A turnabout in the 4-H focus was inevitable. The advent of industrialisation and urbanisation in the first half of the twentieth century as well as the later rise of agribusiness was accompanied by population decreases in the rural areas and increased immigration to metropolitan centres.

As the twenty-first century approaches, urban public schools suffer from insufficient financing and lack of general support. Children in poor households are less likely to find books, magazines and computers at home to compensate for fewer public resources. The overall results are low literacy rates, high numbers of high-school drop-outs, and the de-skilling of the future labour force, all of which further exacerbates the concentration of poverty. Under these circumstances some 4-H programmes have been established in urban areas. Los Angeles County's 4-H, administered by the University of California, has pioneered an after-school programme that is directed to youths who live in public housing developments throughout the county jurisdiction. Funds to support the programme are from the city of Los Angeles (LA), the city's housing authority, private foundations, individual gifts and the Union Oil Company of California (UNOCAL), the local corporate sponsor.[1]

About fifty children attend each 4-H centre in LA and participate in physical fitness, nutrition, gardening, plant science, computer time, arts and crafts and leadership development programmes. The centre serving the Flats area in Boyle Heights is as much a place for 7- to 13-year-olds to participate in programmes as it is one for them to form cliques, tease one another, do their homework, eat snacks, play games, carry out chores when they are too rambunctious, cry, pout, seek consolation, practise drill team moves, and dance at the St Valentine's Day party. Most of the children who attend live in Pico Gardens, the public (a.k.a. council[2]) housing development that lies across the street that becomes a freeway on-ramp. These children are from families whose income qualifies them for residency in one of the city's twenty-one federally subsidised public housing developments. The average household income for public housing residents is between $6,000 and $7,000 a year. Most of the chilren from Pico Gardens attend a neighbour-hood school where the test scores in basic skills in spring 1996 were abysmal. Fourth graders averaged three times lower than national averages in reading and learning, a third lower than the national average in mathematics and well below Los Angeles schools as a whole for reading and learning.

For about fourteen weeks our three-member team worked with children who attend the Pico Gardens 4-H centre, and who expressed interest in learning about cameras and taking photographs. The ones who participated received about an hour of instruction in using a disposable camera. Afterwards, their first tasks were to attach a label with their name on it to the camera and then ask someone to take their picture, ensuring that the first frame on each roll was a picture of themselves. The children were allowed to take the cameras home on three separate occasions, each time for a couple of days, and they were able to keep all their developed photos while we retained the negatives. All the children were excited about 'owning a camera' and all the cameras were returned, mostly on time and with the entire roll of film used.

A means of documentation and representation

The use of visual techniques is one way to document an environment that is frequently stereotyped or ignored (Buss 1994). For example, Native American children were involved in a similar exercise and their published photographs show their world as they see it (Hubbard 1994; *Aperture* 1995). Photographs are also a means of communication for those who may not have access to a more complex written text or may have little or no standing in the community (Dewdney and Lister 1988). Too frequently identified as behaving 'badly', as in media images, or excluded from scholarly studies, the world of children of colour appears to be little known by the dominant society (Graff 1995; Bernie *et al.* 1996). We approached this project then with the assumptions that the opinions of poor children of colour, of elementary school age,[3] are overlooked and that photography is a means of learning about them and their preferences in the environment. That children can document their world also drew from theories about grounded research and feminism, which were used by the senior author in previous work with adults where primarily African-American tenants told their stories about surviving landlord abandonment and forming limited equity co-operatives in New York City (Leavitt and Saegert 1990).

For this project we also suspected that photography might serve other purposes such as encouraging basic literacy skills when combined with producing a written product; for example, a journal or newpaper. Additional impressions emerged during the course of the project as a result of the children's temporary ownership of the cameras and possession of the developed photos. To begin with, acquiring a camera distinguished those who participated from those who did not. The child as photographer was able to choose a subject and select whom to include or exclude. Taking pictures became an independent act with tangible accomplishments. Although about 92 per cent of US households are reported to own at least one camera, it is unlikely that poorer housholds will use their scarce resources to purchase a disposable camera or, if they do, turn this over to a young child. Obtaining a camera – and the children's joy in receiving them would seem to bear this out – may provide a child with a sense of importance and may lead to increased self-esteem. This may have been particularly true for those children whose developed photos were not blurred, whose shots were consistently well framed and who received positive comments from us. Finally, and whether consciously or not, the children may have used the cameras as a means to focus themselves, arrange a sense of order in their immediate environment, and provide more intimate snapshots of an environment that an adult or an outsider might not enter at all or not be able to capture as well.

Participation and replication

Attendance at any 4-H centre fluctuates as school programmes and family circumstances compete for attention, and special projects attract a self-selected audience. During the first part of our project, 'How Kids See the City', a subset of ten to thirteen boys and girls came to twice-weekly sessions. Five Latino boys were initially part of this group but they dropped out and we worked more closely with girls – four African-Americans and three to four Latinas. Three of the five boys were closer to 13 years old and usually attended another nearby 4-H centre. 'Commuting' the block and a half, combined with the age-difference, may have contributed to feelings of differentness and their attendance tapered off.[4] Of the other two boys, one darted in and out over the course of the project, more on a teasing or opinion-stating expedition, while the other boy just didn't appear.

The all-girl core group produced 'Kids Talk Back', a newspaper written in Spanish and English that includes autobiographies, accompanied by their selected photos, and interviews and photos of neighbourhood heroes. The paper, a one-off event, will be distributed to other 4-H centres throughout Los Angeles, accompanied by a detailed set of lesson plans. These cover twenty-six sessions and are divided into four major sections – skills and concepts, the child's environmental autobiography, the social environment in terms of neighbourhood heroes, and the future community – as well as recommended materials and equipment needed for each session, and descriptions of exercises on perspective, scale, measure, distance and so on. Thus the newspaper product and the process document may encourage replication by site co-ordinators at other 4-H centres.

Dominant themes in the photography

Four themes emerge strongly in the children's photos. One is the immediate environment around the centre, the micro-world of the after-school hours. Close-ups of grass adjacent to a wooden garage at the back of the children's centre (Plate 6/1) and palm trees in the distance seen from the second floor of the centre are quintessential images of the city of Los Angeles as façade, a stage-set that does not reveal everything. Like the city where strips of green yard surround single-family houses and mask the overall low ranking of open space per capita, the children's photos of foreground and background take on a different meaning when seen in the larger context. The abundance of grass is seen as only a small area at the farthest end of the traffic island and the trees on the landscape are unreachable across six traffic lanes of the Santa Ana Freeway. Despite such man-made obstacles, the children's photos repeatedly include the natural world as it exists for them. Even in scenes of the housing development, an 11-year-old and a 13-year-old boy show mature trees and grass in photos that reveal the low density of the housing complex (Plates 6/2 and 6/3). These are particularly poignant given housing authority proposals to demolish the complex, lower the

Plate 6.1 Grass at the back of the children's area:
4-H Program, LA

Plate 6.2 Low density housing complex:
4-H Program, LA

Plate 6.3 Greenery around housing centre:
4-H Program, LA

number of replacement units, increase density and parking, and reduce the amount of open space.

A second theme, reflected in photos by two African-American girls who are cousins, one 8 years old and the other closer to 9, is the world at and beyond the centre. The younger one concentrated on art, perhaps unsurprisingly given that one of her brothers was the artist for the Virgin of Guadalupe mural. She, an instinctual archivist, catalogued variations in the murals that mark the neighbourhood as one of the richest in this art form in LA. Her picture of the Virgin captures the top half against a blue sky (Plate 6/4). In her photos, building façades are the canvas on which scenes have more than a flat meaning. The full shot of a second mural on the side of a public housing building is dedicated to the mothers and fathers of the 'projects'. The muralist has portrayed parents and at the juncture where the heads join, symbols of peace and protection for the child flow out, reminders of the fifty-odd killings and blood spilled by youngsters in this neighbourhood. A mural on the side of a market wall juxtaposes history and reality, the symbolic Aztlàn icon sharing space with postmodern dis-investment embodied in the 'for rent' sign. This contradiction is also present in photos whose semiotics is clear cut: 'stop the violence, help the children, help yourself', its venue a building bearing scars of exterior neglect and another 'for rent' sign. Photos of pastoral scenes in arches above the doorways of a tortilla-making factory are also seen in relation to doors with bars over them, on buildings with 'for sale or lease' signs (Plate 6/5).

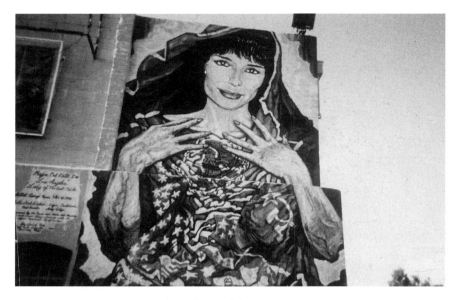

Plate 6.4 Virgin of Guadalupe mural:
Ashley, 4-H Program, LA

Plate 6.5 Tortilla factory doorway:
Ashley, 4-H Program, LA

The older girl takes us behind façades to capture scenes of a friendlier landscape in neighbourhoods that are stereotyped as crime-infested and dangerous: the schoolyard is a shady oasis, whose fence creates safety from the cars ringing the block, a place in which to play; cartoon advertisements on a side of a truck are innocent images that lure us to line up and order Mama Flip ice-cream cones; the inside shot of a corner market shows a young man posed, staring into the camera, in front of freezers selling everything from milk to beer, pin-ups of women on the walls, an interior world at once connected to global consumption and hinting of items children should not be able to buy. Even here, an open door beckons us to move outdoors, to taste the life that unfolds beyond the façade of the posed shot and the advertisements. Similarly, this child's photo of the interior of one residence is multi-dimensional as she foregrounds a toddler facing away from a television set on whose screen a programme is frozen, while outside the window we see a benign view of grass, a tree and other buildings.

The girls' portraits of people, a third theme, take the outsider behind the barriers of the buildings and into homes, with people in groups, amid their furniture, decorations, pictures and knick-knacks on the walls (Plate 6/6). At least four of the girls, two Latinas and one African-American, ranging in age from 8 to 11, portray a woman's world. Boys and men appear in numerous photos although girls and women dominate in the group see in its entirety, be it as babies, friends, mothers, teachers or coaches. The many pictures of Robert and Carlos, the 4-H site co-ordinator and his assistant, are the exception.

Plate 6.6 Home portraits:
Juana, 4-H Program, LA

It may be presumptuous to draw definitive conclusions from these photos; fourteen weeks is a short period of time even when observations are refined with insights that Robert and Carlos shared with us. The children's world may be seen through the photographs that they have taken. The photos do not eradicate the realities of their material conditions but the views offered offset the overwhelmingly bleak conclusions embedded in the statistics. Certainly, the girls' photos show consistent trends both in quality and subject-matter and offer some clues as to what they like or dislike about their environment.

More elusive is what these young people are thinking about themselves. In the literature, when elementary school girls of different racial and ethnic groups were compared, '55 per cent of white girls, 65 per cent of black girls and 68 per cent of Hispanic girls reported being "happy as I am" ' (AAUW 1995). These percentages drop sharply by high school, particularly for white and Hispanic girls: 22 per cent of the white girls, 30 per cent of the Hispanic girls, and 58 per cent of the black girls report high levels of self-esteem. But black girls lack high levels of esteem in issues related to school and evidence suggests that this may be partly caused by teachers who treat students differently by race and ethnicity. Such breakdowns do not appear as distinct among the core group of girls who worked with us. Both 8-year-olds, one a Latina and the other an African-American, are well behaved at the centre and good students. The 10-year-old Latina sister and the 9-year-old African-American cousin are far moodier. The sister didn't make the school's drill team because of her poor grades. The cousin had trouble reading and writing but excelled in photography and drawing in this project and when she reproduced one of her drawings from the exercise on perspective received an honourable mention award at school.

The girls who participated in this project chattered away on a variety of issues as they worked on the newspaper, replicating a 'coffee klatch' as they critically commented on an older girl's child-rearing practices or some event. Perhaps shaded by our own experiences as women, we were acutely aware of the girls' self-depredation of their physical characteristics. All seemed conscious of weight. One girl who wore glasses referred to herself as skinny and four-eyes; another spoke of being skinny and having asthma. Indeed in both cases the girls were thin, one did wear glasses and the other did have asthma. While a realistic statement, more significant is the general awareness of their bodies, a point the literature repeatedly makes (Brown and Gilligan 1992; Orenstein 1994; Pipher 1995). Another girl described herself as ugly in one of her drawings but underwent at least a temporary change of heart and described herself as beautiful under one picture in the newspaper. One girl frequently took the brunt of what seemed to us brutal teasing that concerned her manner and her clothes, with others poking fun by sniffing the air around her. She, in turn, was one of the girls who called herself ugly and attacked a picture of herself with a sharp implement that left scratches on the print. The two 8-year-old girls were noticeably different in their demeanour, more serious and well behaved. The African-American photographer of neighbourhood art made asides on how silly the others were – the boys but also the girls.

Babies are part of the children's life (Plate 6/7) and photos show mothers in traditional roles – in the kitchen, holding children, taking in laundry. There are other signs, albeit indirectly, about the ways in which the girls learn about the world of women. Death and physical harm are not strangers. On the first day of the project, unprompted, one girl told us about repeated dreams that replayed an attack on a sister's girlfriend. Later we were told that she has flashbacks about her father who died. Another girl's brother committed suicide last year. The photos reveal the close quarters in which the girls live and oftentimes the female sensibility reflected in the décor of individual houses. But no single view emerges of the women in their lives. A few of their mothers are active in the community and the girls selected one of their mothers, Pam, to spotlight as a hero in their paper. In the interview, after eliciting that Pam is a gang consultant for the housing authority, one of the girls asked her: 'What are your hopes for the kids in this community?' Pam responded:

> I think I have dreams for the kids in the community. I hope that they are able to accomplish goals that they set for themselves in life. For instance, if you want to be a girl scout, then my goal is to support you and help you to accomplish that. I think that all of us have gifts that God gives us and I think that we need a support person to help us, including myself. I have people who support me. So my whole dream is that you would become whatever makes you happiest and that you accomplish whatever you set out to do.

Plate 6.7 World of women:
Juana, 4-H Program, LA

In response to her daughter's question about any last thoughts, Pam thanked everyone for the invitation and expressed her appreciation for 'your thinking of me as your neighborhood hero. It feels like you gave me a big gold medallion.'

A final theme in the photographs is the ways in which some reveal the negative parts of their world; here we see the lack of fulfilment promised in federal legislation of 1949, that each family should be provided with decent, safe and sanitary housing. These photos demonstrate the results of the housing authority's failure to maintain play equipment, fix the kitchen whose ceiling shows signs of leaks, or renovate the antiquated sink and replace the open shelves with cupboards. Fearfulness or hopelessness may be interpreted in a few pictures such as the juxtaposition of two photos of eyes, one a young boy's and the other a dog's (Plates 6/8, 6/9). The lack of money is evident in some homes that are noticeably empty of decorations and where large paper cartons substitute for chairs. The few pictures of youths who may belong to gangs are more likely taken because of coincidence – the children receiving their cameras at the same time as two young men drop in at the centre[5]. Overall, neither the girls nor the boys dwelt on scenes of poverty. Such negative images as there are appear more as a backdrop to life at the centre and in the family and neighbourhood.

Sceptics might conclude that these last photographs discussed display the 'real' views of these children's world and that the others were 'camouflage'. We think that the photos and the newspaper the girls produced indicate their resilience and suggest that young children can live under circumstances

Plate 6.8 Eyes #1: Ebony, 4-H Program, LA

Plate 6.9 Eyes #2: Ebony, 4-H Program, LA

that reflect systemic problems of poverty and have the ability to see nature, art and the material reflection of people's dreams. Their photos show us their neighbourhood and through their eyes we gain a unique view about differences.

Notes

1 Contradictions in global capitalism are such that UNOCAL supports this domestic programme while undertaking development in Burma where its practices are alleged to damage the lives of women and children. See, for example, Evelyn Iritani, 'Mynamar project fueling international controversy', *Los Angeles Times*, 24 November 1996.
2 Differences exist between public and council housing as to tenure, eligibility requirements and financing. None the less, similarities include the primary role of the state as landlord and the preponderance of residents drawn from the lower income and non-working population.
3 Compulsory US elementary school education, which includes pre-school and primary, usually begins at 6 (depending on the state). A child moves on to secondary education either at grade 7 or grade 9, when aged 12–14. Most of the children whose work is described in the chapter were in the age-range 6–10.
4 In a project with seven boys at Compton Avenue Elementary School in the Watts section of Los Angeles, one girl dropped out after a few weeks. The ostensible reason had to do with the greater pull on her interest in dance, but she may also have been pushed out by feelings about being the lone girl.
5 Since this chapter was written, the housing authority has proceeded with plans to demolish and rebuild. This 4-H Centre was closed and some children 'commute' to one nearby.

7

Watching the detectors

Control and the panopticon

Rosa Ainley

Morals reformed – health preserved – industry invigorated – instruction diffused – public burthens lightened – Economy seated, as it were, upon a rock – the gordian knot of the Poor Laws are not cut, but untied – all by a simple idea in Architecture!

(Bentham 1995: 31)

Jeremy Bentham's description of the uses and advantages of the panopticon has the excited tone of an early form of advertising copy – all this can be yours, an unmissable bargain. The notion of the panopticon has excited many imaginations apart from mine and since the time of Bentham's writing, in the late eighteenth century, there have been many ideas in architecture and related disciplines that have, initially at least, set themselves up as solutions to some social 'gordian knot' or other. If we take architecture as a system of representation (Colomina 1992: introduction), it becomes useful to discuss it in relation to other such systems and so I want in this chapter, looking also at some more modern examples of architectural control (in photography, film and the built environment), to examine some ideas about developments and interrelations of photography, architecture and social control. Or, to put it another way, what exactly is this bargain and what does it cost?

Panoptic means 'all embracing, in a single view'. This sounds considerably more benign than the actual purpose of the panopticon structure. The panopticon was an ingenious construction consisting of a central tower surrounded by individual compartments – for patients, prisoners, pupils, workers, any group whose isolation and surveillance might lead to the benefits promised by Bentham's quote above. Through a complex internal structure of screens, blinds and lighting, the inhabitants could not see or communicate with each other, nor could they tell whether the inspector, who inhabited the central tower, was observing them. But they were led to believe that he might be at any given time. From his tower, the inspector could see into all the prisoners' (and maybe also the guards') compartments. The intricate lighting system intensified these effects, and a speaking tube system allowed him to communicate with any inhabitant without any other prisoner being able to hear the content of the exchange.

The plan of the panopticon itself looks, at first glance, quite similar to a late twentieth-century warehouse conversion or an intriguing amphitheatre structure; it is not necessarily sinister, until you peer at the key to discover the purpose of all the subdivisions and compartments inside. Cells. Foucault's description of the panopticon as a 'laboratory of power' (Foucault 1979: 202) or Soja's 'concretization of power applied through architecture' (Soja 1995: 26) come considerably closer in conveying something of its purpose, and explain the unease that the contemporary reader might feel on consideration of this naked exercise in social control through solitary confinement. Of course, many modern examples of social control through architecture exist, and all the institutions – schools, prisons, hospitals, factories – that Bentham believed could usefully be housed in panopticon structures now exert their institutional control in a myriad of ways, although we shall see whether they are more covert ones.

Bentham's belief in the social force of architecture was, perhaps thankfully, not borne out in the practice of the working panopticon. Thomas Markus, writing in *Buildings and Power*, asserts that, with the exception of Edinburgh's Bridewell prison (built in 1791), no panopticon has ever been built (Markus 1993: 145). There is in fact disagreement about whether a true panopticon has ever been built and therefore whether it may be judged successful or not. Bentham's writings are, so the back cover blurb of the Verso edition informs us, 'frequently cited, rarely read', just as the panopticon is frequently written about but possibly never built. Resiting the study of an architectural form to the medium of imagery, in this case a line drawing, makes it immaterial to the study of panoptic control whether an authentic model has ever existed. The panopticon becomes itself an image, which we may consider alongside other images, a representation of an all-seeing power.

John Ryle, writing in *The Guardian*, describes his visit to a panopticon, built in 1932, on the Isla de la Juventad (Isle of Youth), 30 miles south of Cuba, once inhabited by Fidel Castro and finally demolished on his order (Ryle 1996). Ryle mentions the Millbank Penitentiary as another example, noting that the prisoners there rioted. He offers no evidence to suggest that the riots resulted from dissatisfaction with the design of the penitentiary rather than, say, brutality or bad food, although the reader is led to surmise that this was the reason. Millbank Penitentiary stood on the site now occupied by the Tate Gallery, where people now go mainly to look at artworks, rather than to be observed, and to engage in a communicative act, instead of being deliberately prevented from any interaction. The site then remains a building for viewing but has changed from a place of incarceration and surveillance to one of contemplation and an altogether different kind of gaze.

Foucault makes a distinction between separation and classification as methods of control in relation to the management of disease and contagion (Foucault 1979: 195), using the management of leprosy and the plague as his models. Whereas people suffering from leprosy were separated from the rest of society in order to maintain its pure and untainted nature, in the case of plague systems of minute classification and segmentation were used to contain the 'disorder' of the disease.[1] He describes plague management as 'a compact model of the disciplinary mechanism' (Foucault 1979: 198) and sees the panopticon as the architectural form of this attitude to discipline.

As Foucault says, the panopticon plan compartmentalises the crowd's numerous variables. Initially the cruelty of the panopticon – the isolation from society and peers, the constant torture of the random but ever possible gaze – does not seem compatible with Bentham's utilitarianism. Exploring more deeply into his writings on the subject it becomes clearer. For Bentham, 'punishment is a spectacle', says Bozovic (Bentham 1995: 4) intended as a form of instructive deterrence for the wider, non-transgressive audience, while actual reform or rehabilitation can relate only to the small number judged in need of punishment.[2] This then becomes more consistent with utilitarianism: contributing to the greatest possible good of the greatest possible number.

It is the principle that inmates could never know when they were being watched and the knowledge that this could be at any time that made the idea of the panopticon effective, forcing self-vigilance through fear and uncertainty. To talk about its effectiveness being its spectacle perhaps makes it lose some of its harshness.[3] In his introduction to *The Panopticon Writings* Miran Bozovic writes that the inspector had to present evidence of the power of his position (both in terms of hierarchy and location) only once to a single prisoner to make it effective against the bad behaviour of any of the others (Bentham 1995: 16). In this context Soja talks of the interactive nature of the relationship between surveillance and power (Soja 1995: 23), but it is not clear that this goes beyond one of cause and effect. Once an example of the inspector's all-seeing gaze has been displayed, he can then 'peacefully devote himself to his book-keeping' (Bentham 1995: 17), which was his other function. Even the all-seeing have to do their accounts apparently.

If this one-off demonstration by the inspector were truly effective then there would in fact be no need for the inspector to be present at all. Markus also raises the question of whether the inspector too is trapped within the structure, the notion of the guard being imprisoned along with the prisoners (Markus 1993: 148). This is a flaw in Bozovic's argument – the inmates had no possibility of knowing or finding out what had happened to any other. The question remains of how this knowledge, essential for the functioning of the panopticon model, would come to the inhabitants. Perhaps we might take this as a kind of precursor to the urban myth.

Contemporary attitudes to surveillance – classifying all of society, as in occupants of public space, as potentially 'diseased' – acknowledge the uncertainty and film the variables. Closed circuit television (CCTV) is the current panacea for all public order ills, an electronic panopticon, albeit one without spectacle, and this is increasingly installed in public spaces.[4] Soja says: 'Every city is a carceral city, a collection of surveillant nodes designed to impose a particular model of conduct and disciplinary adherence on its inhabitants' (Soja 1995: 29), so the population becomes composed of surveillants, adherents and recalcitrants. The centrality of the panoptic gaze as distinct from the dispersed nature of CCTV is directly related to the spectacle value of each, and the wide dispersal of CCTV is said to mirror the fragmentation of contemporary urban life. This sounds dangerously close to another kind of argument in current crime 'debates' that asserts that life used to be friendlier, calmer, safer, cleaner. The gaze of CCTV may be as disembodied as that of the panopticon inspector, but its apparatus can always be seen as an architectural detail. Sometimes its installers see fit to add cages around it, against the possibility of vandalism. While commentators on the built environment debate CCTV's uses, its efficacy and the moral issues around it, this intrusion into public space is generally accepted unquestioningly as an (architectural) feature – and by some as an essential – of modern life, although there is little information available at source about why the recording is being made, by whom and for what purpose (Women's Design Service 1996: 1). Describing this continuum, John Ryle cites the panopticon as 'the first ancient monument of the age of surveillance' (Ryle 1996). Other commentators include the prevalence of CCTV in a more ominous and inclusive vision of the future:

> We have arrived on the verge of the *carceral city*, a world of perpetual commodity production and consumption, a *panoptic society* of observation and discipline where the technologies of order and normalisation are physically and electronically integrated into social life.
>
> (Charley 1996: 61)

Twenty years ago in *On Photography* Sontag wrote about how the proliferation of photographic equipment and technology had led to a culture of the photography of self-surveillance – in domestic sex films for playing in the bedroom, wedding videos, taping and playback of therapy sessions, conferences, interviews and so on. She also anticipated the growth in the use of the camera for public surveillance: 'Our inclination to treat character as equivalent to behaviour makes more acceptable a widespread public installation of the mechanised regard from the outside provided by cameras' (Sontag 1983: 365). Contrasting this with surveillance in China, whose internalisation of the practice 'suggests a more limited future in their society for the camera as a means of surveillance' (Sontag 1983: 365), she notes that the monitoring of behaviour is quite a different matter from altering it: 'Social change is replaced by a change in images' (Sontag 1983: 366).

Like Foucault she makes an opposition between surveillance and spectacle: 'Cameras define reality in the two ways essential to the workings of an advanced industrial society: as a spectacle (for masses) and as an object of surveillance (for rulers)' (Sontag 1983: 366). The proliferation and presumable popularity of 'real life' television offerings from crime reconstructions and disaster/rescue re-enactments to 'fly on the wall' documentaries and confessional shows like *Oprah*, *Ricki Lake* and *Vanessa* as well as the reports of CCTV tapes being made available to the residents on whose estates the footage was filmed suggests that the attractions have a mass audience even if not limited to the 'masses'. Laura Barnes's piece *Cruising* (1996) suggests another related attraction, the excitement of voyeurism (see Plates 7/1 and 7/2). The video installation, shown originally in a security office, catches two women cruising each other in a public space, watched by a third woman. This kind of (enjoyable) communication may be captured by a security camera but will probably not be read as such, and tempers the view that the intrusion of surveillance is inherently bad; as Barnes said (1996), 'Surveillance systems can be used by women for their own ends.'

To return to the crime scene, it is of course highly debatable whether CCTV stops anyone actually doing anything; it merely displaces problems to other locations (as Jacquelin Burgess notes in Chapter 9 of this book) and helps apprehension after the fact, in some cases. Its apparatus has become ubiquitous and this silent policing seems less likely to impose self-vigilance. CCTV also has a range of auxiliary uses, from the benign, in searching for lost children and school truants, or as a cost-effective means of examining buildings for maintenance requirements, to the more questionable, such as checking employees' timekeeping and opening up new possibilities for harassment and stalking. Even where the ugly hardware, once installed, is operative – and in many cases the cameras are empty boxes like so many burglar alarms[5] – CCTV requires an enormous amount of personnel time

Plate 7.1 From *Cruising*: Laura Barnes

for it to be effective. This point is not lost on television and film writers who provide endless examples of crimes undetected by sleeping or otherwise absent security staff. The mechanism of vigilance is also one of leisure interest – monitors used for videos, surfing on the Net and computer games. The message seems to be one of throwing up the moral hands in horror in an acknowledgement that we cannot control, we can only present the illusion of control through the ability to watch – perhaps Gil Scott Heron was wrong and the revolution *will* be televised.[6]

As another architectural detail of surveillance we might consider gargoyles, which first occurred to me while studying Brassaï's famous series of photographs of gargoyles on Notre Dame cathedral. Gargoyles appear to be the master of all they survey from their vantage point – another spectacle, for they can see nothing. Generally grotesque rather than ugly, they are often found on Gothic churches, where they can seem in unsettling contrast to the Christian iconography and nature of the rest of the building. They are also functional, but form does not here follow function. Actually a waterspout, part of the drainage system, a gargoyle looks as though it ought to be a piece of surveillance equipment. Perhaps an early monument of the age of *apparent* surveillance – the empty CCTV box, the non-functioning security device, and another example of spectacle-as-surveillance.

The gargoyle *seems* to be able to see into the windows and buildings it faces, perched in its vantage point on the roof gutters. And maybe that is the point, apart from the channelling of rainwater: a stone representation of the all-seeing eye of the Church. One of God's little sentinels perhaps, extending

Plate 7.2 From *Cruising*: Laura Barnes

the sense of his omniscience through this piece of architectural decoration as CCTV falsely suggests the omniscience of its various controllers. Gargoyles, though, are more suggestive of hellish imps and hideous hybrid animals – bogeymen – than earthbound extensions of the heavenly vision.

There is a similarity here with the inspector of the panopticon. As with the gargoyle, the inspector's location gives him the possibility of seeing all the detainees at any time, even though this is not physically possible. The gargoyle, which appears to be constantly scrutinising although it can see nothing, is similarly more to do with spectacle than actual vision. Miran Bozovic's heavily ironic introduction extends this connection to the point of hilarity: 'There is perhaps no other work of human hands, no icon, that can bring God closer to us, through which God can reveal himself to a greater extent than through Bentham's panopticon' (Bentham 1995: 11). The omniscient gaze of God holds some similarity to that of the inspector, who also hides his face and disembodies his voice or at least 'throws' it through the conduit of various earthly representatives.

An echo of Bentham's ideas about real and apparent suffering and surveillance in relation to the force of the panopticon message is contained in current safety debates, which respond to the public's perception of danger, rather than the likelihood of danger itself. Perceived threats to safety are different from, although not necessarily less harmful than, 'real' threats. This makes more sense of the collective embrace of responses that can in no way be said to tackle root causes of violence and crime that people fear – the illusion is acceptable enough. An image of safety can provide a feeling of security. Issues of safety are often subsumed under crime prevention, and security is reduced to a matter of hardware, alarms and ironmongery, a visible effort at least. The focus is then firmly on the danger of outside forces, not 'the enemy within' – Margaret Thatcher's slur on striking miners in the mid-1980s struck a resonant chord. Concentrating on the 'them not us' model brings us again to Foucault's leprosy and exclusion model.

The notion of 'natural surveillance' has had as much currency as its electronic counterpart in discussions of how to combat feelings of unsafety through architectural and town planning practices, especially in relation to residential developments. Natural surveillance results from designing and grouping houses or buildings so that common areas such as courtyards, playgrounds or pathways can be overlooked and monitored by residents. In this way, children may be left to play, apparently unsupervised; outsiders/intruders cannot go unnoticed; vandalism, petty crime and car theft are more likely to be witnessed and so on. The measure of control that, illusory or not, may be gained from this kind of set-up, can help to allay fears about safety, again by concentrating on the spectre of trouble from the outside.

Neighbourhood Watch schemes are run on precisely this principle and – mirroring Foucault's 'leper' model – members of the scheme are pure, while anyone outside is potentially contagious and therefore worthy of suspicion. It is an interesting paradox that, in an age obsessed by individualism and privacy, people are content to be forced into accepting the kindness of strangers to guard their property. Supporters of these schemes contend that a heightened community spirit is another benefit. In this context I think 'community' is used as a euphemism for 'territorial' – it is rather the shared fear of losing property that brings people together. The situation may become polarised into a very tribal one, actually anti-community, anti-society.

The 1980s – that anti-society decade epitomised in Thatcher's infamous and prophetical quote, 'There is no such thing as Society', said on 31 October 1987 – saw the rise (and fall and rise) of Alice Coleman's ideas about designing out crime through architectural means (Coleman 1985). Her thesis was that certain types of design, especially 'unowned' communal spaces such as open green areas and walkways, allowed, even fostered, criminal behaviour, in particular on housing estates, which had earlier been seen as the technical solution to the problems of slum clearance, and housing and land shortages[7] – just as the panopticon was considered an architectural mechanism for the imposition of forms of behaviour. Her 'solution' involved cutting out communal areas as far as possible and reorganising the space so that it became individual territory, which would, so the theory went, then be guarded as private property.

This notion of 'defensible space' featured strongly in the work of housing theorists of the time: that if areas – individual gardens instead of green spaces – were 'owned' by individuals then they would respect rather than damage them.[8] Clearly this is an overly deterministic attitude and completely denies the importance of other considerations, from the architecture- or housing-related factors such as space standards (diminishing) and densities (rising) to the more widely social ones such as access to services and existence of facilities, or the plainly economic – availability of regular well-paid employment: 'the first precondition for reducing crime is to ensure that the Government's policies balance the need for a competitive economy in world markets with the needs of social justice' (Hough 1997). By contrast the 1990s have been marked by a focus on the establishment of 'community', a word which is often a euphemism for underfunded and poorly resourced, and the notions of consultation and participation are paramount as Maher Anjum and Lesley Klein discuss in Chapter 3 of this book.

Prescriptive design and building of this type are of course not limited to the 1980s. Attempts at social engineering through the location, layout, design and proximity of leisure, schooling, child-care and shopping facilities of housing developments have been well documented, as have their short-comings.[9] Housing history is littered with examples of architects trying to ensure the continued purity of their designs by preventing tenants from altering, for instance, interior décor. This sounds superficial and, literally, is – a coat of paint. But here too there is a sense of ownership in how a resident wants a living space to look, and an uncomfortable sense of coercive design and prescriptive interior decoration. A kind of class-based form of colour theory – make the colour scheme tasteful, restrained, in a middle-class way, and the residents will have calmer, less chaotic lives.[10] The phrase 'architecture as "congealed ideology"', coined by the team who authored *Strangely Familiar*, springs to mind here (Borden *et al.* 1996: 5).

One famous example of architectural intrusion is Eileen Gray's house, designed by her, E.1027, of which more later; less exalted examples include attempts by local authorities to prevent children playing on green spaces in public housing developments, and banning the hanging of washing outdoors.

Many of these examples relate to social housing and often to attempts to regulate or contain a largely low-income, predominantly working-class population. These may lie anywhere along the covert/overt axis from the setting-up of zones and ghettos to estates of single household dwellings without access to play areas or green spaces. In *Sliver* (Noyse 1993), a B-movie Sharon Stone-vehicle, by contrast, the regulation is of an exclusive condominium development, housing high-earning professionals. The owner of the block, who is able to view all the apartments on his state-of-the-art surveillance system, plays the role of the panopticon inspector, even taking it to the extent of punishing individual tenants for their transgressions: an unseen enforcer. His mastery of technology – including e-mailing Stone virtual red roses (who said romance was dead?) – is initially part of his charm but speedily tips over into something altogether more menacing as he assumes also the roles of judge and, literally, executioner. Stone is tempted by the power, dazzled by the technology, almost seduced into the role of co-voyeur that he offers her and ultimately disgusted by his justifications and judgements. She also plays the part of the frightened, vulnerable single woman, scared by the stories of murdered previous tenants, as well as the dynamic publishing executive. The intrusion of CCTV – in *Sliver* the hardware is not visible to those monitored – into tenants' supposedly private spaces and the fact that its human monitor uses it to feed his own sociopathic tendencies, belie his protestations that 'it's for their own good'. New equipment, same old story apparently.

Berenice Abbott's photograph *Court of the First Model Tenement* (Plate 7/3), can be read as an example of the intrusion into public space of what are considered to be private, sometimes forbidden, uses, and of natural surveillance. The hardness and austerity of the housing blocks – some might say their integrity – is tempered by the lines of washing strung from a central pole back to the walls. In visual/aesthetic terms the lines of washing are pleasing. The perspective gives the blocks an overbearing, monumental air but the washing brings the gaze back into the centre of the picture, disrupting the hardness of the lines of the buildings by bringing the domestic, the intimate (underwear) sphere into the public domain. I don't know whether the central pole was provided for the purpose of stringing washing lines to it, or if it were appropriated by, presumably, women tenants against the rules.

This visual working of 'washing your linen in public' functions as a

Plate 7.3 Court of the First Model Tenement in New York City:
Berenice Abbott (Baltimore Museum of Art)

depiction of the domestic, the interior, the feminine, spilling out –
threateningly? although it is the buildings which really threaten – into the
public sphere. The pedestal position of privacy is demolished by bell hooks:
'it really becomes a screen for a profound narcissism . . . we're never going
to end the forms of domination if we're not willing to break down the walls
that say, "there should always be this separation between domestic space/
intimate space and the world outside" ' (hooks 1994: 223). The washing is,
in fact, astonishingly well ordered – rows of vests in the foreground and

lines of like-sized articles grouped together behind. The removal of the standard spaces for neighbourly communication – front steps, garden fences, street life – and the sense of community in housing blocks seem re-established here through this apparently small disobedience, the very image of lines of communication.

To return now to Eileen Gray's house . . . Le Corbusier painted a mural *Sous les pilotis* (a.k.a *Graffite à Cap Martin* or *Three Women*) at E.1027 without Gray's permission. He also built for himself a wooden shack right behind the house. In a phrase that cannot help but remind of the panopticon, Beatriz Colomina writes, in her essay 'Battle lines: E.1027': 'He occupied and controlled the site by *overlooking it*, the cabin being little more than an *observation platform*, a sort of *watchdog house*' (italics added). Not only was his gaze architecturally imposed – Gray had chosen the site for its inaccessibility – but Gray considered his murals to be vandalism. Colomina quotes Peter Adam: 'It was a rape. A fellow architect, a man she admired, had without her consent defaced her design'[11] (Adam 1987: 311). But equally important I think is the implicit demand from him that she should organise her living space in a certain way, the attempt to assert control over the space through forcing her to look at his work placed over hers. This kind of violation may be taking the idea that 'architecture is made and remade over and over again each time it is represented through another medium, each time its surroundings change, each time different people experience it' (Borden *et al.* 1996: 5) into another, and unwelcome, realm.

Another film, *Proof* (Moorhouse 1991) gives a different, but related, set of ideas about vision, control and photography. At first, its whole basis seems risible and pitiable; its central character is Martin, a blind man, who takes photographs. He explains that as a boy he 'wanted a camera. I thought it would help me to see.' He photographs his surroundings and a friend describes the picture so that he can then label it in Braille: 'proof that what I sensed is what you saw.' His ability to create an image fills, or helps to fill, his lack, or absence, of vision. The camera gives him the opportunity to witness, even if he cannot see that to which he is witness. A sightless surveillant.

Martin seeks to maintain control through choosing who describes the pictures to him. This control is usurped by Celia, his housekeeper, whose obsession with him is represented through the many portraits of him that cover her walls (which he cannot see, only sense). She manipulates a situation whereby his picture-describer friend is forced to lie about the content of a photograph. Martin later witnesses the two of them having sex and senses two people, apprehending one of them trying to leave, thus echoing his attitude to his photography and underlining his control – what he *sensed* was there. He further re-establishes control by sacking Celia. The unseeing, as well as the all-seeing but unseen, can exert control.

It seems then that neither the panopticon nor any of the more modern methods of control, whether social or more personal, through architectural or photographic means, unties any 'gordian knots'. The costs are high and the 'bargain' non-existent. This is no great surprise – although for Bentham perhaps the fact that offenders were, and remain, a small percentage of the population, is success enough. The panopticon idea apparently took hold of his attention for twenty years; a study of his writings on the subject leads into many areas. Their trajectory is a broad and fascinating one, into the realms of contemporary concerns both empirical and more representational, from housing and safety issues to the operation and force of architecture.

The initial reaction to the panopticon model – that it is some kind of torture chamber based on an illusion, an architectural spectacle – is tempered somewhat by the realisation that its modern manifestation involves turning every public space into a prison-without-walls, and some private spaces into film sets or observation points. Earlier in this chapter I called the panopticon a 'naked exercise in social control'; the ubiquity of the CCTV camera, the many forms of attempted architectural coercion, are no more covert, merely lacking the force of presentation (of spectacle) of an impressive and intricate building. The architectural representations of coercion and control that I have examined all work in this way, whether this ultimately renders them more benign or more chilling.

Foucault ends his chapter on panopticism like this: 'Is it surprising that prisons resemble factories, schools, barracks, hospitals, which all resemble prisons?' (Foucault 1979: 228). We might take this further and add 'housing, shopping complexes, office blocks, public buildings' or as Bentham classifies it: prisons, houses of industry, work-houses, poor-houses, houses of correction, manufactures, mad-houses, lazarettos [ship's storerooms], hospitals, schools, all of which he deemed suited to a panoptic structure. While we may surmise that for Bentham, the spectacle of the panopticon would have alleviated the need for the more pervasively carceral city, many modern commentators believe it is already with us or at least imminent: 'We should be on our guard that the surveillance city . . . does not catch us unarmed, disinterested and incapable' (Charley 1996: 61). But while being alerted to the possible dangers, we might also take care not to ignore any potential pleasures.

Notes

1 Shades of Freud's notion of dirt being 'matter in the wrong place'.
2 In a different relation to 'the spectacle' and the panopticon, Beatriz Colomina in her piece 'The split wall: domestic voyeurism' (1992) writes about Adolf Loos's description of a theatre box as panoptic with only the breadth of its view, its scope of surveillance, making its confinement acceptable. For Loos this represented the point between claustrophobia and agrophobia.
3 Until Bentham talks admiringly about the spectacle of the Inquisition. The effectiveness or importance of ritual aside, this one-dimensional focus on the Inquisition has a similar effect as if presented with the notion of, say, the Ku Klux Klan or the Gestapo as spectacle, which could, chronology permitting, equally have been used as examples.

4 See also the not so contemporary *Photographic Surveillance Techniques for Law Enforcement Agencies* (1972). 'Law enforcement agencies' now means official channels, yet this booklet is plainly aimed at the amateur end of the market and struggles to legitimise its seedy, downmarket audience. As with CCTV its approach is technical rather than moral: advice on positioning surveillance equipment and how to deal with anger towards it. No moral issues are admitted; its stated purpose is 'the observation of *suspected persons* . . . and to record *illegal* activities' (italics added). The principles of surveillance stated here share with the panopticon the same need not to be seen seeing, although here the subject is not controllable, and also share the more modern surveillance principle that everyone is suspect.

5 Another related, 'lying' sign for a piece of surveillance equipment is the roadside sign denoting speed check cameras: by contrast, a likeably attractive ideogram of an old-fashioned box camera, certainly not the equipment to which the sign refers. It lies and yet we like the sign itself.

6 Listen to Gil Scott Heron, 'The revolution will not be televised' – an invocation against the brain candy of television (in the album *The Revolution Will Not Be Televised*, Flying Dutchman Records).

7 Foucault (1979: 216) quotes Julius's description of the panopticon principle: 'solution of a technical problem' in appearance, but in fact 'a whole type of society emerges' (N. H. Julius [1831] *Leçons sur les prisons*, pp. 384–6).

8 See also Newman (1983).

9 See Jos Boys (1989).

10 Not everyone delights in the soothing purity of unadorned white walls. In a memorable passage in Bret Easton Ellis's novel *Less than Zero*, the narrator describes his state of mind during a period of emotional and drug-frenzied breakdown as 'empty rooms and white walls' (1985: 127).

11 It is widely reported that Le Corbusier tacitly accepted credit for E.1027 by *not* crediting Gray for the site of his mural.

8

Having it all?

A question of collaborative housing

Inga-Lisa Sangregorio

'But what would you do if you were free to decide? What kind of houses would you design and build?' The question was asked at the end of a long evening. Nobody seemed inclined to answer it, and the meeting, which had been arranged by a group of women architects, ended with a question mark.

More than twenty years have passed since that evening. Although I am not an architect I had been invited along with other women interested in planning and architecture from a woman's point of view. Most of the evening had passed in complaints about the apparently dismal situation of women architects: lower salaries, slower careers and less credit for their work than male colleagues. Those of us who were more interested in the subject-matter than in other women's careers became impatient. We had heard it all before, from women in other professions. We did not doubt that women architects were discriminated against, as were women doctors, women journalists and women factory workers.

But what interested us in this context was something else. Was it possible to design and build houses and cities that would promote equality and make everyday life less burdensome? One of the catchwords of the women's movement at that time was 'We want it all'. And we did want it all. Careers and children, bread and roses.

Privacy and community

Although that meeting ended without answers, it inspired some of the women to try to explore the question further. A group of ten – architects, researchers, journalists – was formed, most of us with a background in the women's movement and with a growing interest in environmental questions.

We looked with a mixture of astonishment and despair at what was being built at the time. In spite of the fact that more and more women worked outside the home, and in defiance of the oil crisis and a growing awareness of the need to save energy, the prevailing type of new housing was single-family houses sited far from jobs and services, thus necessitating two cars. A combination of high inflation and tax relief favoured the heavily mortgaged one-family house. We felt that it was urgent to find attractive alternatives, better suited to both social and environmental needs.

Plate 8.1 Spring in the suburb of Hallonbergen:
Anna Sjödahl (property of the Museum of Boras)

One night we left the general considerations aside and asked how we ourselves would like to live if we had a choice. The answers were surprisingly similar, in spite of the fact that we were of widely different ages (from late twenties to middle fifties) and living in various kinds of families (married, single and cohabiting, with and without children).

The ideal dwelling, as we saw it, was one that would offer both privacy and community. We were not prepared to move into the kind of communes that were fairly common in the 1970s, where groups of people moved into big villas, sharing kitchen, bathrooms and living rooms, with only bedrooms remaining private. We wanted our own kitchens and bathrooms, and we wanted to be able to shut the door of our private flat. But we also wanted to open that door, in order to solve some of the practical problems of daily life in collaboration with others. We were prepared to give up some private space and equipment in return for space and equipment shared with others.

We named our group *Bo i gemenskap* (Live in community), abbreviated BIG, and set out to create a housing model that would be both desirable and feasible. What we were looking for, like many women and some men before us, was some kind of *cohousing*. I use this handy term coined by two American architects (McCamant and Durrett 1994) rather than the clumsier 'collective housing' with its slightly bolshevik connotations. By cohousing I mean housing with common facilities and shared solutions to practical problems like child-care and cooking.

The old type of cohousing

During this period the residents of the few surviving examples of an earlier type of cohousing were fighting a losing battle to save their homes. The first house of this type was built in central Stockholm in the middle of the 1930s, after an intense public debate. The initiative came from a group of radical intellectuals. This first house had fifty-seven flats, most of them rather small. There was a restaurant and a nursery, and a sun terrace on the roof. A staff of more than twenty people catered to the needs of the residents. Meals could be eaten in the restaurant, or in one's private flat. A special feature of the house was the 'food elevator' used for sending the hot food up to the kitchenettes of the private flats, and for sending down the dirty dishes after the meal. The children were cared for by a staff of professional people in the well-equipped nursery and could even pass the night there when their parents were having an evening out. There was also a laundry and a cleaning service. The residents could throw their dirty laundry down the laundry chute and get it back washed and ironed.

Today this sounds quite absurd, but at the time the alternative would probably have been fifty-seven housewives and/or fifty-seven maids. Public day-care did not exist, and housekeeping was more burdensome than today. The truly revolutionary idea behind this house was that women are entitled to some free time. Instead of coming home to a second workday, the working wives and mothers would have the same privileges as most men have always had: finding their dinner ready, their children well cared for, their clothes washed and ironed, and their home clean. I once met a woman doctor who lived in the house as a young wife and mother. Even fifty years later she blessed it for saving her from having to take on the duties of the housewife. The idea that men might take any part in domestic work seems to have been a thought so revolutionary that not even the most radical of the radicals could think it.

There was, of course, the problem of 'upstairs and downstairs'. But to give some kind of context, the 'upstairs' was not very luxurious, since the people living in the house had reduced their private dwellings to the absolutely essential, and the staff 'downstairs' were probably better off than they would have been doing the same job in private homes.

From service to collaboration

A handful of houses with shared facilities and a paid staff were built in the following decades. They were bigger than the first house, since experience had shown that more people were required to share the costs of the staff. In the best-known of those houses, the so-called family hotel at Hässelby (1955), there are 328 flats. On the whole these houses were a success, and people who lived in them became warm proponents of this type of housing. When I myself was struggling to combine a full-time job with two small children, I used to envy the happy few who lived in these mythical houses. However, there were so few of them that they loomed like mirages over the desert, and they had virtually no impact on what was being built in the following decades. They did not fit into the ideology of either the right or the left.

In the middle of the 1970s came the final blow. The new owner of Hässelby and another similar house decided to close the restaurants. To him the restaurant was simply a complication he did not want to be bothered with, but to the residents it was much more than a purveyor of meals. It was the heart of the house, a place where people met without having to plan it, in an unpretentious daily contact that was the basis of everything else that made Hässelby a very special house.

The residents decided to fight not only for their own house but also for the very idea of cohousing, organising a PR-campaign and a series of public meetings. Since they thought it essential not to give up the restaurant they themselves took over the cooking. It was seen as a temporary solution, but much to their surprise they found that it had many advantages. It proved much less difficult to cook for many people than they had imagined, and they found it was fun to work together. The meals became cheaper, and the residents themselves could decide how long they wanted to keep the dining-room open at night. The potential clash of interest between the staff and the residents had disappeared: there was no longer an 'upstairs' and a 'downstairs' (Sangregorio 1995). Without intending to then, the Hässelby people thus became the first to try out a new type of cohousing, based on collaboration among residents rather than on service from a paid staff. Let us call it *collaborative housing*.

The 'BIG model'

To the women of the *Bo i gemenskap* group the Hässelby experience was an important source of inspiration. We had contacts with the Hässelby people and followed their struggle to save the restaurant. We also visited and were inspired by Danish cohousing units (*bofællesskaber*), which usually consist of a group of small houses with a bigger common house with facilities like dining-room, children's playroom, laundry and workshops. What impressed us in the Danish experience were the unbureaucratic solutions. Whereas Hässelby and its sister houses had been run by the owners, who organised the service and had the final say on most issues, the Danish *bofællesskaber* were organised and run by the residents. No outside authority could decide on whether they could have their meals together or how the common house was used. It was all organised from below, by the residents themselves.

Gradually there was a change of consciousness in our group. We felt less and less attracted by a house with a paid staff providing service to the residents. 'The BIG model', as it has become known in Sweden, emerged: cohousing based on collaboration rather than on service. There were basically three kinds of consideration guiding our search for better solutions to the problems of everyday life.

- One was purely practical: the small nuclear family trying to cater for too many needs and perform too many duties simply is not a very intelligent solution to the practical problems of modern life. Even couples intent on sharing housework and child care tend to be caught in a zero sum game.
- The second consideration had to do with resources. The size of the average household was rapidly shrinking. It seemed absurd that each small household, often consisting of only one person, should have within its own walls not only a growing number of square meters but also all the equipment that one needs only occasionally. Why did one have to own a lot of things privately when having access to them would do just as well and perhaps better?
- The third consideration grew out of the first two. Sharing some space and equipment would give more for less, and taking turns on daily tasks like cooking the evening meal would make everyday life easier. But working together would also lead to natural contacts between neighbours.

The BIG model is based on the extremely simple idea of maximising resources or getting 'more for less' by sharing and collaboration (Berg *et al.* 1982). Residents have their own private flats, complete with kitchen and bathroom, but they also share some common space and equipment and collaborate on daily tasks. In the years before and after the book was published we met with groups of people in different parts of Sweden interested in cohousing. We wrote articles, gave speeches and even appeared on television. We also interviewed people in positions of responsibility trying to find out what the obstacles were. There seemed to be none, formally at least: it was all in the mind.

The book the group published contains examples of how the common areas can be used and how the collaboration between residents can be organised, but an important part of the idea is that it is, indeed, an idea, not a house. Or rather not *one* house, but many different houses, built and organised according to the residents' needs. At that time the first house fitting the description already existed, a converted multistorey house named *Stacken* ('The ant hill') located in the suburb of Bergsjön outside Gothenburg. The dream had come true, although in a not very dreamlike suburb.

Two factors contributed to the creation of *Stacken*. One was the personal interest and professional competence of Lars Ågren, then professor of architecture at the Chalmers school of architecture. For several years BIG members had close contact with Lars Ågren, exchanging ideas, information and mutual inspiration. Without his contacts and knowledge of how to overcome different bureaucracies it would no doubt have taken longer to implement the idea. The other factor was that at the time there were empty houses in Gothenburg, and the house that became *Stacken* was one of them. The owner, a public housing company, did not run a great risk, since the alternatives were worse.

Bergsjön, where *Stacken* is located, is a rather low-status suburb, but the idea of cohousing proved attractive enough to overcome this handicap. A group interested in collaborative housing was formed, with Lars Ågren being one of the members, and the house was renovated according to the wishes of the group. The result was a house with thirty-three flats, a restaurant-type kitchen, dining-room, several workshops and a co-operatively run day-care centre. The residents took turns cooking five nights a week and also took over most of the maintenance and management of the house, thus keeping rents low.

The very existence of *Stacken* blazed a trail. It proved that collaborative housing was a feasible idea and that bureaucratic difficulties could be overcome. Anyone interested in the idea could visit the house and talk to the people who lived there.

The idea put into practice

Since then between forty and fifty similar houses have been built in different parts of Sweden, and more are on the way. In a recent book members of the BIG group present and compare fifteen cohousing projects (Lundahl and Sangregorio 1992). We chose houses that differ considerably, in size, ownership and organisation, located in different parts of Sweden, and in city centres as well as suburbs. They all have common facilities and some kind of collaboration among residents, but in other respects they are quite different.

Among the shared facilities found in most houses are a well-equipped kitchen, a big dining-room that is also used for other activities, guest-rooms, workshops, laundry and sauna. Many but not all have day-care in the house. Most people living in the houses agree that workshops are not essential, whereas a common kitchen and a dining-room are. Still, it is nice to have access to a designated area and good tools for, say, carpentry or for developing photographs. One house has a music room, others have computers, fax machines, photocopiers and are linked to the Internet. Others have gyms and solariums. Pooling resources gives people with moderate incomes access to what would otherwise have been impossible luxuries.

Normally the common space is 'paid for' by somewhat reducing the size of the private dwellings or by choosing a smaller-size flat. A woman who lives alone describes it like this: 'I have 37 square meters of my own, and I have access to 350 square meters that I share with 43 new friends' (for the idea here expressed see Lundahl and Sangregorio 1992). Residents take turns preparing evening meals, in some cases every weekday, in other cases less often. They take care of the common facilities, and in some cases they have taken over most of the maintenance and management of the house. This allows them a substantial rent refund every year, which is normally used for investments like garden furniture, a big screen television, a greenhouse and so on. One of the houses recently bought an expensive encyclopedia for the library.

1 Entrance hall
2 Kitchen
3 Dining room
4 Library, multi-purpose room
5 Weaving room
6 Laundry
7 Workshop

N

0 1 2   5

Figure 8.1 Plan of major common spaces of the ground floor of Färdknäppen:
architect Jan Lundquist, Arkitekter AB

11   Sitting room

Guest room   10

1–9

Sauna, Large bathroom,
Photo lab., Storage

Figure 8.2   A-A section, Färdknäppen: architect Jan Lundquist, Arkitekter AB

Men and women participate in the work on equal terms, as individuals. With shared work everyday life becomes less of a burden, and people get to know each other well, which in its turn creates positive spin-offs. A member of BIG, divorced with grown-up children and a management job with long hours and frequent travel, moved into one of the houses in the summer of 1994. She has a pleasant flat of her own, just as she had in the 'normal' house where she used to live, but she adds: 'The great difference is that here I feel at home as soon as I enter the front door. The whole house is my home.' In her house evening meals – very good meals – are served on Monday through Friday. The residents take turns cooking and are responsible for the cleaning and upkeep of the common areas, as well as for the small garden in front of the house. She has calculated that she dedicates an average of two hours a week to the collaborative work.

> One week out of six I am responsible for the cooking, together with five other people. We plan the meals, buy the food (except staple goods), cook, wash the dishes and clean the kitchen. The other five weeks I don't have to think of cooking weekdays, unless I want to, I come home to a good meal and good company, and I can bring guests if I want to. I also belong to the garden group, since I love plants and flowers and making things grow.

There is a growing interest in ecology amongst residents in the houses, shown by composts and greenhouses and also by buying vegetables, fruit and sometimes meat and other provisions from producers using ecologically sound methods of production. With shared space and equipment resources are saved too – four washing machines instead of forty, the sharing of cars, fewer packages. Since most of the houses are in cities or dense suburbs there is not much room for growing one's own vegetables, but outside some of the houses residents have planted herbs, berries and fruit trees.

It would be a lie to pretend that there are no conflicts. In some cases they have been quite serious, causing people to leave in anger. But on the whole residents have managed to find forms of collaboration that are acceptable to everybody and that make life easier and warmer.

Who, then, is attracted by the idea of cohousing? What kinds of people live in these houses? There is a tendency to consider collaborative housing a middle-class idea, and it is true that you do not find many 'blue-collar' working-class members in cohousing. If, however, 'working-class' is taken in a broader sense, including, for example, hospital workers and other predominantly female low-income workers, the picture changes. In most, perhaps all, of the houses there are more people working with ideas or with other people than with things, but since the houses are quite different their residents differ as well. Even if one could say that some of the houses have residents who are on the whole more 'privileged' than those of others, all collaborative houses have one important thing in common: a surprising and stimulating mixture of people who would not normally have come into such close contact with each other.

It is also important to understand that these small communities are not static but, on the contrary, very dynamic. People move, houses change and are influenced by developments in society as a whole. Unemployment and the economic crisis in general have had greater impact on houses located in suburbs like Bergsjön. Today's *Stacken* is less prosperous than the *Stacken* of fifteen years ago – but it has preserved its vitality.

Collaborative housing has attracted many parents, both couples and single parents (mostly women but also some men), with small children. Being a child – and a parent! – in a house like that is no doubt more enjoyable and easier than in an ordinary house. There is often day-care in the house, and the informal contacts make finding a babysitter easy. Some people felt they would prefer a house where there are not quite as many 3-year-olds disturbing the peace and took the initiative to build a similar house for 'the second half of life', with a lower age limit of 40. This house, *Färdknäppen*, in the centre of Stockholm, has proved a great success. It is not a house without children since children visit there but they do not dominate as much as in some of the other houses. About half the people in *Färdknäppen* are professionally active, the others are retired but very active in other ways.

A realistic model

Why, then, did the seemingly impossible become possible? Why were housing companies willing to try out what they had formerly refused? The main reason is that this is a more realistic model than the old type of cohousing. The two models have important characteristics in common: sharing space and equipment, organising some of the daily tasks on a collective basis. But whereas the older houses required a staff of specialists, which led to bigger and bigger houses in order to get a sufficient number of people to pay their salaries, the new type of houses are based on collaboration among the residents, which favours fairly small houses and considerably increases the options. Thirty or forty flats can be fitted into an infill project, or into a renovated older building. The owner takes no great risk and does not have to launch into unknown fields. He provides only the housing, not the cooking. Residents of the new cohousing projects have proved to be strong but competent tenants, taking good care of the houses and leaving housing companies with practically no losses due to empty flats.

An interesting fact is that some of the best cohousing projects are to be found in renovated houses. Houses built from the 1920s to the 1960s have been converted into well-functioning collaborative houses. One would expect new houses, designed for the purpose, to offer superior architectural solutions to the needs of cohousing, but so far this has not always been the case. One reason may be that future residents have had more say in the process of remodelling older houses, another that it is perhaps easier to imagine what the result will be when starting from something tangible like an existing house.

Another interesting thing about the Swedish experience in cohousing is that most of these houses are built and owned by public housing companies. It is true that rented housing is common in Sweden, but traditionally housing companies have been quite paternalistic and inclined to make decisions over the heads of the tenants. The cohousing experience has proved that tenants can have great influence over and take great responsibility for their housing, in spite of not owning the houses.

This undoubtedly is a way of living that encourages domestic equality between men and women. Once you move housework out of the nuclear family, hidebound traditions disappear. Men and women do their share as individual adults. In the old type of cohousing, with a paid staff, gender conflicts were 'solved', or rather hidden, by having the housework done by somebody else, mostly by other women. Perhaps the fact that collaborative housing promotes equality in this way explains why the idea seems to be more popular among women than among men. It is true that several men have played an important role in promoting cohousing. But it is also true that there is a majority of women in virtually all the cohousing projects. This, however, seems rather to reflect prejudice among men *not* living in this type of housing than disappointment among the ones who do. Perhaps the reluctant men fear that they would lose some privileges by choosing cohousing, whereas men who actually live in the houses are as enthusiastic as women.

Looking back it is easy to see that collaborative housing fits into a long tradition of women's dreams and practice. Evelyne Sullerot, *grande dame* of French feminist research, once asked young career-oriented women students what kind of housing they would prefer. Much to her surprise many of them mentioned the kibbutz. This was in the 1960s, and the kibbutz was probably the only form of 'cohousing' they had heard of. But Sullerot, who in her book *Demain les femmes* ('Tomorrow the women') compares women's position in different types of societies, maintains that communal solutions are more favourable to women as a group than more individualistic ones (Sullerot 1965). She does not deny that some women may benefit more from individual solutions, but her comparative studies show that women as a group have more to gain from collective solutions.

Dolores Hayden has studied men's and women's utopias in her book *Seven American Utopias* (Hayden 1976). The male utopias of the type described there are often completely new societies, embracing all aspects of life and created in new places, whereas the ideas promoted by the 'material feminists' presented in her *The Grand Domestic Revolution* (Hayden 1981) are more pragmatic and based on taking small steps towards a better society. 'For six decades the material feminists expounded one powerful idea: that women must create feminist homes with socialized housework and child care before they could become truly equal members of society', Hayden summarises, 1981: 3). Few women could or would leave everything to create a completely new society from nothing; they would rather try to improve things where they lived, changing daily life in a more modest and therefore more realistic way.

The collaborative houses of the BIG model belong in this latter tradition. They are no grand solution to all our problems, but they are a step in the right direction, and they show the enormous potential of co-operation on a neighbourhood basis.

III

OUTSIDE POSSIBILITIES: CULTURAL PLANNING

De La Warr Pavilion, Bexhill-on-Sea, Sussex:
Rosa Ainley

What role do women play in the construction of spaces of cultural enjoyment; how do perceptions of safety limit their use and enjoyment; what are the limitations on the pursuit of leisure through restrictive practices and discrimination; and what paradoxes are encountered in an attempt to provide lesbian cultural and social 'safe space'? This group of chapters visits and provides a commentary on various sites of pleasure/ leisure as well as looking at representations of space.

Tracey Skelton's work on the representation of women in ragga in the mainstream media of the United Kingdom challenges perceived norms of gendered behaviour in Jamaica, while the historical context in Jamaica gives this contemporary trend a transcendence of time and space. Focusing on the performers Lady Saw and Patra she uses newspaper and film/TV coverage of 'women in ragga' to show a picture of deliberate disruption of the music's misogynistic tendencies, and parody of and rebellion against them.

Moving to Sydney, Affrica Taylor charts the deepening fissures that appear in the notion of 'lesbian community' once the highly charged question of who is to be within/excluded from such a community arises. Ultimately, the instability of the terms 'space' and 'lesbian' becomes gapingly apparent as the attempt to fix identity in place runs aground. 'Identity politics is', she demonstrates, 'not firm ground on which to build or maintain a permanent physical space.' Her account grasps the full import of spatial metaphor, as used to attempt to shore up two highly volatile political concepts.

Urban woodlands, while highly valued and fiercely protected, do not always offer a site for easy enjoyment and recreation. Jacquelin Burgess looks at how fear of crime and feelings of unsafety inhibit the possibility of this pleasure, using the Woods Project as a case study. The project explores experiences in a range of focus group discussions and produces recommendations which could allow a wider cross-section of the urban population to enjoy using woodland spaces.

'But is it worth taking the risk?'

How women negotiate access to urban woodland: a case study

Jacquelin Burgess

The 1990s are witnessing a revival of professional and political interest in soft urban landscapes: the parks, gardens, greenways, commons and woods which fill the in-between spaces of cities. These spaces have suffered sorely from a combination of development pressure, neglect and disinvestment over the last thirty years. One important factor in the revival has been a sustained campaign by a coalition of groups fighting to retain or enhance a place for nature in cities, and a recognition of the personal, social and cultural benefits that accrue from everyday contact with the natural world (see Harrison *et al.* 1987; Ageyman 1988; Cooper-Marcus and Francis 1990; Greenhalgh and Worpole 1995). One element in the new greening strategy has been the establishment of twelve community forests, a national land-use and landscaping initiative involving the Countryside Commission, local authorities and private sector partners, to create extensive wooded landscapes on the fringes of large conurbations in the UK. Of particular concern is the extent to which public perceptions of risk might impede the welcome local communities would give to new woodlands (Walker 1993). In 1989, the UK Home Office Working Group on fear of crime had recommended that 'public sector and private environmental projects should only go ahead if it is clear that the reduction of crime and fear has been properly addressed' (1989: 43). As far as I am aware, the Woods Project I want to discuss in this chapter was the first time a substantial commitment has been given by a public agency to gain a better understanding of how fear of crime might hinder community acceptance of a landscape initiative.

More naturalistic settings, especially woodlands, are among the most highly valued landscapes, in terms of personal pleasures, sense of well-being and contact with nature they afford people. But they are also the setting in which many people feel anxiety either for themselves or their loved ones (Schroeder and Anderson 1984; Talbot and Kaplan 1984; Burgess *et al.* 1988). At the same time, evidence from crime surveys and police records suggests that parks and green spaces are settings where criminal events are least likely to occur (Mayhew and Maung 1993; Mirrlees-Black *et al.* 1996). How are we to account for this ambiguity: that the landscapes which give people so much pleasure should also be construed as the least safe to be in? And what might be done to lessen people's anxieties so as to increase potential access across all social groups? This is the theme of the chapter. The argument is based on the premise that what is perceived to be real, is real in its consequences. In the worst case, people will be totally incapacitated by their anxieties and unable to use green spaces at all. In the majority of cases, individuals have developed coping strategies to help them access the pleasures of being in greenspace. Two aims of the Woods Project were to facilitate a better understanding of the barriers and constraints to recreation in woodland landscapes; and to produce recommendations for landscape designers and community forest managers which could increase the opportunities for a wider cross-section of urban communities to enjoy being in the woods.

Access to greenspace: methodological questions

Access to greenspace involves more than physical accessibility: there are also significant economic, social and cultural factors in play which help explain whether different social groups are able to use and enjoy urban greenspace (Harrison *et al.* 1995). Among these factors, anxieties about personal safety seem to be playing an increasingly important part, corroding the pleasures that people experience in parks and green spaces. The methodological challenges for work on perceptions of risk in greenspace are not insignificant since public concerns vary by geographical location, by gender, age and ethnicity; and by the extent to which green spaces are embedded in the spatial patterns of everyday life. There is growing consensus that observational techniques, experimental methods such as landscape preference measures, statistically representative social surveys and theoretically informed case studies need to be combined to give a more complete understanding of what is a highly complex issue (Lee 1991; Carr *et al.* 1992; Greenhalgh and Worpole 1995). In our work on popular meanings and values for urban parks and green spaces in Greenwich, for example, we triangulated results between four in-depth discussion groups with people living in localities chosen for their different quantities and qualities of greenspace; a formal questionnaire survey of residents in the borough; and structured interviews with providers to explore the extent to which local people's values and concerns resonated with their own understanding and priorities (Burgess *et al.* 1988).

In designing the Woods Project, my experiences in Greenwich led me to believe that single-gender, group discussions would be a suitable forum for people to discuss a range of anxieties they might have about woods and other environmental settings. But, at the same time, it was important to acknowledge that many people might not have personal experiences of walking in woods, so there was a need to provide that opportunity as part of the research programme. I therefore decided to begin with a 'site-visit' (in this case, a walk of about an hour through a local wood), followed immediately with a focus group discussion; bringing people together and 'grounding' their discussions in a shared, landscape experience. There is also the not insignificant factor that for the majority of women and young people, the normal way in which they would experience a woodland landscape would be in the company of others.

I will provide only a brief account of the methodology here (see Burgess 1995 and 1996). Recognising the importance of locality and geographical context, two sites were chosen for the study: Bestwood country park on the edge of Nottingham, and Bencroft-Wormley Woods just north of the M25 on the edge of the Lea Valley Regional Park in London. A total of thirteen woodland visits and group discussions were conducted, seven in Bencroft and six in Bestwood. The groups were chosen to represent a range of different social and cultural experiences, as well as different class and geographical backgrounds. In total, there were nine groups of women, differentiated by age and ethnicity, and four groups of men, differentiated by age. The project entailed many hours of discussion with these different groups – users and non-users of woodlands; women and men; young people and those in later years; women of Asian and Afro-Caribbean communities as well as white women. Their voices and stories ground the account that follows.

Fear of crime in public places

> But if there are two Asians, a man and a woman, then you do get these looks from the white community. Whereas, when I was walking there – all of us together – I was feeling as if I was walking in my own village back home. . . . But I don't think I would go and take my children there. Maybe it's because I'm worried about the safety of my children and the safety of myself. Because no matter what I do, I can't change the colour of my skin. And I might be picked up. You never know, there might be a few gangs who all come to the woods, and I might be picked up for 'fun's sake', or something like that. But I would like to go there and take my children out for a walk.
> (Asian Women's Group, 20–50, Bencroft Wood)

Environmental criminology seeks to establish patterns between types of criminal activity and the spatial distributions of crime, together with work that seeks to understand the relationships between specific built environmental features and criminal activities (Smith 1986; Evans *et al.* 1992; Herbert 1993). Criminologists have long been concerned with relationships between crime and the city. The literature is overwhelmingly concerned with urban populations and built environments; the spatial distributions of specific types of criminal activity in different urban neighbourhoods or 'hot spots'; and the extent to which it is possible to design out crime in urban environments (Newman 1972; Geason and Wilson 1989). The results of these studies confirm that the neighbourhoods with the highest crime levels are the inner cities and poorer council estates. It is widely recognised, however, that crime statistics can give only a partial picture of the true incidence and location of criminal acts. Not everyone will regard a crime as important enough to report; certain groups within the population may feel themselves unable to go to the police; and the willingness to report specific types of crime, such as rape, for example, will vary over time and with the amount of publicity given to those particular crimes.

The British Crime Survey (BCS), funded by the Home Office, carries out three-yearly surveys of very large samples of the population in the UK (see Mirrlees-Black *et al.* 1996). The results show a consistent pattern in which crimes against property form by far the largest category (75 per cent in 1996) while cases of violent crime were steady at approximately 6 per cent of total crimes recorded. As the BCS and other studies show (Pawson 1993, for example), the spaces where women are actually most at risk of physical assault and rape are domestic spaces, and the people they are most in danger from are men known to them rather than strangers. The BCS statistics show that the absolute incidence of crime in parks, commons and open spaces is extremely low – so much so that it falls within the bounds of statistical error (Mayhew and Maung 1993). For the same reason, of the 3,500 projects completed under the UK Safe Cities programme, only a handful have focused on parks (see Burgess 1995; Greenhalgh and Worpole 1996). On this evidence, parks and green spaces are some of the safest spaces in the city. Still, both large-scale social surveys (Hough 1995) and small-scale qualitative case-studies reveal strongly held beliefs that women and children are more likely to be victims of violent crime than men, and that public spaces are more dangerous for them than domestic settings (Garofalo 1981; Stanko 1987; Pain 1991, 1995; Ferraro 1996). So, might it be argued that physical spaces are unfairly stigmatised as being dangerous, or are there other factors contributing to women's anxieties which are not being captured effectively in some of this research? Both physical and social factors contribute to anxieties about personal safety in green spaces. I shall deal with each in turn.

Physical dimensions of risk perception in urban greenspace and woodlands

JB: We walked through the bit where the broom grows right over the path, and some of the girls thought it was really quite scary.

Kathie: I always think that's really pretty. If ever I'm surveying a walk and I come across a wood and there's an arch with everything growing over, I always walk down it. It's beautiful. I've got to use that path.

Brenda: But for me, it would feel restrictive. I would appreciate the beauty of it, but the sense of security . . .

Kathie: Perhaps you could only go down it with other people.

Irene: If you can see your way out of it, if it's not a long pathway, it might be possible.

Jessie: I think the key to it all is sight, being able to see all around you, not just in front. . . . A lot of these trails again are straight and they've got banks at the side, perhaps overgrown – there's no way out, is there? There aren't lots of paths like there are here, where you can perhaps turn a corner and find somebody. It's a lot more enclosed, isn't it?

JB: So you need to be able to get away?

Jessie: Yes, you need the space.

Brenda: I think that's why the footpaths give you a sense of confidence here, because they are wide.

(Mature women, 45-65, Nottingham)

Research shows that the fear of crime is partly to be accounted for by aspects of the physical design of the built environment. The Safe Cities projects completed in Canada, the USA, the UK, Europe and Australia show how important it is to design spaces so people do not feel enclosed or trapped; and where they can exercise control through effective surveillance of their surroundings (Newman 1972; Grant 1989; Valentine 1990; Safe City 1992). Lack of sightlines impedes the visual permeability of the urban environment while small, confined areas such as stairwells and cul-de-sacs are particularly threatening as hiding and entrapment points. Poor lighting is the major problem in public open space, garages, subways and so on, and has a fundamental effect on the extent to which people can read clues about strangers and maintain personal control (Painter 1991; Gardner 1994).

In the Woods Project I had the opportunity to explore just how people responded to the physical qualities of a wooded landscape and so ascertain why those qualities might give rise to feelings of anxiety. The fundamental physical quality of woods and forests which distinguishes them from all

Plate 9.1 Enjoying parkland in company, focus group participants, Lea Valley Regional Park: Jacquelin Burgess

other landscape types is that of enclosure. Enclosure is a characteristic of features such as the density of tree growth/planting schemes; tree species; the height of trees; the thickness of the tree canopy and the density of the understorey. These natural and physical properties create different strengths of lightness and shade, and a closure of views. Of themselves, the physical characteristics of woods have no meaning, but they cannot exist independent of the language, discourses and practices through which societies construct meanings for nature. Thus, for example, qualities of enclosure will be understood and used by a forester to achieve a particular set of goals – perhaps the thinning of trees to allow the regeneration of native flora at ground level. A landscape architect will seek to create a particular aesthetic response through the manipulation of different densities of planting. In both instances, these professionals are also members of a society which imputes certain negative attributes to woods and forests that they may well find difficult to understand.

For the women, men and teenagers who participated in the Woods Project, woodland enclosure was experienced as offering many different places where individuals who might constitute a threat to personal safety could hide. At the same time, people interpreted qualities of enclosure as preventing or inhibiting possible escape because routes are blocked by vegetation, there are inadequate paths, and people cannot see far enough to orientate themselves. Finally, one of the main recreational strengths of woodlands is the capacity of the landscape to absorb much higher numbers of people without its feeling 'crowded'. But for many people in the project, feeling enclosed obscures the presence of other people and makes individuals feel more isolated and alone than they might really be. How strongly individuals react to feeling enclosed by the wood provides one important key to unlocking different levels and intensities of fears about being in woods and forests. It helps account for the extent to which individuals experience a sense of adventure and desire to explore the wood; and how much woods and forests are experienced and appreciated for their 'naturalness' and 'wildness'. And it was clear, listening to the group members' discussions, that similar feelings are aroused by overgrown, dense shrubby spaces embedded in the urban fabric, as well as larger parks and wooded settings.

Thus, the three features which connote the most fearful and most dangerous spaces of the built environment, especially for women, are intrinsic qualities of the physical character of woods and forests. Woods are darker than open settings and visibility is considerably reduced; trees, bushes and tall shrubs are all potential hiding places while narrow paths blocked by thick or prickly vegetation to the side can create the sense of entrapment. Most people spend most of their lives in cities, and have developed a finely tuned sensitivity to built environments. One part, therefore, of women's responses to woodland environments reflects their practical consciousness of how to remain safe in city streets and open spaces. At the same time, to 'design out' the intrinsic woodland features to enable them to feel safer would mean destroying the character of the wood. This is the crux of the physical problem. Experiencing the special qualities of woods is very important for the psychological and social well-being of very many different groups of people, especially those living in cities. It is similar to the problem recognised in the context of large, urban parks. 'The ability to escape the city in parks, including ravines and other forms of urban wilderness, is essential to many urban-dwellers' health. The issue is to create a choice and for the user to be in control' (Safe City 1992: 40). The key is the creation of choice – and for individuals to be in control rather than feeling they are vulnerable to unprovoked attack. Much can be done through good landscaping and design (Storey 1991; Burgess 1995).

But design and landscaping must be supported by much higher levels of maintenance than currently exist in many green spaces. People like to see 'natural' untidiness like fallen logs, tree stumps and brambles in woods. What both offends and disturbs them are the 'environmental incivilities' such as litter, graffiti, abandoned or burnt-out cars, drug needles, broken fences and vandalised buildings which signify a lack of social control and 'ownership' of public space (Herbert 1993; Greenhalgh and Worpole 1996). But the relationship is not as deterministic as implied in some studies: perceptions of risk will not be ameliorated entirely by design and physical management interventions alone. The environmental setting is part of the context but I now go on to argue that social factors are much more significant in understanding anxieties in naturalistic settings. I will discuss three themes that emerged from the Woods study: encounters with

Plate 9.2 A powerful reminder of threatening visitors in countryside areas, Bencroft Wood, Herts: Jacquelin Burgess

strangers; the significance of 'flashing' in risk perceptions in public space; and the role of communication networks in disseminating and amplifying people's anxieties about personal safety.

Encounters with strangers

Penny: I love the forest and I'd love to go, but I'm frightened of going in there by myself. I really am, and my brothers don't always want to come with their little sister, so I can't go.

JB: What are you frightened of?

Penny: Well, I don't often see people when I've been in the forest. Like you might see the odd person walking their dog, but I've never seen a ranger. I don't know if this wood's got any, but I've never seen anyone looking after it. If I did meet a big man there, I mean it would be so easy to do things to me because there's no one around. I think that's very frightening.

(Penny, 16, Bencroft Wood)

Stanko (1987; Stanko and Hobdell 1993) make an important general point that recorded levels of fear of crime and risk of victimisation should alert us to general levels of threatening and violent behaviour by men against other men, as well as women and children. Strangers have become more threatening in public spaces over the last two decades for a number of reasons. Alcohol is now widely available and often consumed in parks/ green spaces; increasing numbers of mentally disturbed individuals are being 'cared for' in the community and often the local park will be the only place they can go to during the day; and at the same time, high levels of surveillance in the city centre, especially the privatised spaces of shopping malls, are driving so-called 'undesirable' people into the largely unpoliced parks (see Burgess 1994; Greenhalgh and Worpole 1995). Verbal abuse and the invasion of personal space is a routine and common experience for women and people of colour in public spaces. 'Insults, mockery, racial slurs, harassment and flirtatious sexual comments that assault a person's sense of order, propriety, and self respect awaken feelings of danger even when they contain no threat of actual physical violence' (Merry 1981: 143). Painter (1992) argues that local victim surveys show that women are not only proportionally more likely to be the victims of a wider range of crimes than men, but that women are subject to particular crimes and threats by virtue of their gender. She is not alone in arguing that sexual harassment is a common experience for women and that it creates particular anxieties for women and young girls when in open spaces.

All the women's groups in the Woods Project talked explicitly about their fears of being attacked by a man, or men, while the teenage boys and mature men also discussed their concerns about women's safety. The aggressors are usually described as 'maniacs, weirdos, nutters' with the clear implication that these are men who are out of control. Dealing with someone who is apparently not behaving rationally raises the level of risk and uncertainty because it is not possible to predict how he will behave. The mature women's group in Nottingham thought that some of the aggression against women was alcohol-related – a view which gained support from one of the young mothers who lived on the edge of Bestwood and often watched 'drunks go up. They take their bottles and you see them come back and they are drunk. That is one thing that does worry me – with the children coming home late.' The explanation offered is primarily that woods attract men who are not mentally stable, either through some kind of psychological deficiency or through alcohol, who are then able to take advantage of the cover provided by the woodland vegetation to prey on lone, vulnerable women and children. This line of reasoning is also advanced to account for the presence of men who expose themselves to women and children. But in this instance, there is a marked disagreement between men and women about the seriousness of this type of incident as I shall discuss in the following section.

Flashing: a crime of public space?

Perdita: It is such a horrible feeling though. It is so traumatic and dreadful. You don't want to bother risking it for the sake of having a walk.
Sophie: It is imposing on you and your space.
Sarah: It is as if they have got no control at all.
Gina: They take one look at you . . .
Sophie: Men have got some urges, but they have got a little bit of control, surely?
Jane: I've been flashed at – when I was working (in the park). The man was masturbating when he was flashing at me. It made me feel sick.

(Young mothers, 21–35, London)

Incidents of males exposing their genitals to women and children are not often reported to police, neither are they regarded as serious enough to figure in surveys such as BCS, even though flashing appears to be a widespread and common experience in public space. Feminists argue that such behaviour signifies the extent to which green spaces and the countryside are male territories, and that any women who have the temerity to use them are 'asking for trouble'. As Jeffrys writes: 'The real effects of flashing are *expected* to be a restriction of the freedom of women. The legacy of flashing in childhood is anxiety and fear, of strange men, of open spaces. In adulthood the message is the same' (quoted McNeill 1987: 107). In her study of 100 women in Leeds, McNeill found that 63 per cent recalled having seen a flasher, and 43 per cent more than once. Similar proportions were found by Valentine (1992), and would also accord with women's experiences in the Woods Project. McNeill also notes that of 233 incidents, only 14 were reported to the police.

In terms of time and location, most incidents of exposure reported in these studies took place in the afternoon/early evening, and primarily in streets, parks and wider countryside. There were variations in the appearance and behaviour of the men involved: some were totally nude, some jumped out at women from a hiding spot, and some tried to speak to the woman before exposing themselves. Evidence suggests that the context in which the event occurred was significant in how the women dealt with it. If one of the women was on her own, in a deserted place, and if the man was masturbating, the sense of fear and panic was heightened. McNeill argues that the primary fear women have in these situations is not of rape but death, and the shock and outrage felt are a reminder that they are so vulnerable.

In the Woods Study, women spoke angrily of their disgust, shock and fury at being assaulted in this manner. But these feelings are overlain by risk and uncertainties, especially in terms of how 'sane' did the man appear to be? Were there people around to hear a call for help? What were the options for escape? Men tell women that flashers are 'harmless' and, in a case of repeated flashing in the Nottingham wood around the time of the research, the rangers had not thought it necessary to take any action. But if such individuals are deranged, then how can one guarantee that they will not one day become dangerous? At the same time, for the authorities to do nothing is to signify that such men have the right to invade women's personal space and destroy their sense of security in public spaces. Further, the immediate male response to stories of flashers is to laugh about them which disparages the sense of outrage women feel, and to suggest that women do not really mind, either. In the following extract, for example, the men's group in Nottingham, some of whom are voluntary rangers, described their experiences with another flasher. The group had also acknowledged that the 'problem' got worse in the summertime when children are at home from school and therefore more likely to be playing in the park.

> Ted: He would leap out at lady joggers. . . . [laughter].
> JB: He would leap out at lady joggers?
> Ted: Yes, just run alongside them, you know . . . [gesticulates/laughter]
> JB: Now you're laughing!
> Ted: Well they took it as a joke, actually. I weren't laughing, 'cos I was chasing the bloke, but he was running through nettles and brambles starkers, and I was near ripped to pieces with my clothes on!

It was often the case that women would giggle in recounting a flashing incident in the group discussions but this is best interpreted as a nervous reaction used in the retelling of events as a way of diminishing their stronger emotions. This is the response so often misinterpreted by men who would seek to trivialise flashing. But these incidents are not trivial in terms of their impact on women's behaviour in public spaces; many say they stop using parks and green spaces altogether. How much more frightening to be in woodlands where the vegetation offers so much more cover for the aggressor and there are so few people around? It is against this background that women must negotiate access to greenspace, and deal with the consequences should something happen to them or their children.

Communicative networks:
media and local understanding

JB: But you were saying, weren't you, that you used to walk but then you stopped?

Charlotte: Yes I did, particularly since Rachel Nickell died. I think that's what turned an awful lot of people away. A lot of my friends who, like me were reasonably [fades]. We didn't think about things like that. I think we felt, of all the people it shouldn't have happened to, it shouldn't happen to somebody like her – who was just walking, enjoying the countryside in a fairly well-used area.

Sarah: And with a child. You think – you've got your dog and you've got a child, and you're safe. I mean, you're not anywhere where you should be in any danger. In broad daylight. You're in a place where people are walking all the time.

Gina: It's like order and unity just went overnight.

(Young mothers, 21–30, Bencroft Wood)

The social processes through which local environments become commonly perceived as dangerous and a threat are important. Local gossip and knowledge of local events is of great importance in people's perceptions of risk in parks and green spaces (Valentine 1992). Women across the generations monitor and control each other's behaviour in public spaces. Their knowledge is drawn from talking to each other about things that have happened in the locality, set within the context of reports in the local media about crime, and the national media treatment of certain, highly newsworthy cases. In the Nottingham context, and indicative of the extent to which Bestwood is actually embedded within its locality, all the groups told us stories about dreadful things that were said to have happened in the park. Details were scant, however – a girl *might* have been raped; a body *might* have been found; *apparently* someone was murdered – but there was a sense when listening to people that these events were being reworked into a local myth. Certainly, and somewhat ironically, it seemed that the 'horror stories' in the mass media had more 'reality' and impact on people's evaluations of risk than this background history. By contrast, no one was able to provide any stories or information about what went on in Bencroft. The wood was not 'known' and therefore, not 'owned' in the same kind of way.

The mass media privilege and sensationalise rare, violent crimes against women and children that occur in urban parks and other green spaces, helping to stigmatise more naturalistic settings and reinforcing the sense of fear and anxiety. For example, the dreadful murder of Rachel Nickell who was sexually assaulted and then stabbed to death on Wimbledon Common on 15 July 1992 was mentioned in all the focus groups. The young mothers in London identified particularly strongly with this case as the quote at the start of the section shows. The case was particularly shocking for people because Rachel Nickell was 'obeying' all the 'rules' – out in the morning with a dog and a young child, and still she was murdered in the most brutal fashion. No wonder people feel devastated by these reports, as they further destabilise risk assessments. Has society become more dangerous? Are there more violent crimes against women and children today than there were, say, twenty years ago – or is it more a case of the ways in which the media present these events?

Detailed research by Soothill and Walby (1991) of the coverage of sex crimes in the media shows that during the 1980s such stories moved from being the staple diet of the *News of the World* to the mainstream press, especially the popular press. At the same time, coverage has expanded from just being a report of the court hearing to full-blown accounts of the event, the police search, the court case, and then, occasionally, what happened to the accused after he was found guilty. In the Nickell case, there was further coverage on the anniversary of her murder – *The Guardian* had a photograph of a young woman walking along a wooded path accompanied by a young child and a dog in a reconstruction of the event. Sex crimes are, in fact, no more or less common than in previous decades but the nature of the reports creates a public understanding that strangers have become much more dangerous than before, contributing to a general sense that things have got so much worse. This in turn leads to a racheting-up of risk perception which makes it more difficult for individuals to visit parks and green spaces as freely as they may have done before (Williams and Dickinson 1993). Sensationalist media coverage lowers the threshold at which women themselves, or their male partners, are prepared to jeopardise their own or their children's safety. Hence comments like this from Reena (see also Malik 1992):

> I used to go a lot to the Forest because we live next to it. But because these things are happening in the world, I stopped going there. I'm scared. I'm afraid. Anything can happen, any time. You never know.

Given these profound anxieties and the level of social pressure exerted on women and children, it is perhaps not surprising that access to woodlands is constrained. But people feel angry about the constraints, for the woodland landscapes offer some of the richest and most diverse encounters with nature, as well as maximum potential for children's adventure play. People develop a range of coping strategies to calm their anxieties and reduce the potential risk to which they would be exposed.

Strategies for coping with fear in parks and green spaces

Gill Valentine, in particular, has addressed the processes through which the threat of male violence has become associated with public spaces in the city, and her work is amply substantiated in more recent work, especially the Comedia parks study (Greenhalgh and Worpole 1995). Working with women in Reading, for example, she explores the connections between specific environmental contexts and the coping strategies women develop to

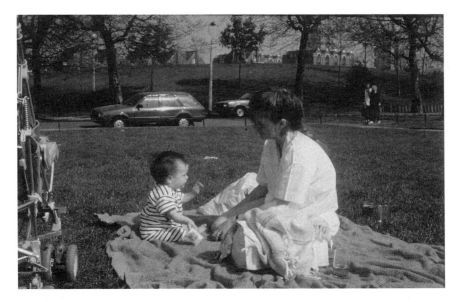

Plate 9.3 Newly created green spaces on the doorstep in inner London, Surrey Docks: Jacquelin Burgess

ensure their personal safety and the safety of their children. As she says, 'the predominant strategy . . . is the avoidance of perceived "dangerous places" at "dangerous times" ' (1989: 386). Valentine's work indicates that women perceive the most dangerous spaces during the daytime to be large open spaces, especially if they are lightly or infrequently used, including parks, woodlands, waste-ground, canals, rivers and countryside.

In the Woods Project, it was possible to identify a range of coping strategies that ease people's anxieties. For women and people of colour living in a predominantly racist society, developing such strategies is an integral part of growing up and learning how to conduct themselves in public space. Coping strategies range from a voluntary self-exclusion and not visiting the greenspace at all to taking a dog, children, a friend, male partner or son, so that one is not going alone. For Asian people, one other person may be insufficient to ensure feelings of safety. For almost everyone, feelings of relative safety are achieved by regulating time-space behaviours in terms, for example, of only using the main paths in the presence of other people; ensuring sightlines are clear; avoiding denser shrubbery/wooded areas if alone; using the space during the daytime, very rarely after dark. Walking in woods, women described high levels of micro-surveillance, continually monitoring their surroundings and maintaining a high level of vigilance over other users and the physical setting. For those with most confidence, strategies included using assertive body language and feeling in control of the geography of the space.

Underpinning these discussions is a sense that it is no longer possible to trust other people who may be present in green spaces. This pervasive feeling reflects a breakdown of one very important element of public life – the ability of women and men, children and adults from different social and cultural groups to be able to negotiate their rights to be in public places without fear of coming to harm. Any man on his own is perceived as a potential threat by women and children. As one of the men in the project said, somewhat bitterly: 'It's not some men they don't trust, it's all men.' One reason for the breakdown in trust is that part of male ideology that claims men can 'lose control' of themselves through excessive sexual 'desires' and/or alcohol, and therefore not be responsible for their actions. At the same time, the under-use of woods, i.e. the lack of people in them, makes those users who remain more fearful because they cannot rely on others to assist them or enforce acceptable behaviour from those who may be transgressing basic social rules of civility.

The Wood research has been able to tease out the specific landscape features which amplify feelings of anxiety and perceptions of risk experienced in built settings. The social processes and, therefore, the mechanisms for ameliorating those fears are broadly similar. People do not want to see drastic interventions to change the intrinsic qualities of woods; rather, in order to feel safe, more intensive programmes of management are needed. For women and their children, the strongest contribution to helping them feel safer would be the physical presence of lots of other people. The new initiatives referred to in the introduction to this chapter recognise the challenge of re-peopling green spaces in and around cities. One major element of the project was to work with Community Forest teams and their partners, to raise professional awareness of the issue and help implement management programmes and policy initiatives designed explicitly to reduce levels of anxiety. Many of the local community forest teams have embraced the findings of the research and are now implementing programmes which will help raise people's confidence in using woods for informal recreation, and thereby enhance the quality of life for all sections of the community.

10

Lesbian space

More than one imagined territory

Affrica Taylor

On the surface, the innocent idea of purchasing some 'lesbian space', of becoming part of the rate-paying public with a stakehold in inner-city Sydney real estate, does not deviate far from the standard Australian dream of home ownership. But a community project in the first half of the 1990s which set out to do just that stirred up a political storm of property and propriety within diverse sectors of Sydney's lesbian community. Ironically, in our attempting to secure a material space in which to 'be ourselves' as lesbians, the inherently unstable symbolic territories of both 'who we are' and 'where we are' were revealed. Cracks in 'the community' appeared midway through the fund-raising stage, when the question of lesbian-identified transsexuals' use of the space was raised. Hostilities escalated, and the eruptions and realignments within the community revealed some interesting fault-lines of identity politics.

This chapter will trace the trajectory of Sydney's Lesbian Space Project as a spatialised narrative of identity and community. In so doing it will explore some of the paradoxes of lesbian space: the transmutability of the symbolic and the real; the centring tendencies of the margins; the destabilising effect of attempting to fix identity both metaphorically and concretely in place; and the inadvertent opening up of new territories of meaning of both 'lesbian' and 'space' while seeking to regulate them.

For me, the physical and symbolic conjuncture of lesbian space simultaneously signifies ghetto walls closing in, and an open field awaiting resignification. Even as the setting of boundaries around physical space seeks to contain, the mercurial qualities of space as a powerful metaphor of freedom dislodge borders and move into hitherto unmarked territories of difference. Theoretically, space offers conceptual agility, room to move. It allows for knowing beyond the already known. Space stretches. It continually makes room. This is what makes it compelling as a metaphor of cultural and political possibility.

But let's not be naive. If visions of travelling beyond are launched in spacey dreams, they often rebound when lines are drawn and limits set. Space will always be claimed and contested as it has undeniable political currency. Securing space, in whatever form, is a political act: whether through invasion of territories; colonisation; dispossession; appropriation;

representation; the disciplining of knowledge; or the purchase of real-estate. The occupying of space is an assertion of power, and continual displacement is power's spatial effect.

So it is with the symbolic space of lesbian identity. The impulse to open up possibilities for lesbians, to defy limitations in order to be whatever we want to be, to keep pushing boundaries, to exceed expectations, is a powerful and a productive one. But this generative impulse is countervailed by the pragmatic restraints of occupying the representation space of a community identity. If we wish to represent ourselves as sharing a common interest because we are lesbians, rather than be defined, ignored or swallowed up by hegemonic heterosexist representations, we have to give ourselves definitional shape and form, communicate what it is that gives 'us' the us-ness. Ironically it is the foreclosure around this us-ness that in turn subsumes our internal differences, reducing the infinite possibilities of lesbian subjectivities into the common denominator of a single community identity.[1] The displacement of internal differences amongst marginalised peoples through the process of consolidating an identity itself constituted through its exclusion from hegemonic social space, is the spatial paradox of identity politics.

Moreover, as they emerge through the positive assertion of difference, identity-based political movements cut across each other's territories, layering the field of identity with what Keith and Pile call 'multiple spatialities' (Keith and Pile 1993: 22), and compounding the difficulty of sustaining a single identity, let alone an uncontested one. Even if I claim that contemporary lesbian identities have emerged at the (often antagonistic) conjuncture of the gay/lesbian/queer movements and various forms of feminism, I must also acknowledge the significance of the colonialist, radicalised and classed underpinnings of these movements. Any attempt to secure the foundations of a cohesive lesbian identity on these multilaminate grounds is, therefore, highly problematic.[2]

Thus cohesion, while it is strategically important for successful political representation, is as impossible to sustain within identity-based social movements, as it is within the dominant social order. Political solidarity does sharpen the boundaries between 'us' and 'them' when the heat is on, but today's 'us' against the wider community, might well be tomorrow's 'us' and 'them' amongst ourselves. This splintering effect within marginalised groups mirrors the dispersion that undermines hegemonic social control. In both cases it is the attempts to regulate differences in order to consolidate the position of 'us-ness' that produce the counter-effect of dispersion. As Annamarie Jagose puts it in *Lesbian Utopics*:

> the reification of the category does not secure a safe space from which to consolidate a feminist initiative; rather it simultaneously limits the field of those subjects it purports to represent while reimplicating them, in the name of their liberation, in the very apparatus of oppression by which they have been constituted.
>
> (Jagose 1994: 19)

It is tempting to read such a repetitive cycle as a vortex of repression, and to surmise that a politics based on identity is doomed to self-destruct. But in 'Contingent foundations: feminism and the question of postmodernism', Judith Butler reframes the paradox, and declares the very instability of the ground of identity politics to be feminism's regenerative force.

> I would argue that the rifts among women over the content of the term [woman] ought to be safeguarded and prized, indeed, that this constant rifting ought to be affirmed as the underground ground of feminist theory.
>
> (Butler 1992: 16)

When the inevitable rifts amongst those involved in the Lesbian Space Project became the focus of debate in large sectors of Sydney's lesbian community, it was not hard to trace moves to regulate internal difference along its fracture-lines. These were attempts to regulate not only the symbolic territory of lesbian identity, by seeking to establish once and for all who the 'real' lesbians are, and thus determine who is entitled to speak, vote, represent, and be represented; but also to gate-keep the physical space, to decide in advance who would and would not be allowed to use the building once it was purchased.

The rifts and the regulators did not surface until the project was early in its third year, by which time it had raised a substantial sum of money and was close to purchasing the property. I began my study not long after these surfacings, when the aftershocks had virtually stalled the project. The headlines of that month's *Lesbians On The Loose* magazine had just declared: 'Lesbian Space up in the Air' (March 1994). In private homes, at coffee shops, within social networks, at community meetings and cultural events, ontological wranglings had become endemic, and the fall-out involved shifts in allegiance, reassessment of affinities, the entrenchment of some new divisions, and reconfirmation of some old divisions in the community. Using Butler's affirmation of 'the underground ground of feminist theory' as a guiding mantra, I plunged into what felt like a seismological study of the Lesbian Space Project.

It seemed to me that it was the struggle to control and authorise the meanings of the couplet 'lesbian space' that had derailed the project, and so I wanted to trace the conjunctive possibilities and limitations of both these concepts through texts pertaining to the project,[3] in order to throw light on the project's rather sad trajectory. I already shared Butler's belief that all attempts to categorically fix gendered and thereby sexualised identities were fraught with contradictions that would eventually rupture their own seams of meaning (Butler 1990). But I was more interested in the ways in which spatialising such identities might intensify the ruptures. While examining many of the texts, I noted the frequent use of the spatial metaphors of scale and distance. In appropriating these metaphors as my own focal point of analysis, I found that they provided me with a critical lens through which to magnify and give perspective to the seismic tremors of this project, and to spatialise the project's story.

Big dreams

Let's start with the scale of events.

At its inception, the Sydney Lesbian Space Project was a lofty one. Under the massive sails of the Sydney Opera House, in December 1991, a concert attended by two thousand women was staged as part of a National Lesbian Conference. It was the taking over of this national icon and its resignification as a lesbian space for that one night that launched both the magnitude of vision and a substantial sum of seed-funding for the Lesbian Space Project. When I interviewed two of the project's visionaries about the inception of the project, I discovered that their initial dreams of lesbian space, as dreams are wont to be, were both high-flying and far-flung.

One dream[4] envisaged the building as solidifying lesbian cultural expression in various ways. The building itself would 'give form' to 'lesbian reality' and thus represent lesbianism. Within this building, 'lesbian reality' would be materialised and therefore visible. Its capacity to accommodate large numbers of lesbian bodies, to 'enable gatherings of up to five hundred women at a time' would be a vital physical indicator of lesbian power. Functioning as a lighthouse, the building would promote and recruit lesbians in the broader community, guide them home, be a 'beacon or focus for others that identify culturally as lesbians, to group and connect'. In its various physical capacities, the lesbian space 'cultural and community centre' would be a public sign of a large, strong and creative lesbian community.

This same dream also encompassed the highly personal and metaphysical possibilities of a material lesbian space. For the individual lesbians who would use it, the building would be an intimate space of psychic and spiritual nurturing. One of the visionaries said, 'It's like a physical form of self . . . when I feel myself turned on, in a sense of alive and vibrant and enthusiastic, then I like to have an interaction with that mirror dynamic.' In this version of the dream, the building would become a house of mirrors, in which each lesbian could see her self-reflection(s). The building itself, as a piece of lesbian architecture, could be the conduit for lesbian identification, or perhaps provide the site for seeing the self/sameness in others. In its largess, this dream maintained a strong belief in the productive possibilities of lesbian and space, and of the relationship between the symbolic and the material. 'The lesbian space project . . . is to home in on and fine-tune and give form to that frequency, that colour, that vibration, because it does not exist very clearly in physical form.' However, this dream limits itself by counting on the repression notion that there is a latent and frustrated 'lesbian reality' trapped 'underground' and hence 'invisible'. In this scenario, the materialisation of lesbian culture through lesbian space would be able to bring forth only that which already exists, but which has not yet been seen.

This particular dream of lesbian space could be described as the alchemist's visioning, where the building becomes a laboratory, a site of energy transmutation, where pre-existing cultural essences are distilled and

Figure 10.1 Advertisement, *Lesbians On The Loose*,
'Opera House Concert', July 1991

transformed from the metaphysical to the material world. In this utopian visioning, the re-emergence of the originary and authentic lesbian will be enabled through the talisman of lesbian space. As well as a laboratory, the building represents the hearth, the home of true lesbianism, the urban sanctuary in which lesbians can be and express their 'true inner selves'.

The wish-list of the other lesbian space dream[5] was similarly grand in its scale, but significantly differently constituted. This one imagined lesbian space as a 'one-stop lesbian shopping mall'. The building was configured as a multifunctional polis: a 'network centre'; 'an information centre'; a 'creative and functional' space; a consumer's paradise; a multi-service centre, where lesbians of all types could provide everything and get whatever they wanted. Circumventing the commercial mainstream, it would plug lesbians into a comprehensive internet of alternative provision. A material space which would be able to provide the scale of choice and access we have come to associate with the plenitude of cyberspace.

In the pluralist expression of this utopian vision, diverse lesbians would harmoniously coexist in the building with 'maturity' and 'flexibility'. There would be room to 'cater for everyone's needs', the space to do so would just have to be organised and negotiated through the allocation of time. There would be a booking system for the space. Acquisition of the building would signify the 'coming of age' of the lesbian community, community ownership and self-provision of services marking a collective rite of passage into independence/adulthood. In fact the 'maturity' factor in this vision was pivotal, both as a declaration of faith in a community to manage its own affairs and negotiate its differences, and as an indicator of the 'end of innocence'. Paradoxically, it was the innocence of pluralist visioning itself, and its assumption that a diverse and just community can be achieved through progress and maintained through rationality, which brought an end to this particular dream.

If the emphasis in the first lesbian space dream was on the reproduction of sameness by transforming a distilled collective spiritual essence into an ultimate lesbian urban materiality, this second dream promoted the unbounded production, dissemination and consumption of lesbian difference within the walls of one inner-city building. These contrasting imaginings of lesbian space as somewhere which could on the one hand open up the bounds of possibility for different lesbian expressions, and on the other hand close in on the essential sameness of all lesbians, represent the inherent spatial contradictions of identity. Even within a generous vision, big enough to 'include' differences, these differences must ultimately be contained at some point by the implication of sameness which hovers around the category 'lesbian'. As Jagose puts it:

> Even given the category's diligent incorporation of the once excluded, what remains problematic is the fundamental validity of that category, the way in which its newly redrawn boundaries reassume fixity and, in a preemptive foreclosure, once again solidify the category.
>
> (Jagose 1994: 18)

Regardless of the positioning of the boundaries, whether they be drawn close in to secure the sameness, or further out to allow for the differences amongst 'us', the surfacing of these boundaries around the lesbian space was inevitable, if not foreseen. Little wonder that the project's actual trajectory took it through some painfully dystopian demarcation wrangles, but it took a while . . .

On the night of 10 December 1993, the second momentous lesbian concert was held in Sydney. It was the Lesbian Space Project's 'grand finale', the climax of one year's fund-raising to reach its quarter of a million dollar target, the ceremonial time of judgement, the announcement of the project's fate. The concert programme declared, 'By the end of tonight's concert we will know whether or not we can go shopping for a building.'

This time the auspicious venue was the Sydney Town Hall. Without the iconic status of the opera house, it was nevertheless deemed sufficiently grand to befit the Lesbian Space Project, for, as the programme pointed out, its large chamber houses the most 'elaborate organ in the southern hemisphere'. The concert declared itself to be 'Coming from a Strong Space'. Size and space signalling the potency of lesbian desire.

There must have been something in that organ. A few weeks later the January 1994 issue of *Lesbians On The Loose* invoked the divine in its euphoric reporting of the project's success. The front page proclaimed an 'ACT OF FAITH' and the editor wrote: 'Dreams have become reality, prayers were answered and dyke power came to the fore as the Lesbian Space Project reached its $¼ million target on December 10 at the Sydney Town Hall.' The magazine's pages were replete with triumphant messages of gratitude and congratulations, with predictions of a glorious future, and with nostalgic reminiscences of the *coup d'état* on the great night. Page four provided a list of names of all who contributed, entitled 'WE DID IT!' The underlying text read: 'and to all the generous, visionary women who gave so willingly at midnight, so that $20,000 was made in 10 minutes, the Lesbian Space Project committee thank each and every one of you for helping to realise this miracle. Lesbians are doing it for ourselves.'

It seemed that this was no ordinary brand of self-sufficiency. Conjuring up Katie King's ironic commentary on lesbian identity as feminism's 'magical sign' (King 1994), this victory seemed to confirm that lesbians have very special powers, and had been signed as the 'chosen people'. In fact it was hard not to be struck by the quasi-religious extolling of lesbian virtue. Something of divine magnitude was being given testament. By these reports, the large congregation of 'visionaries' had performed a 1990s 'miracle' in those mere 'ten minutes' when 'prayers were answered'. Before the altar of the famous 'elaborate organ', the raining of dollar notes echoed the loaves and fishes trick, and climactically signified the consecration of lesbian identity.

With hindsight in the retelling, such pious aggrandisement seems like self-parody. It is a long way back down to earth from the heavenly heights, and 'falling from grace' was to become one of the most dominant tropes of the Lesbian Space Project.

How far can we go?

> There was a point when we were very close, and now we may as well be a million miles away. . . . We now have money and no goodwill. Before we had goodwill and no money. I actually would rather be in a position of having no money and goodwill. It's easier to get money. But once you've lost goodwill, once you've lost the sense of faith, it takes years to recover that, if ever.
>
> (Excerpt from interview 1)

These words, spoken after the rifts in the community had well and truly surfaced, sadly portended distance: the distancing of the project from its original goal; and the speaker's own distancing from the project that she once identified so closely with. 'Falling from grace' had reconfigured desire though distance. The once glorious and hallowed visions had now receded, and from the new/distant perspective, appeared retrospectively to be both myopic and without grace:

> My sense of lesbian space certainly evaporated. I no longer think that a building is a good idea, because there are unfortunately enough women who could make it unpleasant and difficult . . . or women who are different in whatever way. It doesn't even matter how.
>
> (Excerpt from interview 1)

Perceptions of just how much difference matters became fundamental to the project of securing lesbian space. Radio National's *Coming Out Show* team recorded the opening plenary session at the July 1994 National Lesbian Conference in Brisbane, and from this produced a programme called 'Cracks in the Lesbian Nation' which was broadcast in September 1994. Bitter divisions over the presence of lesbian-identified transsexuals, which dominated this conference, were soon to spread south and infect the Sydney Lesbian Space Project. The Brisbane debacle heralded Sydney's great 'transsexual debate'. Despite mandatory lip-service to the principle of difference both at the conference and in the Lesbian Space Project, certain differences were deemed by some to be 'going too far'. This speaker made no bones about her limits:

> My name's Kookaburra and I am a lesbian. I've come over two thousand kilometres to come to this national lesbian conference, I thank the collective for the job they have done, but it is now *our* conference. I have been to all the other lesbian conferences and I have never had to walk into a room and be confronted by, a *man*. That man might be, well he might say that he's 'lesbian identified', but to me I see a man. I came here to be in a safe lesbian space. *This is not a safe lesbian space.* I'm not saying that the transgenders shouldn't have support, I'm just saying that this is not the venue for that support. [Applause] I'm really tired of being made to feel *guilty* for not

including other oppressed groups. *We* are an oppressed group. We have a *right* to have lesbian safe space.

[original emphases]

By emphasising the physical distance that she had travelled, this speaker underscored the categorically gendered distance that she put between herself as a lesbian of the 'natural' kind, and the trany lesbian as a 'man-in-disguise'. Symbolically, distance measured intrinsic corporal differences. The originary, pure and therefore benign lesbian body was positioned at a great distance from the impure, fraudulent and therefore dangerous trany body.

The physical proximity of these proclaimed antithetical bodies in the same space was declared an immediate cause for alarm. Clearly it was the purity of the lesbian bodies that rendered them vulnerable, and hence made it imperative that the physical environment provide sanctuary. The meanings attributed to physical space and its relationship to the bodies that inhabited it, were pivotal to this 'safe space' argument. The presumption was that the physical space would be infused by the bodies, and take on the corresponding inherent attributes of those bodies. According to this conflating formula, physical spaces are essentialised by the bodies that inhabit (or invade) them. 'Natural' environments, made up of pure essences, are always at risk of contamination by impurities. Hence while lesbian bodies purge the spaces they occupy, rendering them pure, perhaps even sanctifying them (witness the reports at the Sydney Town Hall concert), trany bodies defile the spaces they occupy, rendering them polluted and unsafe.

Kookaburra's claim that the contaminating presence of the transsexual in the room not only was deeply affronting to her, but also rendered that space dangerous to lesbians in general, was exemplary of the 'safe space' argument presented by those who subsequently authorised themselves to exclude lesbian transsexuals from the Lesbian Space Project. If 'lesbian space' was initially cast as a lofty dream, it was at this point that it was quickly reeled back in. The desire to open up a 'lesbian space' had been reduced to a tight demarcation of the limited territory of 'safe space'. And furthermore this 'safe space' seemed to be very close to the hermetically sealed space of 'sameness'. Upholders of the 'safe space' argument became the patrol guards and the gate-keepers of the lesbian sanctuary, and they closed ranks to protect it.

Back on the (underground) ground on which political theory and community activism mysteriously converge, the Lesbian Space Project continued to illustrate the very process by which an essentialist identity politics in fact produces a de-centred politics of location, generating new and resistant positions and alliances by its very attempts to regulate the representational spaces of the 'real' lesbian.

Throughout the second half of 1994 the growing political schism between the 'safe spacers' and those who wanted transsexuals to be included waylaid the project. No consensus could be reached about who comprised 'the community' let alone any agreement be made about purchasing a building. At the AGM in December 1994, a contingent of vocal women involved in the Lesbian Space Project and their interstate proxies, staged the inevitable coup, and ensured the exclusion of transsexuals from the project, by amending the constitution and replacing the word 'lesbian' with 'female-born-lesbian'. To this point, the 'lesbian trany' debate had been hypothetical. The Trany Liberation Coalition (TLC) was a financial supporter of the project, but had not sought membership or assurances of rights of access for lesbian transsexuals. A month or so after the constitutional amendment was enacted, Sydney transsexuals were interpolated directly into the fray of the Lesbian Space Project. Unlike those who dreamed of creating utopian lesbian spaces, or those who wished to be protected within a lesbian sanctuary, they had no visions of such a space. According to a member of TLC:

> that's not why we got involved in LSP . . . until they started discriminating against transsexuals, we were financial supporters of it, as soon as they started discriminating against transsexuals we were in dispute with them . . . we said from the word go . . . our only interest was in mending the discrimination.
>
> (Excerpt from interview 3)

To claim that interventions were purely political and strategic, that the only space of interest was the discursive space of anti-discrimination, belies an awareness of the probability that some lesbian transsexuals may have actually wanted to be part of the physical lesbian space, and that one of the main premises of anti-discrimination intervention is the need to open up spaces of possibility for those hitherto excluded. Nevertheless it was clear that those who sought to authorise and regulate the symbolic space of representation by essentialising the category lesbian as 'female-born-lesbian' and thus ultimately to control the physical space, had paradoxically and in quite specific ways enabled contesting positionings of lesbian transsexuals and their supporters. These contesting positions were seeking to rupture the closures of a tightly demarcated symbolic and physical space.

Within the now rather damaged community of Sydney lesbians, itself constituted in its resistance to the heterosexist discourses of the broader community, the pattern of regulation and resistance was being repeated. The centring tendencies within this marginal group were producing its own new margins. Identity politics was perpetuating a struggle of demarcation and displacement at the marginal edge, resulting in the kaleidoscopic effect of ever-shifting boundaries, and new territories of meaning.

The Trany Liberation Coalition, well aware of the paradoxes of identity politics, already had a declared intention to shift the boundaries which contain sex/gender in their binary categories, and to replace this dichotomous distinction with the notion of a gender continuum.

> One of the things that we do in our theoretical world is that we resolve the sex/gender distinction. We do that by making biological sex irrelevant. We

just say it's just another constructed category that's mobile. If that's the case there's no point in distinguishing between sex and gender. We do have in our society a gender system that operates very punitively on a whole load of different people for different reasons and that's the thing we should be focusing on.

(Excerpt from interview 3)

While this quick rendering irrelevant of the categories of biological sex might seem rather glib,[6] the desire to challenge constricting determinations of gender would seem to be very much in line with most expressions of feminism:

this is something that an awful lot of transsexuals have difficulties with, and I think quite reasonably. They just cannot understand why the feminists, or some people who claim to be feminists, are so down on transsexuals, when it's so obvious to transsexuals from their everyday experience that they are doing something to seriously fuck up the gender system, and they're getting punished for it on an everyday basis. . . .

I can not think of two groups that have more closely aligned interests than transsexuals and dykes. All our social issues are the same – discrimination, sexual harassment and violence, denial of the legitimacy of our lifestyle choices. Exclusion, marginalisation, invisibility. And some transsexuals have issues around reproduction. . . . We have a common enemy which is heterosexist culture. . . . We all find these impositions intolerable, we all have a common interest in getting rid of them, we all have a common enemy. I mean what more commonality do people need? I mean do they have to be cloned?

(Excerpt from interview 3)

This upholding of political allegiance as the prime criterion for determining affinity and the affects of proximity/distance, is a position aligned with the contemporary politics of queer coalition. It foregrounds the ways in which determinations of proximity/distance are strategically employed for political reasons, and can be continually (re)negotiated.

For the 'female-born-lesbians' who believed that in order to maintain the 'safety' of lesbian space they had to exclude lesbian transsexuals, it was biology alone that established the ultimate criterion of affinity once and for all. This sort of biological determinism (which borrows and slightly twists the heterosexist logic that anatomical sex determines gender which in turn determines sexual desire[7]) is obviously non-negotiable, and has been taken up by the politics of lesbian separatism. Following the logic of this politics, pre-determined and fixed categories of difference establish once and for all, who can and who can't enter lesbian space.

Rifts over territories of meaning of lesbian in the Lesbian Space Project, were carved out in response to the question 'How far can we go?' Clearly the parameters of desirable difference were aeons apart. The rifts provided a seismic measure not only of just how much difference matters, but also of what sort of difference matters. The fault-lines that shook this project have been located between the lofty imaginings of lesbian community and the bitter reality of struggles over the representation of lesbian identity.

Bewildered by the internal divisions amongst those lesbians who could be represented as 'female-born' (and should therefore have shared a natural affinity) the November 1995 newsletter of the Lesbian Space Project doggedly insisted that it was the struggle to keep the wolves at bay that had stalled the project:

> Materialising Lesbian Space on this planet continues to offer extreme challenges. The creation of man-free space seems to trigger some very primal fears and insecurities – amongst some lesbians as well as society generally and globally.

What does constitute 'extreme'? Even in the biggest picture imaginable, the events of the Sydney Lesbian Space Project are not world-shattering. There is no lesbian in space yet, and this is not star wars.

Scale has its own ironic proportions. Support for the project declined with the perceived extreme positioning of some of those involved. Many distanced themselves from it. A small number closed ranks around the now reduced imagined community that they sought to regulate. For those remaining, firmly standing their ground in the diminished space, the imagined enemy out there looms large. And by its own logic, so it must be.

Identity politics is not firm ground on which to build or maintain a permanent physical space. Space itself is far too mutable and volatile to guarantee any firming-up of boundaries around identity. What we have here in lesbian space are two highly unstable political concepts, each provoking the contestation of the other, and producing ongoing upheaval. This is the best they can offer us. Not materialisation of an imaginary formulation, but underground rumblings that disturb and realign conceptual and political foundations.

Postscript

Since my writing of this chapter, the project has moved on and stalled again. Four and a half years after the project was launched, and following a decision to take out a substantial mortgage to supplement the funds raised, a building was purchased in the inner-city suburb of Newtown. The Lesbian Space cultural and community centre opened in May 1996, and the June edition of *Lesbians On The Loose* proclaimed 'LSP: mission accomplished'. If the purchasing of a building was the ultimate measure of a successful mission, this story would have a happy ending. But large mortgage repayments, personal conflicts, inadequate management resources, persistent community divisions, under-use of the centre, and, rather ironically, a fire in 'the healing room', have all reconfigured the dreams of the now highly problematic materialised lesbian space. A decision was made early in 1997 to lease out all but a small space within the building, in order to meet the mortgage repayments and thus avert the loss of the Sydney lesbian community's asset.

Notes

1 Stuart Hall's writing has consistently emphasised the political role of closure in the determination of identity. When recently reconsidering the question 'Who needs identity?' he reiterated: 'The unity, the internal homogeneity, which the term identity treats as foundational is not natural, but a constructed form of closure . . . constructed within the play of power and exclusion' (Hall 1996: 5).

2 In *Gender Trouble*, Judith Butler takes issue with a form of politics which seeks to 'locate a common identity as the foundation for feminist politics' (Butler 1990: ix). Her (Foucauldian) critique of the political construction and regulation of categories of identity has enormously influenced feminist/lesbian/queer theory.

3 These include promotional material produced by subsequent Lesbian Space Project (LSP) committees; an ABC Radio National show, produced by the *Coming Out Show* entitled 'Cracks in the Lesbian Nation' and broadcast on 17 September 1994; issues of the Sydney lesbian monthly magazine *Lesbians On The Loose* between December 1991 and December 1995; and interviews with three key people associated with the project. The first two interviewees were both involved in launching the Lesbian Space Project, the third interviewee is a member of the Sydney lobby group, the Trany Liberation Coalition (TLC). I simply refer to them as Interview 1, Interview 2 and Interview 3.

4 The description and analysis of the first dream are based on my interpretation of Interview 2, recorded in November 1995. Those words in quotation marks have been taken directly from the transcript.

5 The description and analysis of the second dream are based on my interpretation of Interview 1, recorded in August 1995. Those words in quotation marks have been taken directly from the transcript.

6 For an argument that claims any such political programme to degender society as 'hopelessly utopian', see Moira Gatens's 'A critique of the sex/gender distinction' (1990).

7 See Butler (1990).

11

Ghetto girls/urban music

Jamaican ragga music and female performance

Tracey Skelton

I've been on my own since I was 14. I'm raggamuffin sexy, taking it to a different level. I'm still single. I'm setting an example to the ghetto girls. And I'm doing it because it's real.

(Patra interviewed by O'Brien 1995: 12)

Patra is a female dancehall/ragga star from Jamaica, now residing in New York and being interviewed by Lucy O'Brien for *The Guardian* in London. Whenever she appears on television or is interviewed in print she firmly locates herself within the urban space of Jamaica. Patra aligns herself with the ghetto – its culture, its music and its people. Patra is a ghetto girl, a performer of urban music. She is a Jamaican dancehall star – she reflects the struggle that women in urban Jamaica face on a daily basis and at the same time she is a success story. For Patra, along with other women within dancehall music, dance or fashion, has created a space for herself within a musical genre which has been strongly associated with male performance, prowess and heterosexual patriarchy (Skelton 1995a).

In this chapter I wish to discuss the ways in which contemporary Jamaican[1] female dancehall performers are creating and establishing spaces for themselves in which they debate, contest and subvert the socially constructed gender roles and relations of Jamaican society; to consider the ways in which the women are playing around with gender and constructions of space. First though, it is necessary to discuss what I mean by the term 'dancehall', a very interesting one in cultural geography. It means the actual place/space where ragga music is played and at the same time is also the name for a specific Jamaican cultural production. Dancehall then has a physical entity. In Jamaica the dancehall is invariably an open air space where a stage is constructed and sound-systems set up – it can be any open space where ragga performance takes place. However, the term also defines a musical genre which is called ragga and encompasses a style of dance and fashion which are both firmly associated with the musical form. Throughout the chapter I refer to ragga when I explicitly discuss the music, and dancehall/ragga when I refer to the wider context of this cultural production, namely dance, fashion and the actual space of the dancehall.

Figure 11.1 Jamaica: Linda Dawes, Department of International Studies, Nottingham Trent University

To date there is relatively little written about women, Jamaican dancehall and ragga music apart from media commentaries. There are notable exceptions such as the work by Carolyn Cooper (1993, 1994, 1995) and also the film *The Dark Side of Black*, directed by Isaac Julien, which had a specific section devoted to the issues of gender and sexuality within ragga music. There are also useful comparisons to be made between women and ragga music, and women and rap music; to this end I will be drawing upon the work of Tricia Rose (1994) and Beverley Skeggs (1993). Such comparisons can be justified for two reasons: first, because of the analysis based on women's experiences within these new urban musical forms; second, because there already exists a debate on the interconnections between Jamaican ragga music and US hip-hop and rap:

> [T]he most obvious influence on Jamaican music in recent years has been from hip-hop. . . . More recently, following the success of cross-over artists such as Shabba Ranks, collaborations between US singers and Jamaican deejays have been promoted by record companies in a calculated manner. . . . [B]ut dancehall/*ragga* has had a remarkable impact on African-American hip-hop artists as well, and the Jamaican presence is now firmly established . . . on black-oriented radio in cities like New York and Washington, D.C.
>
> (Bilby 1995: 179; original emphasis)

Such intersections between the musics mean that some of the academic analysis of the role of women in the US musics of hip-hop and rap can be useful as a context for establishing discussion on the role of women in Jamaican dancehall/ragga.

Dancehall/ragga music in social, political and economic context

Dancehall/ragga music, dance and fashion are very firmly located within the urban setting of Kingston's 'downtown' areas, or, as they are often referred to, both pejoratively and with a sense of fierce pride and identity, 'The Ghetto'. These areas are spaces of extreme urban poverty with very high rates of unemployment and also of street violence. If a person has a 'downtown' address then opportunities for secure employment are non-existent. The physical appearance of the ghetto areas is striking in its complexity and density. Narrow, bare-earthen alleyways are defined by boundaries of corrugated metal sheeting (usually referred to as 'zinc' or 'galvanise') and wood. The ghetto areas can be likened to a labyrinth or maze, each corner resembling the last. Behind the 'walls' are mostly small wooden shacks, many of them consisting of just one room, densely clustered around a shared yard space. Where there is electricity it will feed just one light bulb and possibly a single socket; cooking is commonly done in the yard outside on a coal-pot burning charcoal or on pieces of galvanised sheeting over a small open fire.

To
Ocho Rios,
Port Antonio

Padmore

Bowden
Hill

Freetown

Red
Hills

Swain
Spring

Jack's Hill

Irish
Town

Constant
Spring

A3

Industry
Village

Forest
Hills

To
Spanish
Town

Allerdyce
Gardens

Barbican
Heights

Six
Miles

A1

Washington
Gardens

Barbican

U p t o w n

Dallas
Mt.

Liguanea

Mona
Heights

Papine

A1

Half
Way
Tree

New
Kingston

Beverly
Hills

Three
Mile

D o w n t o w n

Cross
Roads

Hermitage

Tinson
Pen

Trench
Town

Long Mountains

Hunts
Bay

Jones
Town

A3

Tivoli
Gardens

The
Parade

A4

To
Portmore

Kingston Harbour

Harbour
View

Port
Royal

The Palisadoes

To
Morant
Bay

The Palisadoes

C a r i b b e a n   S e a

N
W   E
S

Ghetto, **downtown** areas with
dense, poor quality housing
and yards

0   2 km

Area broadly defining **uptown**
with spacious, leafy suburbs
built on the more pleasant hills

KINGSTON

LMDTS.597

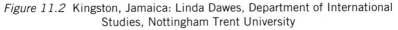

Figure 11.2 Kingston, Jamaica: Linda Dawes, Department of International
Studies, Nottingham Trent University

The neighbourhoods are dense, and, as individuals and television directors (Zabihyan 1995) testify, tensions and animosity between people can often explode fatally. Guns are commonly used, but for the very poor acid-throwing is a vicious and painful weapon. If a victim survives an acid attack it is usually with appalling scars burned deep into the skin. Gang cultures exist and innocents are often caught in the 'crossfire', frequently all too literally. The policing of the 'downtown' areas is brutal, heavy-handed and brings with it its own abuse of power and authority (Zabihyan 1995).

Out of such deprived economic environments, out of places with little political voice or representation, comes a music, dance and fashion form which is part and parcel of the ghetto, which reflects ghetto experiences and life qualities. Just as its forerunner reggae did, ragga music is formed out of 'downtown' life and reflects the experience back to its audience. Ragga music is the culture of the ghetto, it speaks from the ghetto and it tells of ghetto existence. Further, the rhythms and performance of the music mean that it can also transcend cultural and geographical boundaries and scales. So it can speak to people who have no specific memory or experience of the Jamaican ghetto, but who at the same time can identify with the message of the music – either its call for black self-esteem or rebellion and its admiration for male feats of sexual exploitation, or, for the female audience, a woman's voice challenging sexism and patriarchal forces which hold women back. The experience of ragga and dancehall then has several layers of resonance for Jamaican and Caribbean diasporic communities, many members of which may never have seen the specific place of the Jamaican 'downtown' ghetto.[2]

Returning to Jamaica, the experience of the grind of everyday life in Kingston 'downtown' means that the space of pleasure which the dancehall provides on Friday and Saturday nights is central. The opportunity the dancehall provides to wear 'fake' glamour, one's best clothes (many of them designed and worked on by the wearer him- or herself), to dance and perform showing the skill and beauty of one's own body, means that ragga music offers a cultural space away from the deprivation of the everyday life of the ghetto. The dancehall does not offer an escape from reality since the music is formed out of and reflects ghetto experience and identity; it is, in the words of Patra above, *real*. Performers sing of the 'dirty reality' that is ghetto life. Nor is the dancehall always a safe space – gang feuds often spill over into the space of the dance and the police may 'invade' at any given time and carry out random body searches and arrests (Skelton 1995b). Nevertheless, dancehall/ragga speaks to people and it is a popular cultural form in which they invest heavily:

[H]undreds of hopeful young *raggamuffins* congregate day after day in front of Kingston's dozens of recording studios, patiently waiting for auditions . . . Jamaica, after all, is reputed to have the highest per capita output of records of any country in the world.

(Bilby 1995: 180)

Despite the fact that the genre of ragga is male-dominated, as all musical forms of Jamaican music have been – and indeed as most musical forms are – there are notable numbers of women rising to the fore. For the purpose of this chapter I will focus on Patra and Lady Saw, both of whom have gained some recognition from the UK national press and beyond. In the cultural form of dancehall women have always been central through their dance (much of which is highly acrobatic) and the dancehall fashions which they have developed. So women play an important role in the ensemble which is dancehall performance in Jamaica and throughout Jamaican diasporic communities. Indeed the appropriateness of such roles and performances has been the subject of several levels of debate both in Jamaica and the UK concerning whether women should be party to 'slackness' (Brinkworth 1992), or whether 'slackness' is a celebration of women's sexuality and at the same time a defiance against the dominant standards of what is decent (Cooper 1993, 1994).

This is an ongoing debate; what I now want to address are the ways in which Patra and Lady Saw have both created a space for women within dancehall/ragga and been part of a disruptive discourse about women's sexuality, gender relations and male power. These female performers of ragga music are both interrupting and creating this vibrant, dynamic and controversial urban music. Rather than presenting this analysis directly through the music and lyrics of Lady Saw and Patra, I am going to work through their self-representations in mainstream media, such as *The Observer* (Sawyer 1995) and *The Guardian* (O'Brien 1995). I will also draw upon the voices of Jamaican women represented in Isaac Julien's film *The Dark Side of Black* (1994), threading through comparisons with the work of Beverley Skeggs (1993) and Tricia Rose (1994) who both analyse black women and rap music.

Ghetto girls making space for women: Lady Saw and Patra

Lady Saw in *The Observer*

Lady Saw is a Jamaican dancehall star who has remained in Jamaica, a performer of the Kingston ghetto. For the article in *The Observer* (19 February 1995) by Miranda Sawyer, Lady Saw is interviewed in Kingston. The preamble of the article discusses Lady Saw's recent performances, the furore she often stirs up in the Jamaican press and the role of musical production in urban Jamaican culture. Consequently Lady Saw is firmly placed in Jamaican urban space. The front cover of the 'Life' section of this particular *Observer* named Lady Saw as Jamaica's answer to Madonna. Interesting that a black woman from 'downtown' Kingston, who sings a particular musical form firmly located in the place and space of Jamaica, should be compared with US-born, white pop star Madonna. Indeed this comparison is used regularly for female ragga stars: the interview with Patra in *The Guardian* (O'Brien 1995) is headed 'The making of a black Madonna'. Clearly it might be a play on the symbolism of the Black Madonna in the monastery in Montserrat, Barcelona, as well as directly alluding to the pop star Madonna. But in terms of the comparison between Lady Saw and Madonna the only apparent similarity is the way they perform sexuality on stage:

> Lady Saw shakes everybody's hands, smiles demurely for photographs and launches herself bodily into a routine now familiar to the whistling multitudes of skunked-up skankers. Stepping, stomping, grinding, bumping, with plenty of dramatic pauses for hip-height boot ballet and a quick burst of below the belt banter. A performance of Amazonian uninhibitedness.
>
> (Sawyer 1995: 34)

Lady Saw had just been given the Jamaican 'Lady DJ of the Year' award (1995) which was highly significant as she was not even nominated in 1994 (Cooper 1995). She is raw, nasty, sexy and vulgar. Her Jamaican patois has to be translated for the interviewer. She repeatedly fails to make arranged meetings for the interview. Lady Saw becomes firmly defined as a Jamaican, of the ghetto, of the city – she is behaving in an unprofessional way, she is on 'Caribbean time'.

Lady Saw is interviewed in the presence of the man who is her manager, producer and boyfriend – although in his boyfriend role she has to share him with another woman. Lady Saw is therefore in reality one of the women she sings about:

> Oh Lord, please work a miracle for me to fin' a man of my own,
> Because dear Lord I am tired of sleeping all alone,
> Dear Lord I know that good man is very hard to find
> Dear Lord please find me someone who will come home at night
> Me no want no bad man to steal me DJ money
> Me no want no married man lef wife fe take a liberty
> Dey have an odd love affair, but dey not guan get me
> Release me now, oh let me be free
> Oh Lord, please work a miracle for me to find a man of my own.
>
> (Lady Saw, 'I want a man of my own')

She has to share her man, and does not know why he cannot be faithful to her. This is a common lament among Jamaican women and women of the Caribbean generally. African-Caribbean men invariably have more than one sexual partner and often have long-lasting relationships with both or all of the women (Ellis 1986; Skelton 1989). The knowledge that this is a reality for many women of the region does not prevent their individually longing for loyalty and someone to depend upon; nor does it liberate the women in terms of their own sexual behaviour. Women who are not faithful, quiet and patient may find violence becomes part of their relationship, and social censure a severe comment on their morality. The interview with Lady Saw shows her authentic experience: even this nationally famous dancehall DJ cannot be sure of her man's fidelity. When Lady Saw speaks then she reiterates her connection with ordinary people and her commitment to sing for the 'ladies':

> I do speak for other people, on behalf of other ladies. . . . You watch the way people live and what's going on and then you don't do it yourself alone. The talk in the dancehall, that's the talk I use.
>
> (Lady Saw interviewed by Sawyer 1995: 34)

When interviewed by Isaac Julien, Lady Saw makes a similar comment about the ways in which she can use her own musical abilities to speak up for Jamaican women, and also the ways in which her work combines with that of other Jamaican women, the dancehall models, to create a central stage for women:

> Men DJ, right, you get some men and they will go and diss [disrespect] the ladies, but then I am not for that, right, I'm for the ladies, so I go there and defend it and cool it down, right. . . . The ladies are more up front now, you know, they want to be in the limelight – like dancehall models for instance in Kingston here, they are very x-rated on stage and the man go wild for them. So from the body is clean and thing, I think you can show it off.
>
> (Lady Saw interviewed by Julien 1994)

The closing comments made by Miranda Sawyer ensure that Lady Saw's performance and identity remain embedded within Jamaican dancehall culture – she is almost too Caribbean, too Jamaican, too 'downtown' Kingston, too sexy, too hard-core to be able to change cities and spaces to come into 'civilisation'.

> It's doubtful whether Lady Saw's industrial-strength raunchiness will ever be welcome in Britain, where the preferred area of anatomical stiffness is the upper lip. Whether she will be able to shake off the dust from the ghetto sex wars is equally in doubt. The lady herself is keen to spread her wings: 'Send for me, please! I can work for the British people. I know they would love me.'
>
> (Lady Saw interviewed by Sawyer 1995: 34)

Miranda Sawyer's 'Britain' clearly fails to recognise the presence of a Caribbean, and in particular a Jamaican, diaspora who not only do not hold with the stiff upper lip culture but who also create music from their urban experiences. The British Caribbean communities would and do welcome Lady Saw – her lyrics can hold a reality for them too.

The ways in which Jamaican women are creating spaces for themselves in the urban context of Jamaica also has a resonance for those of Caribbean descent in other urban settings. Indeed these created spaces can transgress not only the expected gender roles and relations, but also expected sexual behaviours. Ragga music has an image of intense heterosexuality and elements of the music and some of its performers are very homophobic (Bilby 1995: 240; Skelton 1995a). However, just as ragga music itself is diverse and multi-layered in its rhythmic origins, then so too are the social-relational contexts in which the music is heard. Paul Burston, writing in the *Independent* (1995), talks of gay club nights where black lesbians and gays can enjoy ragga: 'Black gays and lesbians, spurred by the rhythms of ragga, are changing the face of London clubland' (1995: 22). Inge Blackman is a film director interviewed by Issac Julien. She, like some of the people Burston talked to, felt it was important to emphasise that not all of ragga is homophobic, and that not all ragga performers were anti-gay. In fact Blackman discusses the ways in which ragga and dancehall in the UK have given black lesbians a specific space:

> Black lesbians actually do participate in dancehall culture. Dancehall culture, particularly in England, acts as a celebration of black women's sexuality and it's a way in which black women can bond with each other on the dance floor, this is very, very strong. Black women can dance with each other in a very sexual, in a very lustful way on the dance floor in ragga culture. It's not really allowed in any other black popular culture.
>
> (Blackman interviewed by Julien 1994)

What the interview with Lady Saw in *The Observer* clearly establishes and echoes are the ways in which Lady Saw herself feels strongly that she has a role to speak for women and make a space for women in which they can articulate what matters to them in their ghetto lives: whether this is demanding athletic sexual satisfaction, singing about her own sexual abilities, or calling for a change in men's sexual and relationship behaviour.

Patra in *The Guardian*

In the interview with Lucy O'Brien for *The Guardian* Patra is represented, and self-represents, in a context of 'improvement', of 'civilisation'. What is made repetitively clear is that she is 'toned down', she has 'undergone a transition' (O'Brien 1995: 12), and is the 'acceptable' side of urban Jamaican ragga. We are then left with a cultural dichotomy – Patra claims a raw, nasty and raggamuffin style for herself, while the media wishes to show a woman who has matured through her experiences and who has relocated herself away from the ghetto. The reason for Patra being in the media is because of her explicit, raunchy sexual performances, but when we meet her face to face she is represented as a sure-minded performer with business sense.

> This is a serious business. When I first met Patra two years ago she was a slightly shy 20-year-old with a strong Jamaican accent. Now, she sports a slimmed-down-worked-out body, discrete, New York black lycra, killer braids and shiny red talons.
>
> (O'Brien 1995: 12)

The body is controlled, kept in shape, the accent which firmly places Patra as a Jamaican is softening, she is serious – but there is still danger held within this sanitised version of the former raunchy girl of Jamaica, in her killer braids and the dangerous talons. Patra builds on this apparent contradiction to present an image which is positive (and acceptable in the non-Jamaican context) and yet still grounded in a disruptive and resistant (raggamuffin) identity: 'The way I dress is more elegant and classy, whereas in the back of my mind I'm still raggamuffin and hardcore' (Patra interviewed by O'Brien 1995: 12).

When discussing ragga and where she began Patra admits to the difficulty of the battle – the battle to get a space for women performers – and that in some cases that battle was with other women DJs, but mostly the fight was with men, who also often demanded that women become as 'x-plicit' as men:

> It was very tough, a male-dominated field. Getting into the business was like getting through firestones because people fight you left, right and centre. [Commenting on her earlier, often very lewd songs] Back in those days, it was reality, I don't regret it. You call it a start, y'know. It was a gimmick.
>
> (Patra interviewed by O'Brien 1995: 12)

What is clear in this newspaper interview, and in other interviews for mainstream media such as the Channel 4 *Passengers* (1994) programme (see Skelton 1995b for a detailed analysis), is that Patra represents herself as a role model, someone women, including teenage women, can look up to and draw strength from. Responding to a question about her highly sexual performances and the fact that Jamaica has a very high teenage pregnancy rate, Patra describes her own reality and experience:

> I've been on my own since I was 14 years old. My father died when I was three, I had opportunities to mess up. I could have had 10 kids if I wanted. But once you have a goal in mind, you won't think of pregnancy. You have to keep an independent space; a lot of women don't do that. The most I can do for teenagers is guide them the right way.
>
> (Patra interviewed by O'Brien 1995: 13)

The importance of a space for women is therefore central in Patra's definition of how women can succeed and make something of their lives. Elsewhere (as well as in *The Guardian* interview), Patra has admitted that she is not doing anything very differently from what other women in Jamaica are doing but she has the drive and determination to achieve the goal of being a music star, and currently that means moving to the States and specifically New York. However, her self-naming as 'raggamuffin' means that she resists selling out completely and that she still locates her identity within, and as part of, Jamaica.

Creating through resisting: making the connections

What women performers within dancehall/ragga music are doing through their very presence is creating space for women: through the pathways they have made for other women performers; through making a lyrical and musical space which reflects women's lives, experiences, desires and demands; and through being there, on the stage, in the sound, speaking directly to women in the audience. This connects with Tricia Rose's analysis of black women in rap:

> Black women rappers interpret and articulate the fears, pleasures, and promises of young black women whose voices have been relegated to the margins of public discourse. They are integral and resistant voices in rap music and popular music in general who sustain an ongoing dialogue with their audiences and with male rappers about sexual promiscuity, emotional commitment, infidelity, the drug trade, racial politics, and black cultural history.
>
> (Rose 1994: 146)

Women in dancehall/ragga in Jamaica and throughout the diaspora are doing very similar things within their own social, political, sexual and cultural milieux. Rose offers an analysis that contradicts popular media conceptions of the role of women in rap, conceptions that have served to establish a binary division of male/female. This, she argues, delimits the work women in the music have done to simply being 'anti-sexist' or even anti-male. In fact, Rose argues, black women rappers, alongside many male rappers, are 'struggling to define themselves against a confining and treacherous social environment' i.e. white dominant US culture (1994: 148). That is not to deny that female rappers have a central focus on sexual politics and demand some renegotiation of gender relations. Patra is especially sensitive to the latter and clearly feels that showing young women the 'right way' will lead them through exploitative sexual relations (which leave them pregnant at an early age) and assert their autonomy and independence.

Lady Saw's self-presentation, combined with descriptions of her musical performance, finds an echo in Skeggs's work (1993) where she investigates black women rappers and the ways in which they assert their sexual power and independence by speaking what they should not, and how they refuse to be contained within a particular form of femininity. She discusses the ways in which black women rappers are challenging both the silencing of black women's cultural responses and the silencing of black women's sexuality, and the ways in which they will not play the game of the discourses of shame and honour (1993: 106). In Skeggs's eyes black women rappers are talking back and their target is the

> White-Western civilising system which attempts to contain the expression of women's sexuality through the moralising discourses of conduct: politeness, respectability, caring, duty and responsibility . . . they speak against the power of masculinity [and its attempts] to fit femininity to its fantasies.
>
> (Skeggs 1993: 108)

For women in Jamaican dancehall/ragga there is a slight variation on this in that they are less confrontational against masculine definitions of women but they do call for a change in masculine behaviour. Through dance movements and fashion design the women involved in ragga also show, through the ways they inscribe their bodies on the public place of the dancehall, that they are *not* sexually submissive, sexually available as and when men want them, that they *are* in control of their bodies and that they, as women, *will* celebrate their own bodies and their own sexual identity. Consequently they refuse male definitions of themselves – they create a resistive space.

Alongside the resistance against male definitions women in ragga disrupt and resist notions of 'respectable' female behaviour within the socially and culturally dominant definitions of the Christian Church and 'uptown' Jamaican society. Women in dancehall/ragga are out in the public arena demanding sex, singing of women's sexual desires and pleasures. The women present themselves as confident, aggressive and resistant, they articulate the 'demand discourse' (Skeggs 1993). The following selected quotes from Skeggs's and Rose's work demonstrate the close connections between such a discourse among women in Jamaican dancehall/ragga and women in US (and, to a lesser extent, UK) rap music:

> When female rappers explicitly address sexual practice as direct pleasure and fun they locate themselves against good taste, polite conduct and civilisation. In this sense they are dangerous. They embody a threat to the moral and social order.
>
> (Skeggs 1993: 113)

In the British media's representation of Patra her danger is made explicit because although she has 'changed' she still maintains 'killer braids and shiny red talons' (O'Brien 1995: 12). Patra remains predatory and dangerous. Lady Saw is described as too 'raunchy' to be able to come to Britain, or to be welcomed if she did (Sawyer 1995: 34). While the media exploits the sexiness of both women there is the constant reminder that it should be held at arm's length: perhaps, in a rather unpleasant echo of the racist discourse of empire, colonies and slavery in the Caribbean (Cooper, 1993), because it might 'contaminate' other women?

Rose offers a detailed analysis of Salt 'N' Pepa's video for their duet with E.U., 'Shake Your Thang', and many of her comments could be ascribed to a performance by either Patra or Lady Saw.

> Black women rappers' public displays of physical and sexual freedom often challenge male notions of female sexuality and pleasure. [Salt 'N' Pepa's video] is a verbal and visual display of black women's sexual resistance.
>
> (Rose 1994: 166)

> A primary source of the video's power is Salt 'N' Pepa's irreverence toward the morally based sexual constrictions placed on them as women. They mock moral claims about the proper modes of women's expression and enjoy every minute of it. . . . [The video] focuses directly on the sexual desirability and beauty of black women's bodies.
>
> (Rose 1994: 167)

Hence for black women in rap and, to a probably lesser extent, for women in dancehall/ragga performance, the challenging of perceived and constructed notions of black women's sexuality, both by men and by the established dominant power structures in society, is a central part of the ways in which they resist negative, damaging representations of themselves, and, simultaneously, create positive and strong spaces for women.

This chapter draws upon specific moments and sites of representations of two women in Jamaican dancehall/ragga music and demonstrates the ways in which both envision themselves as 'making space for women'. However, it has to be remembered that these are moments in what is a highly dynamic and fluid musical and spatial expression. Through their very presence both on stage and through their music Patra and Lady Saw actively disrupt established notions of women's 'place' and create images for other ghetto girls to identify with. For them, the placing of their music and the gendered experiences which are constructed in those particular places are an integral part of their performance. They sing 'dirty reality' and through their music they talk about their lives, their dreams and their fantasies. It is this element of the gendered perspectives that the ragga women constitute as part of their music which creates the striking connections with black women rap performers in what they demand and display.

As with all discourses of race, gender and sexuality, the struggle for change and transformation within these social and cultural constructions is perpetual, is ongoing and can never be fully achieved. None the less through dancehall/ragga Jamaican women are offering a culturally inspired public space in which women can resist and engage in dialogic challenges and potential transformations. At the same time women in dancehall spaces have a really great time as they sing, dance and dress in such a way that they are able to leave behind for a while the problems of everyday life in poor black neighbourhoods – in Jamaica or anywhere.

Notes

1 Throughout the chapter I use the term Jamaican and this mostly locates the subject within Jamaica. The term is also used to imply the wider Jamaican Diaspora based mostly in the UK and the USA. A Jamaican is not just someone who currently resides in Jamaica, or has ever been resident there, but can also encompass those who define themselves as Jamaican. This is especially important in a discussion of a cultural form that transcends national boundaries and geographical scales of identity.

2 For a more detailed analysis of the origins and connections between ragga music and other Jamaican music forms see Kenneth Bilby's chapter on Jamaica in Manuel's *Caribbean Currents* (Bilby 1995).

IV

'ALTOGETHER ELSEWHERE': FUTURES

De La Warr Pavilion, Bexhill-on-Sea, Sussex:
Rosa Ainley

This final section looks at once at different uses/aspects of technology and future developments in attitudes to space: the cyberdyke; high-technology industry; technological prosthetics in the construction of identity; the 'space' of theory.

Technology and the advent and development of virtual spaces have changed our relationship to the physical and given rise to new realms of association in work and leisure. As technologies begin to become part of the fabric of the city – for instance, the Malaysian 'Cybercity in the jungle' outside Kuala Lumpur (interestingly being financed and constructed in an international partnership arrangement) – rather than simply employed within the city and by its residents, different sets of relations between cities and technologies in the (not very distant) future become visible (Jacques: 1997).

Aylish Wood looks at the representations and use of technology in *Total Recall* in regard to the construction of identity. Going beyond a simple demonstration of fx, the film uses the relationship between male characters and technology to foreground the possibility of new areas of choice. Female characters are limited by a more circumscribed (literally cosmetic) position to the film's use of technology.

Doreen Massey's chapter exposes an old binary – that of reason/non-reason – active in the culture and working practices in a newer environment: the scientific research sector of the high-technology industry in Cambridge, England, and how this operates within a particular form of masculinity. She argues against the 'framing of life in terms of either/or' whether in relation to transcendence/immanence or work/home and shows how reinforcement of dualisms can result from strategies of resistance to them.

The workings of identity and performance in lesbian cyberspace in the Bay area of San Francisco form the basis of Nina Wakeford's piece on sexuality, place and technology. Characterising cyberspace as a series of performances instead of looking for a definitive description she discusses fluidity/fixity of identity in relation to particular spaces.

Fittingly for a final chapter, Jos Boys begins to map out a future terrain in the struggle for territories and meanings. In rethinking the relationships between gender and space for future work, she takes as a commonplace the spatial as a reflection of the social and exposes the closed nature of feminist theories about women and space, exploring alternative ways of conceptualisation.

12

Blurring the binaries?

High tech in Cambridge

Doreen Massey

An important element in recent feminist analyses of gender has been the investigation and deconstruction of dualistic thinking. This chapter takes up one aspect of this issue of dualisms and the construction of gender. It examines the interplay between two particular dualisms in the context of daily life in and around high-technology industry in the Cambridge area of England. The focus on dualisms as *lived*, as an element of daily practice, is important (see Bourdieu 1977; Moore 1986), for philosophical frameworks do not 'only' exist as theoretical propositions or in the form of the written word. They are both reproduced and, at least potentially, struggled with and rebelled against, in the practice of living life. The focus here is on how particular dualisms may both support and problematise certain forms of social organisation around British high-technology industry.

High-technology industry in various guises is seen across the political spectrum as the hope for the future of national, regional and local economies (Hall 1985) and it is important therefore to be aware of the societal relations, including those around gender, which it supports and encourages in its current form of organisation.[1] In the United Kingdom 'high tech' has been sought after by local areas across the country and has been the centrepiece of some of the most spectacular local-economic success stories of recent years. In particular, it is the foundation of what has become known as the Cambridge Phenomenon (Segal Quince & Partners 1985). The investigation reported on here is of those highly qualified scientists and engineers, working in the private sector in a range of companies from the tiny to the multinational, who form the core of this new growth. These are people primarily involved in research and in the design of new products. They are at the high-status end of high tech. And there are two things we need to know about them here: first, that the overwhelming majority of them are male; and second, that they work extremely long hours and on a basis which demands from them very high degrees of both temporal and spatial flexibility (see Henry and Massey 1995). It was the conjunction of these two things which led to the train of enquiry reported here.

Reasons for the long hours of work

There are three bundles of reasons for the long hours worked by employees in these parts of the economy.[2]

The first bundle of reasons revolves around the nature of competition between companies in these high-technology activities. It is the kind of competition which has frequently been characterised as classically 'post-Fordist': production frequently takes place on a one-off basis, as the result of specifically negotiated, and competitive, tenders. High-up among the criteria on which tenders are judged is the time within which the contract will be completed. Moreover, both during and after production there is a strong emphasis on responsiveness to the customer: in answering enquiries, in solving problems which emerge during and after installation/delivery of a product, in being there when needed – even if the telephone call comes through from California in the middle of the night. It is not so much the inherent unpredictability of R & D as the way in which it is compressed into the spatio-temporal dimensions required by this particular social construction of competition which is the issue. 'Time' is important to successful competition. The results of the investigation should give pause for thought. For these are high-status core workers in what is frequently heralded as a promising flexible future. The demands which this flexibility places even on these workers are considerable.

Moreover, these pressures for long hours are added to by a second bundle of reasons: those which revolve around the nature of competition within the labour market. There are a number of strands to this, but the most significant derives from the market's general character as knowledge-based. It is a market in individualised labour power, valued for its specific learning, experience and knowledge. In order to compete in this labour market (and others like it) employees must, beyond the necessity of working the already-long hours required by their companies, continue to reproduce and enhance the value of their own labour power. They must keep up with the literature, go to conferences, maintain the performance of networking and of talking to the right people, and so forth. This is additional labour which is put in outside of the hours required by the company and its success, but it is equally necessary for the success of the individual employee. Within the workplaces, too, the interaction between employees can produce a culture which glorifies long hours of work. Again, this may derive from competition between individuals, but it may also result from various peer-group pressures – the need 'not to let the team down', for instance, can become a form of social compulsion (Halford and Savage 1995).

But the third reason that the employees in these parts of the economy work such very long hours is completely different. It is, quite simply, that they love their work. Figure 12.1 illustrates some aspects of this; the first four quotations are from scientists themselves, the last two from company representatives. These scientists and engineers become absorbed by their work, caught up by the interest of it; they don't like to leave an element of a problem unsolved before they break off for the evening. The way this is interpreted, or presented, by different groups varies. Thus, company representatives speak of the kinds of people they seek to employ as committed and flexible, as 'motivated', as 'able to take pressure', as not being the kind to watch the clock, and they not infrequently acknowledge that this characteristic may derive from pure interest in the work itself. Some company representatives were quite clear that their search for employees was directed towards finding these characteristics. The scientists themselves often talk of their delight in the nature of the work, of its intrinsic interest. Where these male scientists have partners, however (and all the partners we identified were women), the partner's view of it was often more cynical, more tinged with the observation of obsessiveness, or of workaholism.[3]

A couple of points are worth making at this juncture. First, one's immediate response to the working lives of these employees may well be critical. Certainly, as we carried out the research, ours was so, in principle at least. Yet all of the reasons for this perhaps excessive duration of work also have their other side: thoroughly ambiguous though each is in a different way. In terms of competition, 'putting the customer first' is no bad thing (especially if you are the customer). Yet the demands it places on employees can be enormous. In terms of the labour market, it is usually

---

We don't *need* to work longer – I think people choose to because they enjoy their work, because they own the project . . . and there's also ownership of the client.

The clock doesn't matter at all. The only restriction for me is I don't like to get home too late. The landlady's given me a key, but I don't like to arrive much after midnight.

I've got so much holiday I don't know what to do with it.

. . . because I enjoy it . . . I enjoy the work . . . I enjoy computers . . . I often wonder what I would have done if I'd had to get a job in the days before computing.

One person was sent abroad to a conference because they would not take time off.

But the thing we have discovered over the years is that people who work here, and get into it, become addicted . . . we find the problem of getting some people to leave; they do get very engrossed in the thing. . . . This circuit of people working on the system here, the difficulties are extracting them, for some other thing that may be necessary, like they haven't had any sleep for the last 40 years!

Figure 12.1 Enthusiasm for work leading to longer hours: Doreen Massey interpreted as an advance that one's value is based on knowledge and experience rather than, for example, on lack of unionisation, or the lowness of the wages one is prepared to accept. Again, the individualisation of the labour market must in some senses be an advance, certainly over the treatment of workers as a mass, as an undifferentiated pool of nameless labour power. The idea that we are heading towards an economy and society which are based on knowledge, however unlikely in fact, has always been treated as a change for the better. Finally, the fact that people enjoy their work, and that they enjoy it in part precisely because it is knowledge-producing (in the employees themselves), can only be seen as an improvement over the kinds of jobs which are characterised above all by mind-numbing monotony and a desire to get to the end of the day. After years of exposing the fact and the effects of de-skilling I find it hard to criticise jobs because they are too absorbing and demand too much in the way of skill-enhancement! (Yet this very dilemma may point to the fact that the problem has been wrongly posed. Maybe it is the polarisation between de-skilled and super-skilled which should be the focus of our attention. . . .)

A further point worth noting is that the second and third of these reasons for long hours (the nature of the labour market and the love of the work) – though perhaps less so in its particular articulation, the first (the nature of competition in the sector) – are shared by many other occupations and parts of the economy, especially professional sectors and perhaps most particularly academe. Some of the issues which arise are therefore of much more general relevance, beyond the relatively small sectors of high technology in Cambridge. Certainly, they posed questions to us personally, as we did the research. Yet in other ways, the particular manner in which these pressures function, and the kinds of social characteristics with which they are associated, are quite specific to individual parts of the economy.

Dualisms and masculinities

One of the specificities of these high-technology sectors is closely linked to the *reasons why* the employees are so attached to their jobs and how these are interpreted. The dynamics in play here are bound up with elements of masculinity, *and of a very specific form of masculinity*. Above all, the attachment to these jobs is bound up with their character as scientific, as being dependent upon (and, perhaps equally importantly, confined to) the exercise of rationality and of logic. Within the structure of the economy, these jobs represent an apex of the domination of reason and science. It is this which lends them much of their status and which in part accounts for the triumphalist descriptions they are so often accorded in journalistic accounts. What is demanded here is the ability to think logically.[4] It is, in other words, a sector of the economy whose prime characteristics, for employees at this level, are structured around one of the oldest dualisms in western thought – that between Reason and non-Reason; and it is identified with that pole – Reason – which has been socially constructed, and validated, as masculine (see, especially, Lloyd 1984).

Moreover, in this dualistic formulation science is seen as being on the side of History (capital H). It makes breakthroughs; it is involved in change, in progress. And it is here that it links up to the second dualism which emerged as this research proceeded: that between transcendence and immanence. In its aspect of transcendence, science is deeply opposed to that supposed opposite, the static realm of living-in-the-present, of simple reproduction, which has been termed immanence. This opposition between transcendence and immanence is also a dualism with a long history in western thought. And again it is transcendence which has been identified as masculine (he who goes out and makes history) as against a feminine who 'merely' lives and reproduces. As Lloyd argues, 'Transcendence', in its origins, is a transcendence *of* the feminine. In its Hegelian version, it is associated with a repudiation of what is supposedly signified by the female body, the 'holes' and 'slime' which threaten to engulf free subjecthood (see Sartre 1943: 613–4). . . . In both cases, of course, it is only from a male perspective that the feminine can be seen as what must be transcended. But the male perspective has left its marks on the very concepts of 'transcendence' and 'immanence' (Lloyd 1984: 101). The two dualisms (Reason/non-Reason, and Transcendence/Immanence) are thus not the same, though there are interrelations between them.

The reasons for these characterisations, and for the construction of these dichotomies in the first place, and their relationship to gender, have been much investigated (see, for instance, Dinnerstein 1987; Keller 1982 and 1985; Easlea 1981; Wajcman 1991; O'Brien 1981; Hartsock 1985). There has been a close relation between the constitution of science on the one hand and of gender on the other. David Noble's (1992) history of 'a world without women' tells the long story of the capturing by enclosed masculine societies of the kind of knowledge production which was to receive the highest social valuation.

Such dualist thinking, as has already been said, has been subject to much criticism. However, the nature of the criticism has changed and been disputed. In *The Second Sex* Simone de Beauvoir famously urged women to enter the sphere of transcendence. In recent years, however, it has rather been the fact of thinking dualistically which has been objected to. Dualistic thinking has been criticised both in general as a mode of conceptualising the world and in particular in its relation to gender and sexual politics. In general terms, dualistic thinking leads to the closing-off of options, and to the structuring of the world in terms of either/or. In relation to gender and sexuality it leads, likewise, to the construction of heterosexual opposites and to the reduction of genders and sexualities to two counterposed possibilities. Moreover, even when at first sight they may seem to have little to do with gender, many such dualisms are in fact thoroughly imbued with gender connotations, one side being socially characterised as masculine, the other as feminine, and the former being accordingly socially valorised. The power of these connotational structures is immense, and it is apparently not much lessened – indeed it is possibly only rendered more flexible – by the existence among them of inconsistencies and contradictions.

It was only gradually, though, in the course of considering the interview material and the nature of work in the scientific sectors of the economy, that the issue of dualisms emerged as significant in this research. What people said, the way life was organised and conceptualised, the unspoken assumptions which repeatedly emerged: these pushed the enquiry in this direction.

Thus, for example, it was evident that in Cambridge these scientific employees were specifically attached to those aspects of their work which embody 'reason' and 'transcendence'. What they really enjoy is its logical and scientific nature. They themselves when talking may glory in the scientificity of their work, and frequently exhibit delight in the puzzle-solving, logical-game nature of it all.[5] Their partners comment upon their obsession with their computers, and both partners and company representatives talk of boys with toys (one representative candidly pointing out that these guys like their jobs because the company can buy far more expensive toys than the men themselves could ever afford):

> We have toys which they can't afford. You know engineers, big kids really; buy them a computer, you know you've got them . . . you know [they are] quite happy if you can give them the toys to play with.

This attachment to computers may be seen in this context as reflecting two rather different things, both of which are distinct from the more technologically oriented love of 'fiddling about with machines'. On the one hand these machines, and what can be done with them, embody the science in which the employees are involved. They are aids and stimuli to logical thought. On the other hand their relative predictability (and thus controllability) as machines insulates them from the uncertainties, and possibly the emotional demands, of the social sphere.

The aspect of transcendence comes through in the frequent characterisation of these jobs in terms of 'struggling' with problems, as 'making breakthroughs'; as being up against a scientific-technical 'frontier'. One scientist, reflecting on the reasons for his long hours of work, talked of being 'driven by success' and the fact that he was 'always reaching higher'. Another scientist in the same company, but who was quite critical of the hours worked by others, argued that for some people crisis is part of the job culture: 'It's a sort of badge of courage.' Other words, too, reflect the effort and the struggle of it all: 'If I stagger out of here at 11 o'clock at night I really don't feel like going home and cooking.' There's the quest: 'As a parent I try to spend as much time as I can with [the child] but in my quest for whatever it is I tend to work very hard.' There's the compulsion: 'If you've gotta do it then you've gotta do it.' And, hopefully, there's the triumph:

his wife is much more even-tempered than my wife who says sort of 'what the hell, Friday night we have got to go out and don't you forget it', but [my wife] accepts the fact that if there is nothing on specifically and nothing to be done . . . [then] the chances are that I will disappear, and reappear looking cross-eyed and what not, with a slightly triumphant smile or look downcast.

That quotation illustrates also a further phenomenon: that the self-conception of many of these employees is built around this work that they do and around this work specifically as scientific activity: 'the machine in front of them is their home', 'It is their science which dominates their lives and interests.'

Moreover, this glorification of their scientific/research and development capabilities on the part of the scientists can go along with a quite contrasting deprecation of their ability to do other things, especially (in the context of our interviews) their incompetence in the face of domestic labour. This is work which it is quite acceptable not to be good at. Thus:

Laundry? *'I shove it in the machine.'* Cleaning? *'I do it when it gets too much.'* Shopping? *'Tesco's, Friday or Saturday.'* Cooking? *'I put something in the microwave. Nothing special. As long as it's quick and easy that's good enough for me.'* Gardening then? *'When necessary.'*

There is here none of the pleasurable elaboration on the nature of the tasks which typifies descriptions of the paid scientific work. The answers are short and dismissive.

Such attitudes are important in indicating what is considered acceptable as part of this scientist's own presentation of himself. Not only is the identification with scientific research very strong and positive, but it seems equally important for him to establish what is *not* part of his picture of himself. Domestic labour and caring for his daily needs and living environment are definitely out. It is not just that scientific activity is positively rated but that it is sharply cut off from other aspects of life. This is precisely the old dualism showing its head in personal self-identification and daily life. What was going on was a real rejection of the possibility of being good at *both* science *and* domestic labour. A framing of life in terms of 'either/or'.

In this case, and in some others, such downplaying of the rest of life extended to all non-work/scientific activities. But such extreme positions were not common and seem to be more evident among single men than those with partners, and, even more markedly, than among those with children. Some men were clearly aware of the issue. For one scientist, a new baby had 'completely changed his life' (what this meant was that he went home early almost every other night), and yet the difficulty of balancing or integrating the sides of life was evident:

I feel frustrated . . . when . . . after this baby that's changed my life . . . I go home early every other day (almost) and pick her up at 4.35, take her home, play with her until bedtime, and . . . I find that sometimes that's quite frustrating, and keeps me away from work. I mean – it's fulfilling in its own right, but it's . . . I'm conscious of the fact that . . . I call it a half-day, you know. I find it frustrating.

Finally, some of the comments made about the scientists by (some of) the partners were particularly sharp and revealing. They were:

> *Not very socially adequate.*
> *Better with things than with people.*
> *Work gets the best of him.*
> *Work is the centre of his life.*

One of the very few female company representatives (that is, a member of management, not of the scientific team) reflected:

> Well, when I first joined the company there were twelve people here and they stuck me in an office with the development team and it was a nightmare. I really hated it. They didn't talk, they didn't know how to talk to a woman, they really didn't.

What appears to be going on, in and around these jobs, is the construction/reinforcement of a particular kind of masculinity (that is, of characteristics that are socially coded masculine) around reason and scientificity, abstract thought and transcendence. It is a process that relates to some of the dualisms of western thought and that, as we shall see, has concrete effects in people's lives.

Such characteristics of the employees, it must be stressed, relate to the more general nature of their jobs. These are jobs which derive their prestige precisely from their abstract and theoretical nature, the very construction and content of which are the result of a long process of separation of conception from execution (and of the further reinforcement of this distinction through social and spatial distancing). Jobs, in other words, which enable and encourage the flourishing of these kinds of social characteristics. The long hours which, for the various reasons discussed above, are worked in them enforce both their centrality within the employees' lives and a passing on of the bulk of the work of reproduction to others. In Cynthia Cockburn's words: 'Family commitments must come second. Such work is clearly predicated on not having responsibility for childcare, indeed on having no one to look after, and ideally someone to look after you' (Cockburn 1985: 181). The implication of all this is not only that these jobs are an embodiment in working life of science and transcendence but also that in their very construction and the importance in life which they thereby come to attain, they enforce a separation of these things from other possible sides of life (the Other sides of Reason and of Transcendence) and thus embody these characteristics *as part of a dualism*. By expelling the other poles of these dualisms into the peripheral margins of life, and frequently on to other people (whether unpaid partner or paid services), they establish the dualisms as a social division of labour. The pressure is for someone else to carry the other side of life.

If there is indeed a form of masculinity bound up with all this, then the companies in these parts of the economy let it have its head; they trade on it and benefit from it, and – most significantly from the point of view of the argument in this chapter – they thereby reinforce it. Furthermore, the possession of these characteristics, which are socially coded masculine and which are related to *forms* of codification that resonate with dichotomous distinctions between two genders, makes people more easily exploitable by these forms of capital. There is here a convergence of desires/interests between a certain sort of masculinity and a certain sort of capital.

This is not to say that what is at issue here is simple 'sexism'. Our interviews did not reveal the explicit sexism found in some other studies, including Cockburn's (1985). We did not encounter much in the way of strong statements about the unsuitability of women for these jobs. There were a few such statements but they were infrequent in the overall context of our interviews. Nor was it clear that the male scientists who displayed the characteristics which have been described always recognised them explicitly as masculine (although further probing may well have unearthed more evidence on this score). What is at issue here is not so much overt discrimination or sexism as deeply internalised dualisms which structure personal identities and daily lives, which have effects upon the lives of others through structuring the operation of social relations and social dynamics, and which derive their masculine/feminine coding from the deep socio-philosophical underpinnings of western society.

The work/home boundary

The boundary between work and 'home' has often been seen, and in this case can be seen, as an instantiation of the dualism between transcendence and immanence.[6] At work the frontiers of history are pushed forward; at home (or so the formulation would have us believe) there is a world of feelings, emotions and (simple) reproduction. Lloyd, once again, summarises the complex arguments which have evolved:

> We owe to Descartes an influential and pervasive theory of mind, which provides support for a powerful version of the sexual division of mental labour. Women have been assigned responsibility for that realm of the sensuous which the Cartesian Man of Reason must transcend, if he is to have true knowledge of things. He must move on to the exercise of disciplined imagination, in most of scientific activity; and to the rigours of pure intellect, if he would grasp the ultimate foundations of science. Woman's task is to pre-serve the sphere of the intermingling of mind and body, to which the Man of Reason will repair for solace, warmth and relaxation. If he is to exercise the most exalted form of Reason, he must leave soft emotions and sensuousness behind; woman will keep them intact for him.
>
> (Lloyd 1984: 50)

The fact that all this can be, and has been, severely criticised in terms simply of its descriptive accuracy, most particularly from a feminist perspective, has not destroyed its power as a connotational system. What is at issue in the ideological power of these dualisms is not only the material facts to which they (often only very imperfectly) relate (many women don't like housework either, many female paid employees negotiate a work/home boundary, etc.), but the complex connotational systems to which they refer. The negotiation of this boundary has emerged in our research as a crucial element in the construction of these men's attitude to their work, and in their construction of themselves.

One of the avenues of enquiry which originally sparked my interest in designing this research derived from statements made in interviews in a previous project (Massey *et al.* 1992). That project also was concerned with investigating high-tech firms, in this case specifically those located on science parks, and one of the recurring themes in a number of the interviews concerned the blurring of boundaries. 'The boundary between work and play disappears' was a formulation which stuck in my mind. What absorbed me at that point was the characterisation of everything outside of paid work as 'play' and, especially given the very long hours worked in the companies we were investigating, it prompted me to wonder who it was that performed the domestic labour which was necessary to keep these guys fed and watered and able to turn up for work each morning. (The work of 'domestic labour', who performs it and how, and the complex intra-household negotiations over it, is the subject of another forthcoming paper.) But what the interviewee had in mind was the fact that work itself had many of the characteristics of play: that you get paid for doing things you enjoy, you have flexible working arrangements, you take work home, you are provided with expensive toys. In this formulation, there really is no boundary between paid work and play. In this way of understanding things, 'the home' in the sense of the domestic, of reproduction, of the sphere of emotions, sensuality and feelings, or of immanence, does not enter the picture at all.

How then do we interpret what actually happens to the boundary between work and home in the case of these scientists in Cambridge? There are two stages to the argument.

First, there is indeed a dislocation of the boundary between work and home. Most particularly, this is true in a temporal and spatial sense. Indeed it is a dislocation which primarily takes the form of an invasion of the space and time of one sphere (the home) by the priorities and preoccupations of the other (paid work). This can be illustrated in a whole range of ways. The high degree of temporal flexibility in terms of numbers of hours worked turns out in practice to be a flexibility far more in one direction than in the other. While the demands, and attractions, of work are responded to by working evenings, weekends, bank holidays and so forth – and it is expected that this will be so, this 'commitment', and 'flexibility' are required to be an accepted member of this part of the economy – the 'time-in-lieu' thereby in principle accrued is far less often taken and indeed has to be more formally negotiated, and the demands of home intrude into work far less than vice versa. Or again, spatially, work is very frequently taken home. A high proportion of these employees have machines, modems, and/or studies, in the space of the domestic sphere, but there is no equivalent presence of the concerns of home within the central space of paid work (at the most obvious level, for example, not one of the companies we investigated had a crèche). One of the company representatives we interviewed spoke of the employees being 'virtually here' (in the workplace) even when working at home, because of the telecommunications links installed between the two places. Moreover this raises a third and very significant aspect of this one-way invasion. A lot of our interviewees spoke of the scientists' difficulty in turning off thoughts about work, of not thinking about the problem they were puzzling over, even when physically doing something quite different. The men wondered if they should charge to the company time spent thinking in the bath. A few, both men and partners, spoke of episodes when the man would get up in the middle of the night to go and fiddle with some puzzle:

> He is thinking about it most of the time. He might be digging the garden but he is thinking about it. If he gets back at two in the morning he can go to sleep and just wake up in the middle of the night . . . and he has solved a problem in his sleep, or he will . . . have to go and look at textbooks and things.

Men, partners, and sometimes children, commented on minds being elsewhere while officially this was time for playing with the children or driving the car on a day out. Here there is a real 'spatial' split between mind and body. Here there really is a capsule of 'virtual' time-space of work within the material place of the home. While the body performs the rituals of the domestic sphere the mind is preoccupied with the interests and worries of work.

> I am well aware of the fact that in many areas, that you are better having the 9–5pm and everything like that, but I have never found it at all compatible with trying to work or trying to pursue a bit of research or a bit of development, to have to give up at the magic hour or whatever . . . and I mean you can't say to somebody you will think between 9 and 5pm and you will not think between 5.05pm and 8.55am.

This is eminently understandable, and in many ways an attractive situation – it is good to have paid employment which is interesting, and it is a challenge to resist the compartmentalisation of life into mutually sealed-off time-spaces. But what is important is that once again this works only one way. While domestic time is in this sense porous, work time is not. Indeed, and this is the significant point, in its present construction it *cannot* be so. While it is assumed that one may think about work while playing with the children or while out for the day with the partner, the reverse is not the case. Indeed a reason quite frequently given for working late nights and weekends at the office is that the time-space is less disturbed then – even if other people are doing the same thing there is less in the way of in-coming telephone-calls and so forth. One of the dominant characteristics of this kind of work is that it demands, and induces, total concentration. The above quotation is interesting in its implication that 'thought' is involved only in paid work. Moreover it is the kind of thought which requires a lack of intrusion; it is totally absorbing. Even the reservations to this 'all-work' atmosphere of the workplace in a sense reinforce its truth. Thus one or two workplaces had a gym and elaborate catering facilities on site, the aim being to aid rather than detract from the overall ability to concentrate. And in one company, partners – seemingly in despair at ever seeing their men – came into the office:

> they have children and wives and they are always retailing the complaints from their wives. . . . This is a constant complaint . . . there is a perennial complaint that the partner never sees them and they are always in here. In fact, partners tend to come in here and work in the evenings because that's where the other one is; they have different kinds of jobs but they can bring their work with them and do it here.

In fact, it is hardly an invasion: she is conforming to the norms of the workplace; what she has brought in with her is her 'work', not the sphere of the domestic, and he can carry on with what he has to do.

This does not mean that levels of concentration within the workplace do not vary, or that time-out cannot be taken. Indeed time-in-lieu, trips to the shops, etc., provide occasional windows in the working day. But within the workplace, everything, even the exercise of the body, is geared to the productivity of the intellect:

> I was amazed when I went there – I'd been working at [major corporation]. This huge factory . . . had shut and I came down here to the interview with [smaller company, Cambridge-based] and I walked up the stairway and on every floor there was a series of little offices and ramps around the edge and the middle of each floor was open and there was a ping-pong table or a snooker table and everybody seemed to be playing games and I thought that this is supposed to be a place of work – and then when I saw all the things they were doing – a chap put his bat down and [would] go off and design an IC in a little room in the corner.

What we have here, then, is the workplace constructed as a highly specialised envelope of space-time, into which the intrusion of other activities and interests is unwanted and limited.[7] 'The home', however, for most of these scientists, is constructed entirely differently. Both temporally and spatially it is porous, and in particular it is invaded by the sphere of paid work.

There is, in other words, a great asymmetry of power between these two spaces, home and work. The latter can both protect its own inviolability and invade the former. One element in this differential power is simply the force of the wage relation. The workplace and its activities are associated with market/commercial relations which, as in so many other instances, simply override the affective and non-market relations through which the home is constructed. The inequality in power is also attributable to the ongoing, daily relations between already established genders. Many of the scientists' partners gave up the struggle to defend the space-time of domesticity: 'It's just not worth having a row about it. In the end, I put up with it.'

Yet there are also deeper reasons for this asymmetry of power between the spaces of home and work. Once again they are bound up with the dualisms of gender and of science and their intimate relation to spatiality.[8] These men's jobs are devoted to thought, to R & D, to the production of 'knowledge'. And in western society the production of knowledge has for long been associated with abstraction from the real world: with the classic separation of mind from body. The men's workplaces reflect that deep-rooted philosophy: they are designed to isolate the activities of the mind and they are designed to celebrate those activities. The activities of the mind need a space abstracted from the rest of the world and in turn such spaces become elite because they are of the mind. Their status gives them power.

And yet this explanation needs a further twist. Not all places of intel-lectual work have to be like this. One or two of the female partners we spoke to also worked in intellectual environments, but spoke differently about their workplaces: '[Children] come in all over the place, and make a mess with my computer, and there are also [other] people with children around, and also colleagues will invite children to see different things.'

What seems to be distinct about the culture of high technology which is the focus of this investigation is its (particular form of) masculinity. And the particular spatiality of the places of this work both is a product of long-established intersecting dualisms and, in its construction, helps to reinforce those dualisms. These are not merely spaces where knowledge-production may happen but spaces which in the nature of their construction (as specialised, as closed-off from intrusion, and in the nature of the things in which they are specialised) themselves have effects – in the structuring of the daily lives and the identities of the scientists who work within them. Most particularly, in their boundedness and in their dedication to abstract thought to the exclusion of other things, these workplaces both reflect and provide a material basis for the particular form of masculinity which hegemonises this form of employment. Not only the nature of the work and the culture of the workplace but also the construction of the space of work itself, therefore, contributes to the moulding and reinforcement of this masculinity.

Yet what has been discussed so far is an alteration in the boundary between home and work which consists of nothing more than the spatio-temporal transgression by one sphere (one side of the dualism) into the other. The second stage of the argument, however, is that in whatever manner one interprets this 'blurring' of boundaries it does not entail any kind of overcoming of the dualism itself. Yet it is the fact of dichotomy itself (reason/non-reason; transcendence/immanence) which has been criticised as being part of that same mode of thinking which also polarises genders and the characteristics so frequently ascribed to them. What, then, can be learned about the possibility of unification from this study of Cambridge scientists?

Resistance

The characteristics which have been described above are traits of *masculinity*, not of men. As already implied there is no simple homogeneity among the men we studied. However, these characteristics are strongly embedded within the culture of this part of the economy (with some variation in detail between different types of jobs). Moreover, the strength of this embeddedness means that these characteristics 'pull' all its participants towards them. Individual men have relations to these characteristics which are more or less celebratory or painful. Many of them recognise the need to negotiate the very different personas they inhabit at home and at work – the scientist with the new baby (quoted earlier) was doing just that. And what he was confronting there was precisely the difficulty of preventing his dominant self-conception as a scientist from completely overriding those other potential sides of himself. Other men actively try to resist this potential domination. Their number is small and their reasons varied. Most commonly resistance is a response to stress or to strongly articulated objections from the partner, or to a genuine sensitivity to the men's felt need to live a more varied life, not to miss out on the children growing up, and so forth.

However, the resistance takes a particular form. It is almost entirely to do with working hours, and with the time and space which work occupies, rather than with wider characteristics of the job. It also takes place almost entirely at the individual level. These workplaces are not unionised. Moreover, at a more general social level, while there are trade-union campaigns and feminist arguments for a shorter working day and week, they have as yet made very little progress. Certainly there seems to have been no thoroughgoing cultural shift, in spite of the increasing proportion of employment which is part-time, in favour of shorter working hours. Indeed, since in these parts of the economy at least some of the compulsion to work long days comes from the interest in and commitment to the work itself, it is not clear how such jobs and others like them relate to the wider arguments about working time. Given all this, it is the scientists individually who decide how they are going to respond to the pressures and attractions of their jobs, and how they will negotiate the work/home boundary and the distinct identities the different spaces may imply.

In this context it is deeply ironic that one of the important mechanisms of resistance, and one adopted by a number of the men, is precisely to insist on the necessity for and the impermeability of the boundary between work and home. Given the fact that the tendency is for work to invade home life one obvious mechanism for resistance is to protect home life from intrusion. This happens in a number of ways. Some men (a few only, but then the resisters in total are not a high proportion of the whole) have decided not to take work home, thereby preserving the space of home and the time spent in it from the intrusion of the demands of paid work. Sometimes this will involve an intrusion in time terms, maybe involving staying longer at the workplace in order to finish a task there rather than take it home. It is here the *space* of home which is seen as being the most important not to violate. Other men, though again only a few, have made themselves rules about *time* and insist on keeping to a regular daily routine and on arriving and leaving the workplace at set times. Over the long term it is possible that this will be detrimental to their careers, but the men are aware of this and indeed in some cases have adopted the strategy because of other problems (personal stress, problems with health or personal relationships) which had been produced by a previous commitment to the high pressure and long hours more typical of these companies in general. It must be emphasised that this is not the only way of coping with the pressures of this work where they are experienced as a problem. Other scientists, and couples, have found other ways of dealing with the demands and compulsions of this kind of work but what is significant about this one is its irony. The 'problem', as we have argued above, has been posed through the working-out in everyday life of some of the major dualisms of western ways of thinking. Yet, in the absence of collective resistance, legislative action or wider cultural shifts, individual attempts to deal with some of the conflicts thus provoked may result in a reinforcement of the expression of those very dualisms. The dichotomies are rigidified in order to protect one sphere (the home, the 'rest of life') from invasion by the other (scientific abstraction, transcendence). The problems posed by the dualisms result in their reinforcement.

The last section concluded on an irony: that those who were attempting to resist the domination of their lives by one side of a dualistic separation most often found themselves reinforcing the divide between the two poles of the dualism. This was one among a number of ironies in the situation analysed here. What such Catch-22 situations indicate is that the way out of the conundrums does not lie at that level. The 'solution' must be sought in a deeper challenge to the situation.

Similarly, the empirical material discussed here raises a number of confusions and complexities around the politics of campaigns for a shorter working day/week. They are issues, too, which relate as much to academe, especially in its present increasingly intensified and individually competitive form, as they do to the high-tech work discussed in the chapter. They are issues which touched me personally as an academic and which made me think about my own life as I did the research. It is a privilege to have work which we find interesting. At a meeting of feminist academics, where we discussed an early version of this chapter, *none* of us wanted our 'work' to be restricted to thirty-five specified hours in each week. While all of us wanted to resist the current pressures on hours produced by the reinforcement of competitive structures, we did not want to lose either the feeling of autonomous commitment or the possibility of temporal flexibility. But neither did we like the actual way in which this 'flexibility' currently works – the pressure towards what can only be called a competitive workaholism and the inability to keep things under control. These are things which we as academics, as well as those in the high-technology sectors discussed here, need to confront. For when an important element of the pressure on time results from personal commitment on the one hand and individualised competition on the other, as well as from sectoral and work-place cultures, how can any form of collective resistance be organised?

In the longer term the aim must be to push the questioning further, to try to find those solutions which may involve questioning the dualisms themselves. That is, instead of endlessly trying to juggle incompatibilities, and to resolve ambiguities which in reality point to contradictions, it is important to undermine and disrupt the polarisations which are producing the problem in the first place. In philosophy, and in particular in feminist critical philosophy, this position is by now well established. The aim in general is not now only to valorise the previously deprioritised pole of a dualism (as Simone de Beauvoir did) but to undermine the dualistic structure altogether.

Such more fundamental critiques may be carried into other areas. Thus, in the early part of this chapter I wrote of the difficulty I had encountered, after years of criticising de-skilling within industry, when finding myself criticising jobs for being too absorbing. Another irony indeed. However, as was hinted there, it may be that the very dilemma points to the fact that the issue would be better posed in another way. Rather than being critical of de-skilling or super-skilling as such, it is the polarisation between them which should be the focus of critical attention. What is at issue here – and it is an issue which again involves us as academics – is the *social division* between conception and execution, between intellectuals and the rest.

What I find more problematical as a political issue is the division of the lives of the scientists described in this chapter between abstract and completely 'mental' labour on the one hand, and the 'rest of life' on the other. In the version of this chapter that was sent to referees I had unreservedly applauded those few attempts which we had come across to resist the compartmentalisation of life into mutually sealed-off time-spaces. At least one referee questioned this, asking simply: '*Why* is it good to resist compartmentalisation?' And I know for myself that one thing I thoroughly enjoy is to sit down in the secluded and excluding space of the Reading Room at the British Museum and devote myself entirely to thinking and writing. And yet . . . do we want lives sectioned-off into compartments, into exclusive time-spaces (Lefebvre's abstract spaces): for the intellect, for leisure, for shopping . . . ?

This dilemma might relate to, and be partially addressed by, considering the major dualism discussed in this chapter – that in which 'Science' itself is involved. It is perhaps that the problem lies most fundamentally in the postulated separation-off of the isolated intellect from the rest of one's being, and calling the product of the working of that (supposedly) isolated intellect: knowledge. That process of the separation-off of spaces of the mind is one with a long history in the West and which, arguably, is also a history of the production of this form of scientific masculinity. David Noble (1992) has documented the long struggle to create a priesthood (more lately, an academe) through which society's knowledge was seen to be produced and legitimised. What he clearly demonstrates is both the long historical continuities which exist between certain early-Christian forms, all-male monasteries, early European univerisities, and today's academy. The sphere of the production and legitimisation of knowledge was, he shows, and in the words of his title, a world without women. But it was not created so without a struggle: it was constantly challenged by those with other ideas about how knowledge should be organised, who could have access to it and who could legitimately be thought to produce it. Moreover, it was also challenged by those who had other ideas about the construction of gender. From early Christian sects, through the Cathars of southern France, through the radical dissenters of the sixteenth and seventeenth centuries, to the arguments of today's feminists, a challenge has been mounted not only to the exclusive possession of this knowledge (and the spaces of this knowledge) by men, but to the nature of the construction both of 'knowledge' itself and of its attendant form of masculinity and of dichotomised male and female. And in this long historical engagement spatiality has been a crucial term: the struggle to construct elite and excluding spaces celebrating and augmenting the separateness and the status of the activities of the (scientific/masculine) mind (see Massey forthcoming). The spaces of high-technology R & D which have been investigated in this chapter are thus part of a long line of spaces integral to the hegemony of particular sorts of knowledge and particular sorts of masculinity.

If we were to challenge that idea of knowledge which is founded upon the separation of mind from body we should need not only that feminists invade the spaces of its production, but also that we challenge the construction of the spaces themselves. Among many others Ho has argued for an alternative:

> This manner of knowing – with one's entire being, rather than just the isolated intellect – is foreign to the scientific tradition of the west. But . . . it is the only authentic way of knowing, if we [are] to follow to logical conclusion the implications of the development of western scientific ideas since the beginning of the present century. We have come full circle to validating the participatory framework that is universal to all indigenous knowledge systems the world over. I find this very agreeable and quite exciting.
>
> (Ho 1993: 168)

The real irony, then, may be that the long-standing western (though not only western) dualism between abstract thought and materiality/the body may lead through its own logic to its own undermining. And it is on that dualism that much of the separation within the economy between conception and execution – and thus these 'high-tech' jobs themselves – has been founded.

Notes

I would particularly like to thank Nick Henry, with whom much of the empirical work for this paper was done, for much discussion and comment. A first version of this paper, titled 'Masculinity, dualisms and high technology', was presented in a seminar series at Syracuse University. I should like to thank Nancy Duncan for her invitation. She has collected the seminar papers into a book: *Bodyspace*, published by Routledge.

This chapter is an adaptation of that paper and of the one published in *Transactions of the Institute of British Geographers* 20 (1995): 487–99. Thanks both to Routledge and to *Transactions* for permission to publish this version here.

1 Only one aspect of these relations is explored in this chapter. The work forms part of a wider project on high technology and the social relations which surround it. This research was funded by the ESRC: R000233004: 'High-status growth? Aspects of home and work around high-technology sectors' and is being carried out with Nick Henry, now at the Department of Geography, University of Birmingham.

   The project forms part of a wider programme of five pieces of research on the nature and consequences of growth in the south-east of England in the 1980s. The programme is based in the Geography Discipline, Faculty of Social Sciences, the Open University, from where further information, and a series of Occasional Papers are available.

2 The first two of these reasons are explored in more detail in Henry and Massey (1995). As part of the research we interviewed representatives of nineteen companies, sixty male scientists and thirty-eight partners, all of whom were female. 'Partnership' was defined in terms of cohabitation. About one third of the scientists were not cohabiting. The quotations from interviews which are cited in this chapter have been selected as *symptomatic*. They capture, or express with precision, points or attitudes which were typical or widely prevalent or, if indicated so in the text, which characterised attitudes held by some among the interviewees.

3 One result of this absorption in their work is of course that these men have less time over than they might otherwise have for life in the domestic sphere. A future paper deals directly with this issue. In discussions on the present chapter, Cynthia Cockburn wondered 'whether the time stolen by these men to sustain their addictive habit may actually not be stolen from the home (other men don't spend more time than they have to in the home), but rather stolen from pub, club and trade union' (personal communication). There is probably a lot in this. The point in the present chapter is precisely to emphasise that what characterises these sectors is a *particular form* of masculinity.

4 Cynthia Cockburn has pointed to some of the inconsistencies and contradictions even here – see her treatment of the concept of 'intuition', and of the scientists' ambiguous relation to it (Cockburn 1985). Indeed, the very fact that the men 'really love' their work, are 'obsessive' and so forth, touches on realms outside that of pure Reason (see Massey 1996). The attempt to purify the spaces of science is never really successful. But as pointed out in the opening paragraph, consistency has never been the outstanding attribute of the functioning of these dualisms, nor has *in*consistency seemed much impediment to their social power.

5 Similar worlds have been described by Tracey Kidder (1982) and Sherry Turkle (1984).

6 While the home/work distinction may validly be read as an instantiation of this dichotomy it must be stressed that there is far more to the possibilities of 'immanence' than having children and doing the housework.

7 This is broadly true of most workplaces, though to different degrees. The windowless boxes of so many modern factories precisely demonstrate the desire not to let the eye/mind wander 'outside' during working hours. But in the kinds of employment under discussion here, together with some others, it is especially marked.

8 This argument is explored further in Massey (1996).

13

Urban culture for virtual bodies

Comments on lesbian 'identity' and 'community' in San Francisco Bay Area cyberspace

Nina Wakeford

San Francisco has a special place in the lesbian and gay imagination. In his travelogue *States of Desire: Travels in Gay America*, Edmund White suggests that 'The city can serve as a sort of gay finishing school, a place where neophytes can confirm their gay identity' (1980: 66). The city is thus described as if it itself expertly bestows a sexuality on an individual, a sexuality that is withheld from those who are gay or lesbian in other places. The historian John D'Emilio draws an explicit comparison between the urban space of San Francisco and a religious site. He states: 'San Francisco has become akin to what Rome is for Catholics: a lot of us live there and many more make the pilgrimage' (D'Emilio 1992: 74). The San Francisco urban culture becomes part of an initiation whose symbolic heart is the Castro district, a small but frenetic place increasingly segregated from the poorer neighbouring areas by high rents and the volume of gay tourist dollars. In a more sombre reflection on the city's reputation, Kath Weston tells of the psychological and economic risks to 'queer migrants' who arrive with utopian visions of harmonious community only to be confronted with the harsh reality of job scarcity and unreliable support networks (Weston 1996).

Other coexisting utopian discourses simultaneously transform this sexualised city, most recently the venture-capital-led visions of a multimedia future in cyberspace. 'Multimedia Gulch' has transformed the South of Market district into a centre of new Internet and multimedia 'start-up' companies. There is a growing urban culture for virtual bodies. These virtual bodies are the seemingly groundless assemblages of identities which are in fact groups of Internet users situated in the San Francisco Bay Area. In this chapter I will discuss the resolutely local culture of one set of virtual persons: those involved in a lesbian community on-line. This group of users coexists with the day-to-day urban realities of lesbian and gay San Francisco and the surrounding area. To contextualise the comments on the specific forms of identity and community which became apparent in studying this group, I first outline how San Francisco emerged as 'a sort of gay finishing school' and then illustrate the kind of debates about sexuality and gender which are current in some local circles.

The gay and lesbian utopian imagination about San Francisco has a long history. At least since the 1950s, and possibly even before that time, San Francisco's urban culture has included the tolerance of life-styles visibly outside the dominant norms of 'traditional' heterosexuality. Both John D'Emilio and Lillian Faderman in their histories of sexuality in the USA claim that gay urban subcultures were aided by the Second World War and the period immediately following it (D'Emilio 1992; Faderman 1991). They suggest that San Francisco's geographical and strategic position as a major port of departure and return for those in the service, as well as an exit port for those ejected with dishonourable discharges, combined with the relatively liberal California state laws on homosexual gatherings in public places, led to the city's growing reputation as a visible venue for the enactment of lesbian and gay identities. D'Emilio also cites the literary Beat culture as a vital influence in the late 1950s. Some of the earliest lesbian and gay political organisations such as the Daughters of Bilitis (1955) were able to form and in time had local political influence. Eventually the sheer quantity of gay and lesbian votes could be held over politicians as leverage in a campaign, although this did not prevent continual police harassment in bars and of club-goers, and the most famous anti-gay murder in the city's history, that of the supervisor Harvey Milk in 1978 (D'Emilio 1992).

Nearly twenty years later references are still made to 'the lesbian and gay vote' in local elections, although such assumed alliances are made less certain by heightened awareness of the fractures along the lines of race and gender within communities which were previously constructed as a monolithic whole, at least at election time. At no time was this split more evident than in the recent mayoral victory of an African-American hetero-sexual man Willie Brown who beat white lesbian Roberta Achtenburg. Both appealed directly to their impeccable record on lesbian and gay rights, a situation which would be hard to imagine in any other US city except perhaps New York.

San Francisco retains its image as being on the leading edge of recon-ceptualisations of gender and sexuality, both in public and private worlds. Contemporary Bay Area cultures of sexuality are both diverse and complicated. Nevertheless, the city retains its reputation for tolerance and acceptance of virtually any subjective definition of sexual identity. A recent advice column featured a letter (signed only 'Dickless in Frisco') which illustrates the kind of intricate reconfiguration of body, desire and vocabulary in this local context. In the first phrase there is a comparison to 'bioboys', a term defined later in the column as 'boys born boys, as opposed to girls made boys':

> You bioboys think you've got problems . . . I'm a female-to-male transsexual who since my accession to sentience has been wild about boys. For years I tried to be happy as a straight female, but it never worked, I wasn't a female and I wasn't straight. What I was, and am, is a guy who is into gay S/M

leather as a master/top. I've been on testosterone a year and a half and pass as male most of the time, and in daily life my gender is not problematic. . . . And since I'm also a drag queen, I like being able to still look good when I go out en femme – which is not the same as reverting to female: I mean drag in corset and fishnets. Deep down, I think I'm a she-male dominatrix trapped in the body of a FTM tranny.

(*SF Weekly*, 11–17 June, 1997: 89)

Several current debates within the classification of the diversities in the city's non-heterosexual population are illustrated in this description. The labels of transsexual, femme, female, etc. are not presented as incompatible markers of separate identities, but are combined into a complex web of self-characterisation. The transsexual/tranny is aligned with the gay in opposition to the previous straight identity. The S/M vocabulary signals a sexual community which has thrived in San Francisco's Folsom Street area, at least relative to elsewhere. The drag queen is collapsed into a femme/ butch dynamic which resists clear gender categorisation. The resistance to assimilation of such a subjective classification is substantial. The most that can be said is that the writer is not (and has never been) a 'bioboy'. Yet the terms are also local and historically specific, signalling years of political and cultural work which have made this kind of hybridity intelligible to the local population.

Although this writer never mentions lesbian identity, there are parallel debates about the kind of sexualities which can be known as lesbian, and these draw upon the same distinctions of male/female, gay/straight, 'bio-'/transgendered. San Francisco continues to be the site of many such definitional battles, although as important a process of labelling to many commentators on lesbian communities in the Bay Area is the sheer range of lesbian identities which coexist or clash. In Arlene Stein's introduction to *Sisters, Sexperts, Queers: Beyond the Lesbian Nation* (1993) she describes the lesbian diversity with the following opposition:

In San Francisco today, the hottest lesbian club hosts a once-a-week splash that unabashedly features go-go dancers on pedestals and patrons clad in leather miniskirts. Across town sixty or seventy women gather each week in a dusty church basement to discuss the legal ins and outs of donor insemination, foster adoption programs, power of attorney contracts, and parenting. There are many other signs of lesbian life in this great gay Mecca, but few seem to capture the spirit of the moment so completely as the femmes strutting around in their lipstick and high heels and the prospective mothers worrying about the quality of the school systems.

(Stein 1993: xi)

Much of this lesbian activity happens in the wider Bay Area outside San Francisco itself since the high cost of living in the city forces those on lower incomes or without employment to migrate to less expensive cities within a 50- to 60 mile radius. Although each place has a specific manifestation of lesbian and gay urban culture, much of the feeling of San Francisco also permeates the cities of Oakland, Berkeley, San Jose, Palo Alto, Santa Cruz and others nearby. Debates and experiences are refracted through an image of 'The City' and the variation in what it means to claim the label 'lesbian' is equally wide elsewhere. Stein writes of her experience teaching an undergraduate class at University of California at Berkeley 'where the differences among women who identified themselves as lesbians were often as great, or greater, than those between lesbians and women who called themselves straight' (1993: xvi).

One of the most visible public displays of lesbian style is in the bars and clubs of the city. In the late 1980s and early 1990s the most popular San Francisco lesbian club experience was Club Q. Deborah Amory's study of this club in terms of style, age and ethnic profile described the clientele as 'hot young urban women', and identified them as transforming lesbian identities, influenced by black popular culture (in particular through the funk music preferences of DJ Page Hodel) and an enactment of the 'comeback' of butch/femme style (1996: 158). Amory rejects the blanket characterisation of the 'lipstick lesbian' to capture this transformation, particularly if the subject is assumed to be white. Insisting on the local and specific forms of this new image among many young San Francisco lesbians, she comments: 'The women at Club Q took the notion of the lipstick lesbian and worked it, right across the colour spectrum' (Amory 1996: 148).

The current and constant reformulation of what it means to be a lesbian in the Bay Area appears to confirm Stein's assessment: lesbian culture is decentred and up for grabs (Stein 1993: xvii). What does on-line lesbian activity signify in this local context? How are lesbian communities formed and their activities made intelligible where there are initially few clues to physical identity? As stated above, cyberspace has become the latest utopian discourse to confront San Francisco's urban culture. Yet it encounters an urban experience which is already sexualised. More generally the concepts of 'cyberspace' and 'the lesbian' have both been engaged in similar visions; cyberspace promises utopian otherness through technology, the category 'lesbian' through the invocation of identities and communities which reject the dominant orders of masculinity and heterosexuality. The group which I have studied – the Californian network of 'Bay Area cyber-dykes' (BACD) – is at the intersection of these visions. Their experiences speak to, and further complicate, evolving notions of the nature of lesbian identities, communities and the creation of places in cyberspace for those who are not bioboys.

Formal theorisations of 'lesbian' which function utopically suggest that this identity can be a way out of present conditions, or in Jagose's words 'designate a site exterior to the mechanisms of power: a space, system or economy that is altogether elsewhere' (Jagose 1993: 276). She describes the basic characteristics of such a site as 'its excess of cultural legislation, its alterity and exteriority', and this leads her to the characterisation of some definitions of the word 'lesbian' as necessarily 'altogether elsewhere'.

The phrase 'altogether elsewhere' mirrors much of the current framing of the word cyberspace, from its science fiction origins of 'a consensual hallucination' (Gibson 1984) to popular media conceptions of the liberating fluidity of identity based on an escape from the identificatory exigencies of the here and now. Exteriority to contemporary social relations is also promised in theoretical accounts (Benedikt 1991; Kroker and Weinstein 1994). Benedikt predicts 'New, liquid and multiple associations between people . . . new modes and levels of truly interpersonal communication' (Benedikt 1991: 123).

Much of such writing on cyberspace invokes gender as one of the constraints from which we might be liberated, yet does not associate this possibility with feminist political utopias; for instance, lesbianism as a utopic site. Accounts with a feminist focus include 'cyberfeminist' visions which merge utopias of cyberspace and feminism to promote increased interfacing of women and machines. Sadie Plant, the most well-known cyberfeminist, states:

> Complex systems and virtual worlds are not only important because they open spaces for existing women within an already existing culture, but also because of the extent to which they undermine both the world-view and the material reality of two thousand years of patriarchal control.
>
> (Plant 1996: 170)

Despite the anticipation that cyberspace is a way to avoid patriarchal control, it is unclear from the textual productions of cyberfeminism how the everyday practices of those in cyberspace who identify as lesbians might be theorised, particularly as it cannot be assumed that all women have an equal relationship to this 'material reality' of 'patriarchal control'. A summary of the debates circulating around cyberspace and the lesbian as independent concepts is necessary here to contextualise my comments on the activities of the BACD participants.

Defining cyberspace(s)

In popular culture the concept of cyberspace is suffering from over-excitement, over-exposure and under-precision. Consuming current media accounts prompts questions of the following kind. Is cyberspace the same as the Internet or does it include computer networks outside the Internet such as independent Bulletin Board Systems? Does it include every activity available over computer networks from electronic mail, to interactive chats or games, to browsing the World Wide Web? Does it include mediations of communication which have been around much longer than the term itself such as the space within which we make a telephone call? The competing definitions of the territory might better be resolved by characterising cyberspace as a series of specific performances, rather than searching for one underlying totalising definition (Wakeford 1995). Focusing on the local practices of those who are constructing spaces in self-proclaimed cyber-spaces suggests that a strategy which schematises the variety of spaces and activities may be more useful than continual (de)territorialisation.

In practical terms, in order to develop an epistemology and methodology for data collection we need a classificatory system of cyberspaces which is plural and multidimensional. Dimensions must include but not be limited to: the extent of synchronicity or asynchronicity of communication, direct and indirect costs of participation, cultural skills required (e.g. language, literacy, keyboard skills), the specifications of hardware and software configurations used. Each dimension works towards increasing specification, yet the recognition of continual change is best achieved by resisting the idea of a final or complete classification. The classificatory system is a work-in-progress for a wider research project on women in a diverse set of cyberspace situations.[1] It includes two dimensions which will be elaborated here as they relate directly to my discussion later of the Bay Area cyberdykes. First, the extent to which each space or activity is thought to be a site for the fluidity (or fixity) of identity can be used for categorisation. Second, the same investigation can be schematised in terms of the rhetoric of community.

Identity

Popular accounts of cyberspace have propagated a 'moral panic' around the presentation of self, or more specifically the *mis*representation of self which appears to be possible. Reports have suggested that on-line men pretend to be women, women pretend to be men, and heterosexual men try to adopt female personas strategically to attract women who turn out to be other men (Stone 1991). A tentative dimension which deals with identity must acknowledge that embedded within the normative patterns of each space or activity are assumptions about the accountability of the user for presenting a self which is honest or deceptive. Computer-mediated electronic spaces vary widely in the ways in which identity can be hidden or revealed. We expect that e-mail addresses are sent by those whose name appears in the 'From:' line, and this requires relatively advanced knowledge to subvert. However, in some forums, such as certain real-time textual exchanges, it is expected that one will not adopt a 'real' identity, but rather a nickname, and the practice of gender swapping is common (Kendall 1996).

The extent to which identity is treated as fluid in any particular area of cyberspace is complicated by the different levels of trust in 'truthful' representations, and this can cause further complexities. For example, in the real-time chat function over the Internet, called IRC (Internet Relay Chat), it is expected that men will not join lesbian 'channels', which are set up as private women-only spaces. If a nickname is suspected to conceal a male user who refuses to leave the space, the system operator of that channel can set a command to exclude further participation. Users must trust that there are only 'real' women in the space. Yet within the channel, the normative behaviour is to reject 'real' first names, and use mythical characters, lesbian idols, animals, objects or colours. Nicknames may also include adjectives like butch, happy, sexy, etc. Inside the space it is not expected that the identities are truthful, and there is not an expectation that participants need to measure up precisely to the personality traits or features which the nickname might suggest.

Community

One of the key discourses of the development and promotion of cyberspace has been to associate the word with the development of 'virtual communities'. To a large extent this promotion can be attributed to the writings of Rheingold who has been a consistent advocate of the sociability and new community formations which emerge electronically (Rheingold 1993). However, to characterise every cyberspace as being amenable to this kind of rhetoric is misleading. Rheingold's influential comments on his own experiences were initially based on a small Californian Bulletin Board Service, the WELL. The WELL was not the 'global community' of the Internet, although it has been assumed by many taking up his ideas that the 'virtual community' can be scaled up universally in this way, at least rhetorically.

For this dimension the crucial measure is the extent to which each computer-mediated activity draws upon the rhetoric of community, and also how this is related to the forms of activity which happen within that site. Usenet groups have been portrayed as communities (Baym 1995). Similarly some authors have written of the immersive textual environments called MUDs/MOOs as communities, drawing on the observation that users develop evolving personas and build their own virtual rooms in the system (Reid 1995). We cannot assume that any space consists of, or promotes, community merely because interaction can happen. There is a wider political agenda in labelling a cyberspace 'a community'. A crucial task is how each activity or space in the dimension is able to justify use of the word, particularly in terms of the kind of interaction which happens there.

Defining lesbian(s)

Undercurrents of standardisation and marginalisation permeate the discussion of lesbian identities and communities, and here I can only skim the surface of the lengthy debates about whom/what these terms have come to signify. In terms of standardisation of the lesbian identity there has been a tension between the need to stress lesbian identity on a continuum which included all women such as that proposed by Adrienne Rich (1980), and the need to specify 'insiders' and 'outsiders' by clarifying a boundary (e.g. Wiseman 1993; Walker 1993). The latter tendency is clear in some of the direct responses to Rich's lesbian continuum. One reaction to Rich defines a lesbian as

> a woman who has sexual and erotic-emotional ties primarily with women or who sees herself as centrally involved with a community of self-identified

lesbians whose sexual and erotic-emotional ties are primarily with women; and who is herself a self-identified lesbian.

(Ferguson *et al.* 1982: 153)

This kind of definition might be criticised in terms of its totalising stance towards 'the lesbian', particularly with relation to its potential incapacity to take on board the transcultural and transhistorical. Nevertheless there is an increasing recognition that the solution to definitional anxiety is not to simply add an 's' in order to encompass that which is characterised as 'difference', nor to preface words with qualificatory adjectives leaving the central concept unchallenged (Walker 1993). In the last few years the category of the lesbian in feminist and queer theory has been confronted by the mestiza consciousness (Anzaldúa 1987), and drag kings and what *Time Out* referred to as 'hasbians' (has-been-lesbians), as well as reproductions of the debates evident in the San Francisco Bay Area. The result is 'a certain taxonomic crisis' (Jagose 1993: 264) where attitudes of 'fundamental uncertainty of the category "lesbian" are virtually de rigueur in current lesbian criticism and theorising' (ibid: 265).

In an attempt to move on from this impasse, authors such as Shane Phelan stress that working with 'multiplicity' is a way to build politics as well as rethink lesbian identities (Phelan 1994). In opposition to that which she characterises as a previous politics of the unitary lesbian self, Phelan proposes a postmodern politics of 'getting specific'. Central to 'getting specific' is an acknowledgement that defining lesbian identities must begin with everyday concrete experiences. This kind of approach, which argues against a separated utopic lesbian identity and in favour of a contextual construction of lesbian identities, is also the position of Jagose, who asserts:

There is no prediscursive (lesbian) body; there is nowhere some pure (lesbian) body of which discursive constructions of the (lesbian) body are a misrepresentation.

(Jagose 1993: 281)

In refusing any kind of essentialism, strategic or otherwise, it seems that we have moved from 'Any woman can be a lesbian', the slogan of the mid-1970s, to 'Any *body* can be a lesbian' or 'Any *discourse* can be lesbian'. Phelan states that 'our lesbianisms must become more porous and plural' (Phelan 1994: 96). This theoretical position is problematic, and this becomes apparent in the BACD data. Although I find the idea of contextual construction attractive, it potentially underplays the differential power of naming between those who are constructing competing definitions. Phelan believes that we should be more concerned with coalition-building and 'a logic of inclusion' (Phelan 1994: 97) than with defining identities, and seems to suggest that 'others' can be trusted to be gate-keepers of lesbian identity. She states:

Lest anyone fear that this meaning will become too vague to be useful, we must remember that this process is occurring within a society with its own strong notions of what a lesbian is, that *it will police our borders for us.*

(1994: 97; emphasis added)

In the British context legal challenges to identity such as Clause 28 suggest these border police may be far from benevolent, even if their actions do have indirect consequences in terms of strengthening political resistance (Stacey 1991). Players in the lesbian definition game have differing degrees of influence in terms of who may present their contextual construction as the standardised definition and act to include or exclude on the basis of it.

Nevertheless the discursive-contextual production approach does stress the relationality of identity production, and much of the literature on lesbian identity stresses the connection to the notion of community (Ponse 1978; Kreiger 1982; Phelan 1989, 1994; Franzen 1993; Eder *et al.* 1995). Ponse describes entering 'the lesbian community' as one of the steps of 'the assumption of lesbian identity' (Ponse 1978). A decade and a half later Phelan suggests that 'within these communities they [women] are free to celebrate their "difference"' (Phelan 1994: 14), although she considers only some lesbian communities to be productive in terms of wider political campaigns. She criticises 'radical feminists focused on building a "women's community"', for not entering 'the world of modern patriarchal bureaucracies', with the implication that lesbian *communities* cannot automatically be trusted with 'getting specific' about lesbian *identity*.

Phelan clarifies her vision with a description of the four major processes of lesbian communities. First, a community provides insulation from hostility in relation to sexuality. In other words a place 'where being a lesbian is simply not an issue'. Second, a community promotes visibility or, in Phelan's words, acts as 'a beacon for lesbians'. Third, it encompasses a socialising function and provides guidance on behaviour and self-interpretation: the 'how to be a lesbian' function. Finally, the community is situated politically in relation to hegemonic systems. Phelan states that communities are 'the base for or result of political mobilisation'. With this set of measures for lesbian community in mind I turn now to the data on the Bay Area cyber-dykes and investigate the kind of claims to identity and community which are found on-line, and in their off-line activities.

Bay Area Cyber-Dykes

How do those who participate in explicitly lesbian cyberspaces measure up to these definitions of identity and community? There have been very few studies of such spaces. Correll (1995) has reported on an ethnographic study of a Lesbian Café Bulletin Board System (BBS) which connected those living in the eastern and southern regions of the USA. Within this cyberspace posters to the BBS created a fantasy Lesbian Café in which regulars posted their drink orders as they arrived on-line, spoke of their imaginary favourite seats, and used coded language to flirt with other regulars. 'Newbies' and 'lurkers' were encouraged to join in, and male 'bashers' were confronted then strategically ignored. Correll reports that the group did just once materialise by meeting 'in real life', but that only the regulars (about eight women) were involved. In another study, Hall (1996) examined the international lesbian mailing list Sappho and concentrated on expressions of feminist discourse. From a linguistic perspective, Hall describes the on-line screening process for participants which involved conforming to ideals of discursive femininity, an expectation of a female name, an anti-flaming policy (to counteract 'flames', or rude/offensive messages), repeated discussion of overtly 'female' topics, a pro-separatist and pro-women attitude and the use of feminist and/or lesbian signatures. Parts of these signatures frequently contain references to the lesbian body using a textual code called the Muff Diva Index, which allows users to devise a code for their self-image. By using ASCII characters one could rate oneself on the scales of butch/femme, long hair/no hair, love/hate of women's music and so on (Wakeford 1995).

The common theme in these accounts is the gathering of geographically dispersed subscribers in one electronic space. These are descriptions of electronic communities seemingly without situated place. In contrast, the BACD electronic mailing list has 200–220 subscribers (March 1995/ November 1995 figures) who are required to reside in the San Francisco Bay Area in order to participate on the list. Many of the features of the list can be derived from the urban culture in which it is created and maintained.

Technically speaking, the list functions automatically via the computer program Majordomo which distributes messages sent to the BACD address to all subscribers. The communication is non-synchronous, and messages are not subject to vetting before they are distributed, as they are in moderated forums. There is no charge for subscribing to BACD itself, but access to the Internet is available at no charge only for those studying or working at certain institutions or businesses. Through this route many of the BACD subscribers have free accounts, and the minimum cost for others per month is between $5 and $20 for an Internet connection, plus any additional costs of a computer and modem.

Due to the textual nature of mailing lists, and the lack of the need for any fonts or graphics in the messages which are sent and received, the initial cost of setting up a connection and subscribing to BACD is generally lower than other pay-per-minute lesbian on-line activities such as the WhistleStop Café Bulletin Board, or the Lesbian and Gay Chat rooms on America Online. During the period within which these data were collected the volume of communication which the list generated on a daily basis was 5–25 e-mail messages, reflecting the fact that many subscribers were living or working in situations where their computer systems had the capacity to receive this quantity of information, and that they had the time to read (or at the very least to delete) these messages on a regular basis. Although the list runs itself automatically, it also has an owner, or 'list mistress', Amy Goodloe. Amy set up Bay Area Cyber-dykes in November 1994; she handles the requests of those who want to join or leave, and also pays for the

Internet account from which it is run. The total financial cost to her each month is around $50, which is the sum of several Internet Services including a site for her Web pages and computer server space to run nine women-only lists.

Studying BACD through on-line activity, formal face-to-face interviews and participation at social events, it was clear that the theoretical categories of identity and community could be discussed in relation to much of the data collected. Here I present two examples where the two are mutually and inseparably constituted in a way which reflects the local culture of production: the on-line informational list message, and the categorisations of subscribers which occurred during social gatherings.

Information message

In order to find out about BACD, anyone with an e-mail account can send a message to the computer at which the list is housed and will receive back an automatically generated reply containing the 'info message'. The e-mail address for this request is publicized on World Wide Web sites and in the lesbian and gay media reports, and in this way the 'info message' acts as promotional material for the list. From the first section of the 'info message' four passages describe the purpose of the list :

(1) This list is for lesbians and dyke-identified women ONLY* (*for the purposes of this list, dyke-identified means any woman (born or TS) who identifies as lesbian or bisexual).
(2) Unlike the national lesbian lists, like Sappho and dykenet-l, this list is intended ONLY for those who live in the San Francisco bay area.
(3) Unlike ba-sappho, it is NOT a networking list . . . but instead a general chat and discussion list.
(4) Since we all live relatively close to each other, we can also plan on the occasional get-together.

Not only does the 'info message' set the rules for participation on-line, it suggests that 'get-togethers' might happen outside cyberspace. It also indicates the way in which lesbian identity is defined in terms of the concept of identification: 'lesbians and dyke-identified women', 'any woman (born or TS) who identifies as lesbian or bisexual'. These statements display a clear policy of inclusion of categories – bisexuals, transsexuals – which in other cyberspaces are problematised (Wincapaw 1997). For those who frequent several mailing lists with a lesbian theme, particularly ones with a large number of subscribers and postings such as Sappho or dykenet-l, it is common to encounter two key debates which often cause divisions in the list. These debates are about bisexuality (often abbreviated to GBD, the Great Bisexual Debate) and transgender. In her interview Amy suggested that subscribers could mark the passing of time by these debates:

> I mean the three topics which always come up on any list and always cause big flame wars are butch-femme, bisexuals and transexuals. It's like, it

happens every couple of months and you can almost just count on it. It's like, gee we haven't had the Great Bisexual Debate in a while [laughs] [pauses]. It's coming!

She also commented on the specificity of BACD:

> A lot of things come up on ba-cyberdykes which don't come up on other lesbian lists . . . different ways of dealing with things, because of the Bay Area, sort of a different community of lesbians . . . like the discussions of, like, what would be considered on the larger lists when bisexuality or transexuality come up, either topic . . . huge debate, lots of tension, lots of ignorance, lots of um, lots of negative energy. And it tends to be in the Bay Area there is a lot more understanding. Roughly ten percent of the list is transexual. [pauses] That's a lot. [laughs] That's pretty cool!

The local contextual definition of who was to be allowed on to BACD reflected the local cultures of lesbianism in the Bay Area of San Francisco, but was framed largely in terms of the debates, and has also shifted with time. Interestingly, when the list began there was also the requirement that subscribers identified themselves as 'post-op' transsexuals. Our exchange about the change in the policy points to the continual ambiguities over where to draw the boundaries of the list:

> Amy: My policy had been post-op transexual only, so I know, so, a lot of transexual women have made it a point to say that, just to let me know
> . . .
>
> What's the post-op/pre-op thing?
>
> Amy: That's not a policy anymore. That was by vote at the beginning of the list. When I first started the list, people were like, where do you draw the line, you know, at what point do you accept somebody who is a man who thinks he might be a woman, at what point do you say this is really a woman with a penis, so that was sort of, it's an arbitrary marker that a lot of people chose, it's an operation, I'll choose that, um, and some people were kind of suggesting to me that they had to actually have lived full time as a woman for a year, but then what do you do about a person who has been like nine months? So I just said, well, women only. And to identify as women-only you just identify as a woman, I mean you identify as a lesbian or bisexual woman, um, whatever that means!

The logic of self-identification is not unique to lesbian identity in cyberspace (Walker 1993: Wiseman 1993: Lemon and Patton 1997). What does seem to vary in comparison to presentations of self in other arenas is the way that identification must be shown textually in order to gain access to the list at all. To join the list a potential subscriber must e-mail Amy and state that she fulfils the conditions stated above. This is the point at which identity which is theoretically fluid – you may textually attempt to create any identification – becomes fixed and stabilised in relation to a specific local culture, in this case the urban cultures of sexuality of the Bay Area. Fundamentally it is Amy who fixes the definition of the BACD as she judges the discursive productions of lesbian identity, and makes the final decision about who will be sent messages. On the other hand, any subscribers who participate in activities outside cyberspace must present themselves as roughly similar in gender and sexuality to how they have described themselves in their applications. The geographical proximity seems to promote an increased degree of trust that subscribers are being honest in their identifications. This explains the lack of emphasis on an ongoing screening process which Hall (1996) describes in terms of the international Sappho list.

Building diversity at social gatherings

Whereas the text of the 'info message' is at the mercy of Amy's decisions as an individual owner, there are also group activities which attempt to further categorise the diversity amongst participants on the list. This categorisation originated at two social events held at the list mistress's (i.e. Amy's) house. Although from the social functions, the interviews and the on-line discussion it was clear that the list was diverse in terms of ethnicity, age, class, educational level, occupation and computer experiences, there was in general far less discussion about these sources of 'difference' than what I have called 'intra-lesbian diversity'. The best examples of this were two activities which were initiated during events outside the on-line forum.

Both activities might be characterised as party games. The first involved a white sticky identification label on which was written your e-mail address. Most party-goers did *not* also add their 'real' names. Additionally smaller circular stickers were distributed in green, yellow and red to indicate relationship status: green could be read as 'Unattached. Go for it!', yellow meant 'I've got a girlfriend but might be interested anyway', and red warned 'I've got a girlfriend so stop right now!' Later in the evening subscales were also developed and a team of three BACDs started circulating assigning numerical scores between 0 and 5 for the scales of butch/femme and top/bottom, to which the term 'switchable' could be added. Much of this assignment was carried out by the team loudly asking the assembled group what was the collective view of an individual's score. Although these ways of differentiating occurred at the party, they were carried over to the list activity in the following few days, and explained to non-party-goers and refined in an ongoing discussion during which participants would include their increasingly complicated 'identity' at the end of their post to the list.

The other diversity-generating activity was a game at a second social gathering some four months later. This involved playing what might be described as Bay Area lesbian bingo in which certain stereotypes of cyber-dykes were written on a paper grid. Categories included having more than three e-mail addresses, owning certain types of footwear (Doc Martens), having non-visible piercings, preferring particular sexual/erotic activities, keeping particular pets (reptiles). The participant who was first to have all these boxes signed by others with these attributes was the winner, although in practice the game was causing so much mingling (and a great deal of amusement) that it continued for some time after this had happened.

Both these games indicate the use of reflecting and building diversity from what was intended to be a fun and non-threatening perspective, and provide further clues as to the nature of the identities of the BACD group, again reflecting the particular cultural location of the list. The activities of those involved in BACD illustrate an alternative way to experience the debates around gender and sexuality in the San Francisco Bay Area. Just as Club Q is a way in which the stylistics of some contemporary lesbian identities are highly conspicuous, BACD also signals the continual recon-struction of who/what is a lesbian in 1990s San Francisco. Meanwhile participating in the list is simultaneously a means by which users come into contact with urban culture and a network of those self-identified (and accepted) as lesbian, while also negotiating the culture of the Internet and the intersections of on-line and off-line interactions.

How far did the list fulfil Phelan's four-part schema of lesbian community processes? The activities building intra-lesbian diversity both during list conversations and elsewhere seem to fulfil the socialisation function. BACD also promotes visibility, particularly as the list mistress Amy runs the most frequently accessed Web site, www.lesbian.org. Although the list has no overt political stance in terms of organised campaigning, by its very nature it is under threat from the American legislation concerned with 'cleaning up' cyberspace. The most problematic process to map on to BACD experiences from Phelan's outline is the 'insulation from hostility' function. Phelan stated that this was 'where being a lesbian was simply not an issue'. On BACD the intro message suggests that 'not an issue' occurs only after someone has bestowed cyber-dyke identity upon you and allowed you on the list. Before that time being able to claim lesbian identity is the *major* issue.

Despite the approximate reflection of Phelan's processes of lesbian community, the extent of interaction and off-list socialising, and the geo-graphical boundaries around participation, in interviews many participants seemed to be hesitant to call BACD a community, and it was certainly not a highly conscious utopian project. The list mistress herself described the conversation as 'light' and had started another list with a restricted membership of fifty in order to be able to talk in more depth with a smaller set of subscribers. Instead of explicit community building activities, which Correll documents in the shared construction of a BBS imaginary Lesbian Café (with bar stools, a fireplace, a futon), the focus seems to be on the process of building diversity within a space whose boundaries are set out in terms of identification rather than a notion of shared space. This seems curious given the fact that the participants shared a geographic location, but it is perhaps precisely the kind of imaginary space constructed around the Bay Area location which permitted a process of recognising diversity as well as acknowledging the boundaries of the list.

Much of the research on lesbian identity and community suggests that interaction with any 'visible' lesbian culture (traditionally bars, clubs, women's rallies and women's events) is an integral part of lesbian identity development. Perhaps the significance of BACD is not whether the participants believe the list is a community or not, but the process through which their experience of lesbian identities is locally and continually confirmed or challenged. A recent study concluded that accessing geographically situated lesbian culture was not a straightforward process, and there is no evidence to suggest that on-line lesbian culture is any more homogeneous or stable. Gai Lemon and Wendy Patton's study concludes: 'The majority of women experienced trial and error scenarios whereby they would enter a face to face situation and present their interpretation of being a lesbian' (1997: 126). The responses from other women would shape future interactions, strengthening the case for the 'feedback-loop' model proposed by De Monteflores and Shultz (1978). The same kind of encounters were apparent on BACD where responses from others, even though not usually face to face, enabled a newcomer to learn from those who appeared to have more knowledge about the cultural mores of the space.

Virtual bodies learn urban lesbian culture. They also encounter virtual culture and the ways in which on-line identities and exchanges materialise in the interactions of get-togethers. These are lesbians who negotiate part of their lesbian identity as a computer-mediated lesbian identity. Some also participate in off-line gatherings, but there is no requirement to do so. Therefore some cyber-dykes participate in the on-line list without ever experiencing the constraints and opportunities of face-to-face interactions with others in the group. The large international list Sappho has produced many regional offshoots such as BACD, and it remains to be seen how each list will reflect the local culture within which it is embedded. Additionally, since 1994 there has been a flood of new lists about specific interests which have no formal regional restriction: kinky-girls, boychicks and politidykes, for example. What kind of urban (or other) cultures will clash or coalesce for the virtual bodies inhabiting these lists as they cross national and international boundaries? What situated silences will be reproduced? There is a risk that such questions of geographically located experiences and the local politics of boundary markers become lost in the rush to claim the Internet as a vehicle of a global (lesbian) community.

Note

1 The study 'Women's experiences in virtual communities' has been funded by the Economic and Social Research Council as part of their Postdoctoral Fellowship scheme.

14

'You ever fuck a mutant?'

Identity, technology, and gender in *Total Recall*

Aylish Wood

Total Recall is an exploration of the construction of identity. Its main character negotiates a position between a fragmented self and one which is located in a specific cultural and political domain. My concerns in this chapter are with the ways in which technology is centrally employed as an agent in the creation of choices and decisions made in such constructions and negotiations. Debates about the social and cultural impact of technology, and representations of technology, have often invoked either the notion of use or that of abuse. In *Total Recall*, technology is not simply used to enable choice-making by the human characters: the new possibilities created by the relationships between humans and technology are instead defining what choices can be made. This is not to say that *Total Recall* is an unproblematic exploration of the interfaces between technology and identity. The gender differences which emerge within the film remain a significant constraint to its more radical moves.

At the end of *Total Recall*, Mars is explosively altered from a planet with a red atmosphere to having one that looks like Earth's.[1] This event signals the destruction of all the narrative components around which the identities of the film's characters have been constructed. Within the story of *Total Recall* domes were built to provide habitable spaces for the (human) Martians.[2] In turn the identities of the Martians are constructed through their relationship to the inside and outside of the domes, as well as to types of dome, cleanness of air, and access to technology. The cataclysmic shattering of these domes during the creation of the oxygen-rich, and therefore humanly habitable, environment provides a visual description of the inherent instability of the identity positions of the Martian populace.

However, the editing of this sequence is curiously at odds with such an analysis. In a sequence which has spectacularly broken apart all devices that have structured the various identities of the Mars inhabitants, the editing operates against fragmentation. After the release of oxygen and the atmospheric change of the planet there is a series of images of the people moving towards what were the frames of the domes, towards the open air. In the clearing dust Tony, one of the mutant characters, moves from lying on his back to turning and standing upright, looking frame left. His movements are echoed by others of the mutant community in the background. There is a cut to the tourist section, who, also looking frame left, get up from their knees and begin to move towards the open air. After a second shot of the tourists, this time from behind, there is a cut to Melina and Quaid, the hero figures, who also get up from where they had been lying on their backs and move left across the screen. Such editing – continuity tightly established through movements across the screen, the linked looking of the characters, as well as the echoing of their physical movement – creates an illusion of a wholeness in the experience and for the viewer. At the same time, each of the groups – the mutants, the tourists, the heroes – remains in its own space.

The sequence outlined above reveals a central tension of *Total Recall*: that is, the attempt to explore the negotiation of wholeness and fragmentation. This occurs through a concern with constructions of identity. Identity is a hugely debated category, in terms both of the place in which it is physically and psychically located, and of what, in fact, identity means. I am using identity to mean the ways in which an individual assigns herself or himself, or is assigned, to a particular position in culture based on the desire to be aligned, or unaligned, with recognisable movements, practices and belief systems. By movements, practices and belief systems, I intend the ways in which gender, race, sexuality, class (to name but a few) are structured by, or structure, the place of an individual in culture.

In this piece I argue that the narrative of *Total Recall* challenges the ways in which the human subject recognises itself within particular spheres of human existence. It does so mainly through the character of Douglas Quaid (Arnold Schwarzenegger) who functions within the narrative as the site at which knowledge of the self is radically questioned. This theme is not only linked to knowledge and a construction of the self, but also interwoven with questions of recognition and misrecognition of identities by others. Additionally, technology is pivotal in the constructions of identity which occur in the film. Meaning more than a resource to be used or abused, technology functions as an aspect of cultural processes through which identity is constructed.

While such an analysis might suggest that *Total Recall* is a popular text with radical tendencies, an examination of the limit of those tendencies reveals an inherent conservatism in relation to gender. The main women characters are located within stable categories which remain unquestioned. This is especially evident in the plot devices and structures which frequently blur the construction of the male characters but leave the female characters in focus. Furthermore, technology as means of construction of self-identity is available only to the male characters.

Identity and technology

Unstable identities are manifest within *Total Recall* on different levels of the narrative. The instability of the plot structure works in conjunction with the plot device of memory implantation to create a precarious identity for the central protagonist of the film, the white male Douglas Quaid. The use of the body as the site of repetitious cycles of recognition/misrecognition functions to reiterate this issue. Stylistically, the look of the earlier sequences of the film works against such instabilities. The use of strong lines, both across and into the depth of the shot, in conjunction with high lighting effects which minimise shadows, creates a geometry of clarity.[3] Clear angular framing devices are also used as echoes between the connecting shots of the continuity editing. Visual connections are also made through colour. Quaid, while on Earth, wears a work shirt almost the same shade of red as Mars, the planet of his fascination. Such a stylistic economy produces an impression of clear definition against which the more opaque questions of identity are deployed. Once the film plot has relocated to Mars the clarity of identity and the clarity of space are both absent. The repeated sequences of earthmovers connecting and disconnecting tunnels inscribe a shifting geography in which identity is denied a mapped space.

It is not only through the characters whose stories are told in *Total Recall* that doubt is placed around the constructions of identities. The plot itself functions to self-consciously undermine narrative stability as its convolutions insist that the spectator question the authenticity of her or his reading of the story. Superficially, *Total Recall* is about a male protagonist who 'gets the girl, kills the bad guys and saves the entire planet'. But it is also much more than this readily recognisable description. Almost as soon as the plot presents the character of Douglas Quaid as a man who lives on Earth, has a wife, a construction job, bad nightmares and daydreams of going to Mars, it is suggested that Quaid is not himself, that is, Quaid is not Quaid. Within the story-world of *Total Recall* there exists a technology through which it is possible to have memory implants and hence take a 'vacation from yourself'. This technology permits the existence of a single human body through which a sequence of identities is manifest. Quaid, as an identity, exists as a technological insertion into a body. His body is not his own, or more accurately, not only his own. It has been combined with other identities, which through the use of technology have been erased, and replaced by the one that allows Douglas Quaid to know himself as himself. In other words, contrary to the humanist tradition, his body is not himself.

The status of this internal narrative is itself subsequently undermined through the interventions of two characters, Dr Edgemar and Cohaagen. Edgemar (Roy Brocksmith), a representative of Rekall, the controllers of the implant technology, visits Quaid, by this point in a hotel on Mars. Edgemar's entry into the plot serves the function of making the character Quaid question his identity as a secret agent. At the same time it alerts the viewer to the plot subterfuges which are at work within the film. Edgemar informs Quaid that he is experiencing a dream, a free-form delusion while he, his body, is still strapped in the implant chair in Rekall on Earth. For both the character Quaid and the viewer, the question arises as to which version of the story is correct. Which Quaid is which Quaid? The textual play on the doubt surrounding Quaid's identity is made explicitly visible when Edgemar tells Quaid: 'I'm afraid you're not standing here right now.' As he speaks, Edgemar is positioned between two Quaids, one the flesh-and-blood Quaid and a second Quaid reflected in the mirror.

At the end of this sequence there has emerged a crisis of identity for the character Douglas Quaid and a disruption of the narrative expectations of the audience, as the hero protagonist figure that Quaid is becoming may be no more than a guy having an hallucination. After the narrative pause which takes place as Quaid makes up his mind whether to take the pill offered by Edgemar, also giving the spectator pause to consider what is going on in the plot, the generic devices of the action film are mobilised to reassert a degree of narrative coherence. The action fight sequence re-establishes Quaid as the secret agent, and, while this does not resolve the question of whether or not he really is a secret agent, it provides the plot with the momentum to continue. It is not simply that Quaid makes his choice of identity through killing Edgemar, the emboldening of his action hero-protagonist position functions as a recognisable device of emplotment through which the spectator can relocate herself or himself in relation to the continuation of the narrative's trajectory. The two components of generic device and identity characterisation coalesce just subsequent to a moment where extreme doubt is created about the character of Quaid and about the film itself.

Similarly, when the attempt by Cohaagen (Ronny Cox), the mega-lomaniac chief of the agency, to undermine Quaid's acquisition of an identity fails, the plot reiterates Quaid's choice by following it with an action sequence which again solidifies his position as the action hero. The narrative resolution of Quaid claiming the role of the heroic saviour of the disempowered populations of Mars also has the potential to stabilise the identity choice of Quaid. In choosing to remain a part of the rebel cause he denies his access to the other identities and memories that have existed in his body. The final scene kicks space dust back into the face of the spectator as it disassembles all the ploys used in the film to create a coherent sense to the narrative. In posing the question that the plot has only ever existed as Quaid's dream there is a rupturing which re-activates all the moments of doubt about the identity of the story and the characters within it.

The combination of these plot devices and structures raises the question of the impossibility of having knowledge of an authentic self. If an individual is defined by her/his memories, and those can be altered, then what has happened to the original, authentic self?[4] In *Total Recall* Quaid looks for but can never find himself because there is never an authentic being to whom he can return. Quaid almost secures his identity as the hero protagonist but since the story is itself in question, the closure is unstable, and therefore without a fully authorised resolution. The narrative device of mismatching the internal stories constitutes another layer of commentary on the construction of identity. Because the spectator has no privileged position from which to 'know' the story, the viewer is not presented with the plot, or its identity, as a coherent whole. Composing the film in this way may cause the spectator to negotiate the difficulty of assigning an individual a fully realised identity. The ending of *Total Recall* can be read as an acknowledgement of the politics of the necessity to take up a position in relation to an identity. At the same time, however, this position is indicated as being precisely, and only, a deliberate construction.

Technology is central to the troubled acquisition of identity in *Total Recall*. However, the film can be read as more than a simple use/abuse/ misuse scenario. Fred Glass has argued (Glass 1990: 4) that *Total Recall* trivialises technology:

> Conveying an epistemological position on social use of technologies, the toys imply disgust at their trivialisation and, while the mutants suffer, potential wasted. The most notable example is Rekall, Inc., which shrinkwraps an impressive scientific understanding of the intricate relations of psychology and biology into mental home-movies.

Such an argument assumes a particular relationship between the humans of the film and the technologies of the film. The notion of 'social use' implies a dynamic whereby the human and the technological are held apart. Humans make use of technology. A similar separation is established in J. P. Telotte's analysis of *Total Recall*: 'Quaid seems an equally telling example of the roboticized modern being, of a public body primed to be surprised by the self, by a human identity that will not be denied' (Telotte 1995: 159). In this analysis technologisation takes over the self, and that human self 'will not be denied' its presence. The dynamic is again one of domination, though, in this instance, human identity is imposed upon by the various technologies of the film.

An alternative argument is that the human and the technological coexist through a dynamic of interactivities. The human can be defined through technology, and technology, in the same instant, can be defined through the human. The acquisition of identity is established through connections accumulated across as well as within boundaries of humanness and technologiness.[5] As such identity, and its constructions, become sites which are structured through and around categories of race, gender and sexualities which are themselves aspects of a cultural and political process in which the technological is an inseparable part of the lived experience. In *Total Recall*, Douglas Quaid is a visible site of these intersections.

Bodies and Technologies

Above I have discussed how the narrative of *Total Recall* equates the construction of identity with a knowledge of memories. Within the film the body functions as another site through which identity can be stabilised or destabilised. Through the use of holography, technology is again the means through which the body can be altered, to be made to look transiently different, and therefore an unstable category.

The holographic body

As in the case of memory, the ability to be deceptive, to misinform about the body, is linked to the use of technology and the holograph is one of the major devices of such disinformation. The product of the holograph, the hologram, is an image of a human being in which the transcription is so perfect that the image is indistinguishable from the original. The holograph is used as a means to create technologically an image of the self and as such it is an echo of the device of splitting identity through multiple sets of memory being located in one body.

The sequence in which Quaid first finds the holograph consists of a complex interplay between body, identity and technology. Quaid has entered a deserted cement works to investigate a suitcase left for him. Inside he discovers a wristwatch-type instrument, the control for a holograph which projects a hologram of the wearer. Switching the device on, Quaid is confronted with an image of himself which he fails to recognise as himself. Although Quaid can easily rid himself of this double by switching off the technology, he cannot deal so easily with the problem of his identity. The history of the body which he inhabits is still beyond his knowledge. It requires another piece of technology to provide him with a clearer sense of self. From the suitcase Quaid pulls out a video system which plays back a recording from Hauser, who claims to be Quaid – or rather, claims that Quaid is in fact him – and provides Quaid with a history he can believe if he so chooses.[6] Quaid's choice is linked to yet another technological appliance. The identity that Quaid had on Earth as a construction worker is tethered to a tracking device which has been inserted into his sinus. His removal of that piece of technology distances himself from that identity. Quaid's choice-making is engendered through the technologies that surround him and enable him to be aware of the constructions of his identity.

In spite of the range of technological devices used to construct Quaid/ Hauser in the warehouse sequence the scenes in which a human and holograph appear together reveal an inconsistency in the desire of the narrative of *Total Recall* to question bodies and identity through technology. Each time a human gets close to her or his hologram its edges fray and blur. In other words, each time a human enters into the space in which her or his image and her- or himself become visually inseparable the difference is made clear through a technological insufficiency.

The mutated body

The body in *Total Recall* is not only a site of the deployment of techno-centric identity games. It is also the site of an explicit critique of a system in which access to the benefits of technological developments are directly proportional to economic capability, or the ability to pay. The mutants, the underclass of Mars, evolved as mutated because their ancestors could not pay for access to good domes and so the contamination of their environment by 'the rays' resulted in their becoming affected individuals. Without the means to pay for sufficient clean air to clear the rays, they suffered this environmental insult that led to an accumulation of mutations over the generations.

Membership of the community of mutants is ascribed by the possession of a marked body. The visual impact of these marks constitutes one of the spectacles of the film. When Quaid goes to Venusville he is addressed by several strangers on the street, a man, a woman and a girl-child, all of whom have the facial distortions which characterise many of the mutant characters. The other types of mutation include restricted growth and extra growth, such as a third breast. Spatially the mutant community is also marked off both geographically and narratively. Quaid must take a taxi-drive through the tunnels of (red) soil to get from his plush Hilton suite to Venusville while the mutants are visible only within the narrative space of Venusville, the 'red-light' district of the red planet.

The mutants are not simply in the narrative to function as one of the visual spectacles. They are also aligned with the major site of resistance within *Total Recall*; that is, they are aligned with the rebels who are attempting to overthrow the corporate control of the planet. However, as might be expected in a film which is infused with questions of identity the equation between marked body, mutant and rebel is problematised. When the rebel leader, Kuato (Marshall Bell), first appears he is presented as a normal-looking white man called George. Clearly established as a source of authority, he indicates to Melina that she should talk to Quaid when he visits the Last Resort sex-club. The visual duplicity of *Total Recall* and the rebel leader is subsequently revealed when it emerges that he too is a mutant, and, furthermore, that he and Kuato part-share a body. Kuato may appear quite normal, but underneath his shirt is a more complex set of interrelations. This figuration of the bodyshare of Kuato and George reiterates the crises in the assignment of identity in relation to the habitation of the body. In the instance of Quaid, the narrative abandons a simple equation between identity and the body. Similarly, the body which incorporates Kuato and George represents a quite literal partial separation of identity and body. The childlike psychic Kuato and George are embodied together, but can be identified as distinct personas. This latter feature is significantly emphasised through their separate deaths. Though mortally wounded, Kuato sufficiently survives the first ballistic onslaught to have to be shot through the head.

Total Recall also sets in motion questions concerned with the assumption that political alliances are based on simplistic constructions of identity. This occurs through a move which subverts the equation of the mutant body with the rebels' cause. First established as an apparently normal black taxi-driver who gets caught up in the activities of Quaid and Melina, Benny (Mel Johnson Jnr) substantiates his credentials as a rebel sympathiser by revealing that he is a mutant who disguises himself with a clever prosthetic hand. With these actions Benny plays a double game. On the one hand, he demonstrates that he has prevented the recognition of his status as a mutant. He has used technology successfully to disguise his mutated arm. On the other, he then uses this authenticated mutant identity to ally himself with the rebels. Since Benny is subsequently revealed as an agent working for the agency this double misrecognition presents the problem of collapsing bodily appearance into a particular identity position. It questions the assumptions made in assigning an individual's political affiliations based on a restricted knowledge of that individual. The fact that Benny is a mutant does not automatically mean he will be supportive of the rebel cause.

Identity, technology and gender

In the foregoing discussion I have presented a reading of *Total Recall* in which the character of Douglas Quaid is the active site of identity construction. This identity is structured through the relationship of the protagonist to the rebel cause and that of the controlling power. Technological interventions are also used to mobilise questions of shifting knowledges of the self. Additionally, the construction of the plot is itself unstable, augmenting the lack of coherency inherent to the character of Douglas Quaid. However, as I have already suggested, there are limitations to these radical tendencies of the film. Such problems are especially visible when the intersections of technology/body/identity are considered at sites of gender difference.

The mutant body, as discussed above, is marked by visible mutation. That the majority of the mutated individuals are seen only within the technologically impoverished narrative space of Venusville and the Last Resort explicitly links the marked body with the exotic and/or erotic. Although the mutant community is closely allied with the rebels, even within the rebel headquarters the visible body is that which passes for normal. The remarked-upon body remains in the space of exotic adventure. Within Venusville there also exists a gendered demarcation between the exotic and the erotic. While all the mutant bodies are exoticised by virtue of their difference in appearance, not all mutants are eroticised. Within the Last Resort the erotic/available object is a woman. The costumes of the women are clichéd revealing black, red or pink night-club wear. It is the women who dance in cages, and trail their legs across the railings. In contrast the men are dressed more like Quaid, in work clothes, shirts, overshirts, trousers. So when Benny says to Quaid, 'You ever fuck a mutant?' we are meant to hear this as 'You ever fuck a mutated (marked) woman?'[7]

A consideration of Melina (Rachel Ticotin), the main woman character of the film, further reveals the differential constructions of gender. The plot construction inserts her character, like that of Quaid, into the narrative at several points. Her first appearance occurs in the dream sequence which opens the film. Melina is the woman in the space-suit who walks with Quaid along the canyons of the Martian landscape. Her second appearance is as the digitised embodiment of Quaid's ideal woman at Rekall, Inc. When asked what kind of woman he would like in his fantasies Quaid indicates 'sleazy and demure'. In a moment of technological creativity the pixilated image of such a woman resolves and smooths into Melina. Her final insertion into the narrative is as the sex-worker/rebel who works at the Last Resort. As such Melina is the woman who will become Quaid's lover, and, depending on which version of the story is accepted, may have already been his lover. Melina, therefore, exists as three possibilities within the film, none of which is privileged by the resolution. Although as a character Quaid is subject to the same lack of coherent position, the contingencies upon which his construction are founded become apparent to him as well as to the viewer of the film. Ultimately, Quaid has the freedom to make a choice. In contrast, Melina never has an agency which will allow her to account for the different constructions of her identity, her character remains constructed from beyond her knowledge of herself. Furthermore, those constructions are motivated through the waking or dream fantasy scenarios of Quaid.

It is not only through a lack of self-consciousness of her identity that Melina remains unexposed to the destabilising tendencies of the technology/body/identity crossover. The potential impact of technology on her body and identity is also figured differently from that of Quaid. The implantation technology has facilitated Quaid's choices and transitions through the story. For Melina the implantation technology represents a threat which will disempower her further, making her 'respectful, compliant and appreciative – the way a woman should be'. Although this statement, spoken by Cohaagen, is not one condoned by the film, there remains behind it the notion that technology can be used *on* the women of the film. This is not to say that the women characters are excluded from using the technologies of the film. Clearly they are as capable as the male characters in their use of weaponry. Lori (Sharon Stone), Melina and the women in the Last Resort can shoot to kill with skill. Dr Renata Lall is in charge of the Rekall implantation technology. Tiffany, the receptionist at Rekall, can do her nails at the touch of a technological wand. But simply being able to use technology is not the point. What makes *Total Recall* interesting is the incorporation of technologies into the construction of identities. It is the way in which technology becomes active in the questioning of what it means to be someone and to be seen as that someone. That only the male characters figure in such a questioning is a limitation of the film.

The transitions visible in the predominant characterisation of Melina are outside of just such a questioning. Her major narrative location starts within Venusville, not because she is bodily marked as a mutant, but because she is a sex-worker, and perhaps also because she is a rebel. As the plot progresses she leaves both the spatial location of Venusville, and the narrative location of sex-worker. Melina's transitions in identity from sex-worker to rebel activist, as I have already stated, do not mobilise the interconnections of technology/identity/body that accompany the narrative movements of Quaid. Instead, the potential for Melina's character to have radical tendencies lies in a consideration of the conventions of the action genre, as opposed to being located within the film itself. Yvonne Tasker has discussed the role of woman as side-kick to the male protagonist of the action film (Tasker 1994). Typically, the woman-as-side-kick is released from her narrative status through the intervention, often romantically motivated, of the male protagonist. The ensuing journey is one of self-discovery where she learns the skills she requires for her new, more active role. Like the woman police officer Lewis in *Robocop*, also directed by Paul Verhoeven, Melina already has the skills she needs. Her leaving Venusville is motivated not only through her romantic attachment to Quaid, but also through her activist position within the rebel cause. Her aim is to take Quaid to Kuato, the rebel leader so that he can discover what Quaid knows. Melina's narrative transition from sex-worker to rebel activist is further emphasised through a change in costume. She switches from her sex-worker's outfit into a pale khaki-green one which, while still displaying her body, does not reveal it.

Despite her already acquired knowledge Melina is not a fully fledged action hero in her own right. Her movement across the film's narrative spaces dislocates her from her position as a sex-worker and re-places her both as Quaid's action cohort and his lover. Melina is never allowed to become Quaid's equal, it is his actions which finally fully enable her. This is evident in the scene in which she rescues Quaid from Lori.[8] In an action sequence which is choreographed as a 'real' fight, as opposed to a women's 'cat-fight', Melina first shoots dead all three men and then enters into hand-to-hand combat with Lori. Lori is the better fighter and only Quaid's intervention of shooting her ensures Melina's success. This sets the pattern for the remainder of the film. Melina may be a good fighter, but she is not quite good enough to be a real action hero in the mould of Ripley in *Alien*. In certain respects her position is an action film equivalent to the heroine figure who proceeds the Final Girl in the history of the horror film. Unlike the Final Girl who can 'virtually or actually destroy[s] the antagonist and save herself', the heroine can survive but needs another figure to finally save her (Clover 1992).

The impact of the conjunction of technology/body/identity in *Total Recall* is most clearly visible through the character of Quaid, and to a lesser extent George/Kuato, and Benny. Melina, Lori and the women in Venusville function outside of this discursive space. That this distinction is so clearly demarcated by gender is indicative of the categories which can and cannot be destabilised within the film. Perhaps the most revealing moment is the point at which technology fails to enable Quaid to reconstruct his identity. Needing a disguise to get to Mars he has acquired a technological mask which will enable him to cross-dress and pass as a woman. Almost immediately the mask malfunctions, resulting in both the audience's and the film's other characters' recognition that the woman is really a man in disguise. Technology, in *Total Recall*, remains limited to the destabilisation of identity components which are not situated in relation to or across gender constructions.

Total Recall questions the identity of identity. In negotiating between identity as whole or fragmented it privileges the inauthentic technological construction of Douglas Quaid, not as a stable identity, but as one which is contingent on a process of choice-making. The resolution, I have argued above, through undermining the plot of *Total Recall* resists the stasis of the final identity position. It instead advocates the process of choice as ongoing. Technology is the device within the film which enables this process, as such technology is engaged with as a component of the dialogue with lived experience through which identity is chosen and constructed. Through its working and reworking of the theme of misrecognition/recognition of bodies, the narrative further insists on the refusal of static identities. The spectator is continually being reminded of the inadequacies and dangers of assigning identity positions to (male) characters based on what they look like.

Total Recall can be seen not only as a film which problematises the construction of a character's identity. It is also one which attempts a questioning of the narrative structure of mainstream film. As an action film there are certain legitimate expectations placed on it, the most obvious being the hero figure, the side-kick character, and action sequences. A further aspect of narrative structure associated with mainstream film is a linear narrative with clear cause-and-effect associations. *Total Recall* puts these latter narrative structures into doubt through its plot devices. However, it does so in the presence of the recognisable components of the hero and the action sequences, and consequently the potential for destabilisation of the narrative is only partial.

At a deeper level the proliferation of unstable bodies and identities evident in *Total Recall* provokes questions about the limits of representation. The camera can be viewed as a device which disciplines or attempts to regiment the objects it takes pictures of, including the human body.[9] The body, however, exists in excess to the image screened, it will always be more, and mean more, than that which is visible in any one moment, or sequence of frames. *Total Recall* almost catches a glimpse of this through its constant attention to shifting identities and bodies. In spite of this tendency certain categories are left intact, there remains something to be recognised amongst the shifting configurations. That this recognisable figure is of a woman reveals the gendered partiality of the endeavour of *Total Recall* to problematise constructions of identity.

Notes

1 *Total Recall* (1990; USA) was directed by Paul Verhoeven. It is based on the short story 'We can remember it for you wholesale' by Philip K. Dick.

2 A clear question arises about Mars as a colonised space. The 'original' Mars inhabitants are present only through the artefacts of their technology. It is significant that it is they who are referred to as the aliens, and not the human race.

3 This is perhaps most obvious in the sequence where Quaid is first on the run. As he races down the stairs towards the Metro the intersections of the walkways are clearly visible into the depth of the image.

4 Alison Landsberg also discusses the ways in which *Total Recall* problematises the notion of an authentic identity through a discussion of prosthetic memories in conjunction with a proliferation of mediated images. See Alison Landsberg (1995: 175–89).

5 Tiziana Terranova warns against giving technologiness too much a sense of autonomy. As she argues, technologies, even autonomously evolving ones, still have their origins in the human condition (1996: 69–83).

6 Hauser is the character who speaks to Quaid in the form of a pre-recorded video message. The body that was Hauser is also the one that now appears to be Quaid. Although this might seem to be an example of the mind superseding the body as the site of self-knowledge, this position is undercut through the romance narrative in which Quaid has 'feelings' for Melina, the woman who was Hauser's lover.

7 Jonathan Goldberg makes the claim that Arnold Schwarzenegger as Quaid is coded as the object of gay desire in *Total Recall* (1991). However, the more explicit sex objects in the film are the women characters in the Last Resort.

8 Within the plot of the film Quaid believes himself to have been married to Lori. It is suggested that their marriage was part of a memory implant and that Lori was living with Quaid only to ensure that he did not rediscover his previous identity.

9 It is interesting to see *Total Recall* in the context of writings in which the camera seeks to control the body. I refer to Lisa Cartwright's work on the cinema of science, *Screening the Body* (1995) and Linda Williams's work on porn films, *Hardcore* (1990).

15

Beyond maps and metaphors?

Re-thinking the relationships between architecture and gender

Jos Boys

It was nearly twenty years ago that feminists working in architecture, planning and associated fields began to challenge the underlying assumptions of rationalist and modernist city and building design. In writing and in practice they argued against concepts of architectural space as a neutral, transparent and 'obvious' medium and against professional design knowledge as an objective and rational problem-solving activity. They questioned definitions of masculinity and femininity based on a series of simplistic binary oppositions such as home/work, production/consumption, private/public and inside/outside (where one side of the equation was always privileged at the expense of the other) and began to unravel how these concepts were being literally mapped on to the material landscape as hierarchically zoned and functionally separate bands stretching from 'working' city centre to suburban home (Werkele *et al.* 1980; Hayden 1981, 1984; Matrix Book Group 1984; Women and Geography Study Group 1984).

These attempts led to the articulation of many issues previously unsayable. They exposed how middle-class women in particular had come to be isolated in the suburban home and enabled a whole new history to be written about the deliberate construction of gender difference through the allocation of 'separate spheres' for male and female activities in much western thought (Davidoff and Hall 1987). It became possible to explore how some modernist planning and design deliberately attempted to express these stereotyped gender roles in the spatial arrangements of towns and cities; and to examine some of the disjunctures and contradictions between these spaces and the everyday lives and experiences of different women and men (Roberts 1991; Boys 1984, 1986). These moves, however, also left their own silences and difficulties: their authors were limited by prevailing structures of thought and too often caught up in trying to describe a simple logic of oppression. As Soja and Hooper note:

> For the most part, this expanded feminist critique and spatial remapping remained modernist, in the sense of channelling its critical power and emancipatory objectives around the gendered binary men/women. Urban

> spatiality thus came to be seen as oppressively gendered in much the same way that the city was shown to be structured by the exploitative class relations of capitalism and the discriminatory geographical effects of racism, the other two major channels of radical modernist urban critique developing over the same period.
>
> (Soja and Hooper 1993: 193)

The predominantly white, middle-class feminist debates of this period, then, were unable to engage with a number of important issues. Initially, at least, we failed to articulate key differences in how 'common-sense' conceptual spaces framed different groups of women differently, in how this affected the experiences-in-material-space of working-class, black, lesbian or disabled women, for example, compared with 'suburban housewives':

> In focusing on the eighteenth- and nineteenth-century shift in English middle-class values which sought to separate private and public life and to allocate women to the private realm, this work has only investigated one of the many ideals, myths and stereotypes about women and men in popular circulation during the nineteenth and twentieth centuries. Crucially working-class and black women have often been constructed as the opposite of the ideal offered up to middle-class women, and therefore it has had different effects and contradictions for these women.
>
> (Boys 1990: 250)

What is more, argument was frequently structured around the logic of function – delineating experience only in terms of physical *use* of the built environment and space rather than, for example, via experience or meaning. Finally, and perhaps most fundamentally, the focus on merely reversing the values allocated to existing binary oppositions (for example, criticising the suburban home as 'obviously' oppressive to women) severely limited our ability to 'see' let alone challenge the underlying limitations of thought structured in this way.

The new politics of space and difference

More recently, however, there has been a renewed academic interest in the relationships between body, social identity, space and representation across such previously diverse disciplines as philosophy, linguistics, cultural studies, geography, sociology and anthropology (Harvey 1989; Soja 1989; Jameson 1991; Wilson 1991; Rose 1993; Keith and Pile 1993; Lash and Urry 1994; Massey 1994; Grosz 1995). This has led to very fruitful unravelling of older, enlightenment 'ways of seeing' based on the flawed logic of binary oppositions; to valuable critiques of the limitations of modernist identity politics (including these earlier feminist studies of the built environment) which remain contained in binary ordering in both their analyses and plans for change; and to a series of reconceptualisations concerned with framing a 'thirdspace' beyond the simple dualisms and oppositions found in so many western socio-spatial concepts:

In the new cultural politics of difference, the aim is neither simply to assert dominance of the subaltern over the hegemon in a rigidly maintained bipolar order, nor even to foster some specified opposing traits and traditions. It is to break down and disorder the binary itself, to reject the simple structure of closed dualisms through a (sympathetic) deconstruction and reconstitution that allows for radical openness, flexibility and multiplicity. The key step is to recognise and occupy new and alternative geographies – a 'thirdspace' of political choice – different but not detached entirely from the geographies defined by the original binary oppositions between and within objectivism and subjectivism.

(Soja and Hooper 1993: 198)

This rethinking of the space of theory itself thus searches for new categories of position beyond man/woman, home/work and so on. Rather than mutually exclusive territories, defined by their oppositional characteristics, categories of thought are here conceived as more fluid and overlapping; for example, as linked contradictions, borders and margins, or indeterminate and open systems (ibid.: 189–200). Such conceptualisations are then offered back to architecture by some cultural theorists as a mechanism for un-locking relationships of space and identity, for confronting the very nature of architecture as it has been 'thought' – even where the resulting physicality is not yet comprehensible. Grosz, for example, writes of the need to think the 'unthought', to imagine an architecture of the 'outside' – that is, not what is 'the necessary structure of compromise that produces a building as a commodity; [but] what is alien, other, different from, or beyond it'. She situates gender identities at the very centre of this theoretical and material relocation:

The project ahead is to return women to those places from which they have been dis- or re-placed or expelled, to occupy those positions – particularly those which are not acknowledged as positions – partly in order to show men's invasion and occupancy of the whole of space as their own and thus the constriction of spaces available to women, and partly in order to be able to experiment with and produce the possibility of occupying, dwelling or living in new spaces, which in their turn help generate new perspectives, new bodies, new ways of inhabiting.

(Grosz 1995: 135)

In a series of recent conferences and publications, these critiques are being re-engaged with by architects and critics (Colomina 1992; Ghirardo 1991; McCorquodale *et al.* 1996).

Relocating architecture

These forceful shiftings of thinking about architecture away from rationalist problem-solving to elsewhere than concern with function and use, are valuable and powerfully resonant. And yet. In cultural theory's newfound interest in architecture and the city, many unresolved gaps and silences remain. I want to suggest that with many cultural critics the underlying structures of thought about relationships between space, society and the body continue to restrict how we 'think' architecture.

The first problem is that social structures and values are still too often assumed to be somehow literally engraved into the physical arrangements and representational qualities of three-dimensional space. A city or building can thus be literally 'read' as a map of aspects of a society, its social structures and values. The predominant mechanism enabling such a connection is the metaphor – that is, where an analogy is made between perceived qualities in elements of the physical form and specific social values. Such metaphorical relationships can be via aspects of any of the following: location, building type, layout, constructional method(s), materials, appearance, formal 'ordering' and 'setting'. Thus the suburban home, the tower block or the ghetto comes to 'stand for' a specific bundle of social behaviours, which are then applied *as factual description* back to all the occupants of that location.[1] While there are many valuable case studies refusing to rely on such simple analogies as explanations of either social or spatial change (MacKenzie 1989: Hayden 1995), the use of architectural imagery as supporting evidence in analyses of *social aspects* remains endemic. Many contemporary debates – particularly about the changing nature of society in the late twentieth century – are literally structured around analogous relationships between society and its physical form. Thus, arguments concerned with the 'postmodern' propose that we now live in an increasingly depthless and superficial world and use the analogy of changes in architectural style (alongside other cultural artefacts) to support their case (Jameson 1991; Frampton 1983).

The second problem is that where authors do use spatial/representational characteristics as *evidence* of social forms and beliefs (and vice versa) via analogy, these remain structured around binary oppositions. The observer perceives a connection – for instance, that rectilinear and repetitive forms indicate 'rational' social values – and links the opposite form with the opposite values, so that asymmetric and dynamic forms are then assumed to express lack of social ordering. This is not only a closed and self-referential system of thought, it also enables the observer to argue a particular relationship of social and spatial qualities as obvious and transparent and to insist that an alternative view represents an inability to 'see' properly. Such an approach, I would argue, is a key mechanism in enabling what Gillian Rose has called 'masculinist rationality':

> Masculinist rationality is a form of knowledge which assumes a knower who believes he can separate himself off from his body, emotions, values, past and so on, so that he and his thought are autonomous, context-free and objective . . . the assumption of an objectivity, untainted by any particular social position allows this kind of rationality to claim itself as universal.
>
> (Rose 1993: 6–7)

The third problem is the underlying structure of evaluation contained within this framework. Within a system of binary oppositions, either side can be given positive value merely by juxtaposition with its opposite. Thus rectilinear design can be seen as either rational/logical/neutral and 'good' (modernism) or rational/banal/elitist and 'bad' (anti-modernism). Postmodern design can be seen as either pluralist (good) or chaotic (bad). Material space becomes *either* a reflection of society (which can be 'read' off the surface) *or* a 'disguise' which hides the 'real' structure of society, and can thus be interpreted either as more 'real' (authentic) than the space of ideas or as a deliberate distortion and mask of a 'deeper' truth. Within such a circular framework, a piece of architecture can justify almost any view (which the observer insists is objective and obvious) using analogies to support 'universal truths' (even though an analogy, by its very nature, must be partial and temporary; Rose 1996).

I suggest that the continuing dominance of these conceptual 'spaces' in debates about buildings and cities perpetuates our inability to think effectively about the relationships between gender and architecture. We cannot stop linking women to home/domesticity or men to work/public life architecturally and thus conceptually, even when we know the realities are very different. It comes as no surprise, for example, that the American architect Frank Gehry recently explained his own house design as the deliberate juxtaposition of the original tract house (stable, rectilinear, knowable, domestic, *feminine*) with the new extension (unfinished, rough, asymmetrical, *masculine*), or that many critics take this as a valid and 'objective' form of social and architectural comment (Boys 1996).

So, this chapter asks once again, in this new context, that basic question which was so hard even to articulate in the 1970s. What is the relationship between architecture and gender, between space and social identities? This now first requires a deliberate refusal. Material space is no longer to be imagined as a map (however partial) of gender relationships and architectural representation is not to be interpreted as a metaphor of aspects of society. There are then two, interwoven issues. First, how and in whose interests has such a conceptual framework developed? How does it frame our interrelationships with the material world (what is exposed to view and what made invisible)? How has it affected the actual construction of architecture and cities on the one hand and theoretical and popular debates on the other (Boys forthcoming)?

Second, how might we build alternative structures for explaining the connections between material landscapes and social identities? Here I will just begin to examine aspects of these questions through two partial studies; one investigating the economic and social processes through which architectural production and consumption take place, and the other examining how buildings might be analysed so as to incorporate issues of gender and identity at every level.

In these explorations there are several valuable lessons from the best of contemporary work on society and space in geography, cultural studies and related disciplines. First, a concern with difference is essential to these debates, not merely 'added-on' to an existing theory. I take this as an awareness of the specificity of cases, locations, identities and the central need to examine how inequalities are thus produced and reproduced, not the mere relativism of 'plurality' or 'diversity' favoured by some authors. Second, binary oppositions cannot be any longer seen as an *explanation* of society or its spatial arrangements (whether in a real or imagined form) but must be investigated as part of a continuous cyclical process by which in a variety of attempts to delineate gender identities, conceptual structures and spatial settings, the results are themselves transformed or fractured by translation into specific architectural forms (channelled through particular patterns of power) and then re-adapted or challenged through the playing-out of gender identities in these spaces. Finally, our relationship to buildings and cities needs to be conceived as much more than one of simple function or need and its study must therefore incorporate richer notions such as identity, desire and memory.

Beyond maps and metaphors

I have argued elsewhere that architectural production and consumption are predominantly considered through two mutually exclusive frameworks, which in many texts merely sit alongside one another (Harvey 1984). On the one hand, architecture is seen as a *product which reflects* societal structures and values. On the other, it is seen as the *result of a process* based on the economics of development. The first is used most often to 'explain' building design; the second, patterns of urban growth and change. What buildings 'mean' is thus dealt with predominantly via visual representation with architecture visualised as a *container* of symbolic values. This becomes separated from 'non-representational' and abstract issues of resource inequalities where building design is assumed to be the *outcome* of particular patterns of resources distribution. Where architecture is articulated as map and metaphor, it is perceived as a product, with even its relationship to the process which produced it as one of analogy. This not only prevents an engagement with historically and geographically specific processes of production and consumption, it also makes invisible the variety of positions of those involved in these processes.

Here, instead, I want to propose two linked concepts intended to disrupt the binary structure of maps and metaphors and the masculinist rationality it supports: and to bridge the gap between the dualisms of product/process, 'container'/ 'outcome' and access to physical resources/access to 'meaning-making'. These are, first, positionality, which aims to make explicit the 'positions' of different actors in the process of building and city production and consumption: and, second, mechanisms of translation, that is, the analysis of the specific processes by which different positionalities in particular contexts are transformed into material form. I have found Bourdieu's work on the relationships between 'taste' and 'position' immensely useful here. He argues that social groups place themselves in relation not only to financial but also to cultural capital; and that different groups maintain various strategies – both to legitimise cultural capital as a valuable form of power and to contain it within specific forms. His studies thus combine an analysis of power and social 'location' with an exploration of aesthetic preferences. As he says:

> Only at the level of the field of positions is it possible to grasp both the generic interests associated with the fact of taking part in the game and the specific interests attached to the different positions, and, through this, the form and content of the self-positioning through which these interests are expressed.
>
> (Bourdieu 1984: 12)

Positionality is not, of course, neutral, but built within a framework of power relations which supports and legitimises some beliefs and activities and not others. It is also in a permanent process of contestation and transformation. However, the unravelling of these positions and their connected structures for interpreting architectural form does not, of itself, provide an explanation for the shape of the built world. The act of producing and consuming buildings and cities is also mediated via historically and geographically specific environments and processes. These mechanisms of translation include 'common-sense' beliefs (Lawrence 1982), the structure of architectural knowledge, the physical context, the parameters of existing building technologies, the nature of the building industry and the financial structures of production and consumption. Within the requirements of such a complex analysis, issues of gender take on a peculiar, dual aspect: they become simultaneously marginal – as a particular subset within a whole series of events (which are as likely to have unintended consequences as deliberately oppressive outcomes) and resolutely central, as one of the most immediate filters through which we inhabit, connect with and interpret the material landscape. In the rest of this chapter I will initially expand out to the wide view, until gender threatens to become a mere pinprick on the horizon, before returning to focus on the embeddedness of gender relationships and inequalities in architectural form.

Architecture as a mechanism of translation

There is not a huge amount of research into the specific processes by which building and city development take place. Detailed development case studies are restricted by issues of commercial confidentiality, whilst urban economics tends to stay at the abstract level. This chapter relies extensively on the work of Healey *et al.* (1988), Warren (1993) and Adams (1994). Even in these texts it should be noted that architectural and city *design* is dealt with only marginally.

Here, then, I want to outline briefly how the land and building development market – and the patterns of regulation and control within which it operates – crucially frames assumptions about what design is *for* and therefore the mechanisms by which specific resources and 'meanings' are translated into physical form. I want to consider the 'positions' of various actors involved, located within existing economic, political and cultural frameworks of power, and the systems of legitimacy they employ. Only then is it possible to begin to 'locate' gender within the production and consumption processes of architecture. I suggest that three sets of basic bifurcations can be discerned, the first with its roots in what was traditionally known as the 'private' sector, the second within what was called the 'public' sector in Britain and the third framed by structures of professional knowledge across the development, design and building industries.

The production of architecture, where this is perceived essentially as a commodity, can be differentiated between two main arenas. There is, first, the large-scale, mass market, privately organised sector which has an extremely instrumental attitude to design in relation to profit margins and produces, for example, large industrial sheds and 'spec' offices. Second, there is a smaller 'high-design' market based on scarcity value and the 'one-off' where buildings are commissioned or purchased precisely because of their 'uniqueness' (for instance, by the deliberate employment of a famous architect). To this must be added buildings commissioned or bought with the inclusion of some element of 'public interest' criteria (however this is defined). There are also 'public sector' buildings designed entirely on perceived economic efficiencies, but for a client representing 'the public'. The historical development of professional knowledge also straddles a potentially contradictory divide: on the one hand, professional expertise is construed as working for specific clients, so as to maximise their particular interests, while, on the other, many professionals often believe in abstract concepts of the 'public interest', and in an objective and 'disinterested' resolution to any problem (Perkin 1989). These three underlying tendencies are themselves, of course, in a constant state of transformation – because of current changes in the nature of building production both nationally (with the increased use of complex public–private partnerships) and globally; and because of the specific characteristics of buildings as products over other designed items.[2]

Architecture, aesthetics and commodity production

A considerable proportion of land and building development is thus less about the quality of the architectural product or urban space – let alone any intention to 'express' social values – and rather more about the economic return which can be generated from different aspects of the process (such as development finance deals, land speculation and rental revenues). There is no specific interest in qualitative spatial relationships or 'meaning' except in so far as these issues might affect that return on capital. These processes are themselves set within a variety of regulatory frameworks in different societies, locations and time periods depending on the economic, political and social context (Warren 1993).

Town and building development is both a dynamic and an uneven pro-cess where historically and geographically specific patterns of uneven growth and change themselves affect the next 'layer' of development processes. These processes will often have unintended consequences on environments as the sum of individual decisions is played out in the material world. Following Warren, it can be suggested that the current form of the development and construction industry in Britain (and its regulation) has led to a tendency for design to be 'imagined' through one or all of the following: as providing 'off the peg' building design and construction processes to increase efficiency by repetition; as a mechanism for improving speed of turnover or lowering cost (by, for example, improving technology); and as a means of 'adding value' to a product to increase its saleability.

The first and second categories mostly cover situations where buildings can almost be treated as a mass product with small variations (such as retail parks, out-of-town supermarkets and speculative offices). Here the spatial and representational qualities of architecture are often articulated as an *unnecessary* expense (that is, as additional 'decorative' aspects of building form) and architects are used infrequently. The third category is more complex: adding value may operate at the level of standard mass-produced and cost-effective products – whether functional and/or symbolic (such as in the mass housing market), adding to the 'experience' of a commodity (such as fantasy or spectacle in leisure provision) or adding value not by repetition but by aesthetic differentiation from similar buildings and environments (as in fashion). In each of these cases, though, there is the same division between the building as a commodity and a perceived 'added', optional layer of design representation.

At the client-led, luxury and bespoke end of the market, it is these 'designer' aspects which are exploited, precisely because they are perceived to have the scarcity value of a custom-made or 'artistic' object. Here, the client and/or developer is deliberately investing in architecture as a cultural artefact.

Architecture, professional knowledge and 'masculinist rationality'

Overlaying these assumptions, are two – potentially contradictory – beliefs about the design professional's relationship to this market. On the one hand, architects' practices specialising in commercial and private sector business will align themselves with the aims and objectives of their clients. On the other, architects, through their training often believe in a more 'distanced' stance linked to concepts of social justice and the public interest, where design knowledge is deliberately envisaged as being separate from and above the economic nexus. In both cases, architectural expertise is most often offered up as a rational, diagnostic and objective skill for meeting and expressing the clients' needs, and/or for representing appropriate social and public aspects. This is most often assumed through two aspects of the design approach; first that the building should express its 'contents' in its external form and second that the architectural 'language' of the building should be logically consistent in its overall composition.[3] Such a stance is then deliberately set in opposition to the 'look' of commodity production, which adds 'features' emblematically and facilities ad hoc, only where these are perceived to provide added value and therefore enhance saleability.

I have shown elsewhere that the historical development of professional architectural knowledge through the nineteenth century, legitimising the architect's role in providing design in advance, self-consciously developed the belief in 'authentic metaphor' as a mechanism for expressing social content 'directly' in architectural form: a mechanism which appeared to enable the simultaneous expression of individual client characteristics and more abstract, societal values (Boys 1996 and forthcoming). In the nineteenth century many architectural writers argued that while in previous periods this occurred 'naturally', such an act of reflection of society through design could now be undertaken only consciously. *How* architecture might reflect society thus became a major component of radical architectural debates. By the 1920s it had become such a commonplace (to avant-garde Europeans at least) that architecture did/should express the *Zeitgeist* (that is, an abstract representation of society-as-a-whole) that the nature of this particular connection was no longer questioned.

Of course, it is such a 'structure of knowing', delineating cultural artefacts as visual and/or spatial *representations* of aspects of society, that enables (privileged) observers (whether architects or cultural critics) to consider themselves to be making a neutral and justifiable case. Since the building *obviously* 'reflects' society, the architect's/cultural intellectual's claim is that because of specialised knowledge he or she *in particular* has the ability to create/read that reflection truthfully and objectively. As the architectural profession increasingly consolidated itself around providing 'design in advance' at the turn of the century, the claim (over other built environment professionals) to this area of diagnostic/analytical knowledge became increasingly important. It simultaneously enabled architectural professionalism to appear to be 'above' lower-status concerns such as economics, building production processes, client taste and fashion cycles.

Architecture and gender (1): the limits of 'oppression'

How, then, can this very basic outline of the complexity of architectural production processes be interrogated through the filter of gender issues? I have already proposed that the structure of professional architectural knowledge is based on masculinist rationality because it uses a system of binary oppositions and incorporates an assumption of its own 'rightness', which thereby prevents alternative articulations. What is more, the preference for specific social and architectural characteristics historically can be consistently shown to be framed around masculinist images of society. This is not to say, however, (as became common in the Thatcherite period of British politics) that architecture provided through the private sector automatically offers an improved material landscape compared with the welfare state architecture of postwar Britain. The logic of design within commodity production prevents the architecture of towns and cities from incorporating a public or gender dimension except in so far as it overlaps with the profit motive. Thus, in the British case, we have had, on the one hand, publicly provided architecture which has predominantly designed buildings as *metaphors* of society, that is, primarily through symbolic representation, and, on the other, a building market which is hardly able to engage with a social dimension at all. It is here that gender issues need to be placed – within a critique of existing design and development processes – not in simple analogies between architectural space and oppression or in Grosz's dream of an architecture of the 'outside'. Here is the 'space' that most urgently needs to be reclaimed, not just around gender, but as a focus for political and social debate about, for example, the inequalities of land and development economics, about issues of professional knowledge and ethics, about how to enable access to both resources and 'meaning-making' in building production and consumption, and about methods for improving the quality of the built environment.

Architecture and gender (2): positioning identities?

In his book *Postmodernism, or the Cultural Logic of Late Capitalism* Frederic Jameson famously uses the example of the Westin Bonaventure Hotel, in Los Angeles, to illustrate his argument that western society has changed in some dramatic way towards depthlessness and spectacle. He proposes that the Bonaventure expresses this through 'a mutation in built space itself' because of its lack of clear entrances, its reflective glass skin, systems of circulation and huge, disorientating interior spaces:

> I am more at a loss when it comes to conveying the thing itself, the experience of space you undergo when you step off such allegorical devices into the lobby or atrium. . . . I am tempted to say that such space makes it impossible for us to use the language of volume or volumes any longer, since these are impossible to seize. . . . What happens then is something else, which can only be characterised as milling confusion, something like the vengeance this space takes on those who still seek to walk through it. . . .
>
> So I come finally to my principal point here, that this latest mutation in space – postmodern hyperspace – has finally succeeded in transcending the capacities of the individual human body to locate itself, to organise its immediate surrounding perceptually, and to cognitively map its position in a mappable external world. It may now be suggested that this alarming disjunction point between the body and its built environment . . . can itself stand as the symbol and analogon of that even sharper dilemma which is the

incapacity of our minds, at least at present, to map the great global multi-national and decentered communications network in which we find ourselves caught as individual subjects.

(Jameson 1991: 42–4)

Jameson here provides a useful example of the all too easy slippage across conceptual and material space; and between material space and societal structures. To him, this architectural example is of value precisely because it is seen as a map of, and metaphor for, postmodernity. The building is perceived as frighteningly complex, diverse and chaotic and is analysed therefore as the expression of new societal fragmentations *on the surface* and as the simultaneous obscuring and expression of the complex and disordering 'deep' structures of late twentieth-century capitalism.

There have been many valuable, critical accounts of these types of analyses (see, for example, Massey 1996). Here I want to use it as an example of how relationships between gender and architecture might be more fruitfully interrogated than through such simplistic metaphors. This would first unravel a range of positionalities. Initially, for example, Jameson's specific anxieties (the fear of a rational masculinist, perhaps) that the world is becoming unmappable and unreadable and his desire to have the physical form of society express legible 'deep' meanings need to be examined in the context of current academic and intellectual shifts – such as the increasing predominance of issues of culture, new concerns with representation and the invention of concepts of postmodernism. As Featherstone writes:

These changes require careful documentation and explanation in terms of the dynamic of academic and intellectual fields as well as their capacity to respond to and thematize sociocultural changes. They should not be taken just on the level of a paradigm shift or the victory of a superior set of methodologies.

(Featherstone 1991: 30)

Then, other positionalities, such as that of John Portman, who was (unusually) both architect and developer, as well as other actors and agencies in the design and development process, could be explored. Portman combines professional architectural knowledge with a powerful place within commodity production – that is, he bridges the bifurcating tendencies outlined above. This might be linked to specific forms of architectural investment in the building, such as the emphasis on the spectacular, particularly in the huge areas of the atrium and expanses of mirror glazing in comparison with, say, the basic planning of bedrooms and their circulation. This notion of spectacle would then itself need to be examined within a history of capitalist commodification as combining function and meaning in specific building types (where meaning is articulated predominately as visual representation plus emotional stimuli), within the history of competing architectural knowledges (including, for example, the history of hotels as a building type, contested positions within architects and between architects and builders over 'appropriate' socio-spatial concepts, and changing attitudes to architectural imagery such as the various 'meanings' applied to mirror glass and curtain walling by different social groups), as well as being linked to the connected debates in academia on spectacle and postmodernism (Zukin 1993).

It is in this context that the other characteristic highlighted by Jameson – the hotel's separation from its locality and the internalisation of public space – could be studied. Writers such as Davis and Soja, for example, have argued that this building is part of the logic of 'Fortress LA':

> Redeveloped with public tax increments under the aegis of the powerful and largely unaccountable Community Redevelopment Agency, the Downtown project is one of the largest postwar urban designs in North America. Site assemblage and clearing on a vast scale, with little mobilized opposition, has resurrected land values, upon which big developers and off-shore capital have planned a series of billion-dollar, block-square megastructures: Croker Center, the Bonaventure Hotel and Shopping Mall, Arco Center, CitiCorp Plaza, California Plaza and so on. With historical landscapes erased, with megastructures and superblocks as primary components and with an increasingly dense and self-contained circulation system, the new financial district is best conceived as a single, demonically self-referential hyperstructure, a Miesan skyscape raised to dementia.
>
> (Davis 1990: 228)

Here, Davis relies on analogy to link economic and social change with architectural form, where one becomes evidence of the other. Instead the actors in the process need to be articulated within their various positionalities, and the architecture and city development then studied in its particular context as a mechanism of translation. While such a study will necessarily be more complex, it may also enable a richer and denser level of analysis, and one which can incorporate a gender dimension into investigations of the changing relationships of public/private and inside/outside space.

Finally, such a study would need to explore the positionalities of those people not directly related to the development and design process to see how they have engaged with both building processes and products through time. This would need to incorporate issues of legitimacy and marginalisation both in relation to access to resources and to 'meaning-making'. It might include an examination of those who previously occupied the site and those who now inhabit the area – hotel visitors and hotel staff. This is where huge gaps and silences remain in our understanding of how architecture operates. Exploring such positionalities is not merely about 'what people want' or like and dislike, but, as Bourdieu shows, about differential positioning within specific patterns of privilege and legitimacy. This would have three interconnected elements. First, one could explore both the different analogies applied by these 'others' to the building and its locality and the relative importance of analogy as a form of discourse about architecture compared with alternative criteria. Second, the relationship of different individuals and groups to the building's spatial arrangements and settings (for example, what activities are kept together, what are kept apart and what areas there are of symbolic and economic investment) could be unravelled, as well as the tensions, discomforts and transgressions thus generated. As Valentine writes:

> gender is the repeated stylization of the body, a set of repeated acts within a highly rigid regulatory framework that congeal over time to produce the appearance of substance, of a 'natural sort of being'. In the same way the heterosexing of space is a performative act naturalized through repetition and regulation. . . . These acts produce 'a host' of assumptions embedded in the practices of public life about what constitutes 'proper behaviour' and which congeal over time to give the appearance of a 'proper' or 'normal' production of space.
>
> (Valentine 1996: 148)

It is this 'congealing' of specific gender and other relationships through space that needs exposing. Finally, it is important to note that these positionalities are also transmuted through mechanisms of translation, that is, the specific economic, social and personal contexts in which we operate and which have an impact on what is possible and 'appropriate' in particular situations.

Breaking the boundaries

This chapter takes only initial steps in thinking through how to break out of the 'binary' boundaries so as to imagine alternative, more equitable and creative processes for the production and consumption of architecture and urban space. There are three pointers proposed here.

First, architecture cannot be viewed as a simple map of social relations nor through representation as a simple metaphor of gender differences. Architecture and cities are formed as material spaces where processes of production and consumption, theory and practice, belief and experience collide. What is more, this built materiality is not merely the result of these processes but is itself also translated via the specificities of development and design conceptions and physical realisations. There is thus considerable space here for partiality, for variety, for different positions held simultaneously and for confusions and unintended consequences. Here, the study of positionalities might also allow the development of a new politics of architecture and planning which re-engages issues of resource distribution and inequalities (economics) with access to, and control over, 'meaning-making' in imaginary and material spaces (culture).

Second, it is essential to examine processes by separating out, however artificially, the spaces of theory, of social identities and of materiality so that the mechanisms of translation from one to the other can be explored. Only then is it possible to examine in what shape and in whose interest such mechanisms are maintained, and how these are or can be transformed. It is only then that we can begin to see the interrelationships between underlying positionalities and the particular buildings and cities which grow out of them.

Third, architects, theorists and critics need to deliberately disrupt the assumed linking of architectural form with the metaphorical expression of specific social values or relationships, while re-engaging fiercely in public debate about what constitutes appropriate physical arrangements, appearances and settings for the social aspects of existence – and the mechanisms by which these might be implemented. For while architecture does not 'reflect' society, and is only partially shaped by our continuing and contested struggles for identity, the buildings and cities we inhabit remain deeply implicated in shaping our everyday experiences.

Notes

1 Hence the 'shock' when riots occur in non-ghetto locations such as suburban estates or country towns. For a more detailed critque see Boys (1996).
2 For example, buildings are extremely expensive compared with other products. Each is built as a 'prototype', with little or no co-ordinated monitoring or evaluation of use. Each is dependent on specific site locations and typographies both physically and in terms of inherent inelasticities of demand and inflexibilities of supply, as well as on the physical possibilities of structure and construction.
3 As Bourdieu shows, even where artistic avant-gardes deliberately break these rules, they remain framed by them (Bourdieu 1984).

Bibliography

Works cited in the short introductions to the book's four sections are included in the first section of this bibliography.

Introduction and section introductions

Anderson, B. (1991) *Imagined Communities*, London: Verso.

Ardener, S. (1993) *Women and Space: Ground Rules and Social Maps*, Providence: Berg.

Bachelard, G. (1994) *The Poetics of Space*, Boston: Beacon Press.

Bell, D. and Valentine, G. (eds) (1995) *Mapping Desire: Geographies of Sexualities*, London: Routledge.

Bhabha, H. (1990) *Nation and Narration*, London: Routledge.

Bornstein, K. (1994) *Gender Outlaw*, New York: Routledge.

Butler, J. (1990) *Gender Trouble: Feminism and the Subversion of Identity*, London and New York: Routledge.

Calvino, I. (1986) *Invisible Cities*, London: Secker & Warburg.

Colomina, B. (ed.) (1992) *Sexuality and Space*, Princeton, NJ: Princeton Architectural Press.

—— (1994) *Privacy and Publicity*, Boston: MIT Press.

Duncan, N. (ed.) (1996) *Bodyspace: Destabilizing Geographies of Gender and Sexuality*, London and New York: Routledge.

Gale, P. (1995) *The Facts of Life*, London: Flamingo.

Grosz, E. (1992) 'Bodies–cities', in B. Colomina (ed.) *Sexuality and Space*, Princeton, NJ: Princeton Architectural Press.

—— (1995) 'Women, *chora*, dwelling', in S. Watson and K. Gibson (eds) *Post Modern Cities and Spaces*, Oxford: Blackwell.

Harraway, D. (1991) *Simians, Cyborgs and Women: The Reinvention of Nature*, New York: Routledge.

Hayden, D. (1981) *The Grand Domestic Revolution: A History of Feminist Designs for American Homes, Neighborhoods, and Cities*, Cambridge, MA: MIT Press.

—— (1995) *The Power of Place*, Cambridge, MA: MIT Press.

Hite, S. (1993) *Women as Revolutionary Agents of Change*, London: Bloomsbury.

Jacques, M. (1997) 'Where the future is outrageous', *The Guardian*, 22 March 1997.

Koawale, H. (1995) 'Sisters take the rap . . . but talk back', in S. Cooper (ed.) *Girls! Girls! Girls!*, London: Cassell.

Lefebvre, H. (1991) *The Production of Space*, trans. D. Nicholson-Smith, Oxford: Blackwell.

Matrix Book Group (eds) (1984) *Making Space: Women and the Man-Made Environment*, London: Pluto.

Oxford Popular Dictionary (1993) London: HarperCollins.

Parker, A., Russo, M., Sommer, D. and Yaeger, P. (eds) (1992) *Nationalisms and Sexualities*, New York: Routledge.

Rutherford, J. (ed.) (1990) *Identity: Community, Culture, Difference*, London: Lawrence & Wishart.

Sennett, R. (1973) *The Uses of Disorder: Personal Identity and City Life*, Harmondsworth: Penguin.

—— (1994) *Flesh and Stone: The Body and the City in Western Civilization*, London: Faber & Faber.

Watson, S. and Gibson, K. (eds) (1995) *Post Modern Cities and Spaces*, Oxford: Blackwell.

Wilson, E. (1989) *Hallucinations: Life in the Post Modern City*, London: Radius.

—— (1991) *The Sphinx in the City: Urban Life, the Control of Disorder, and Women*, London: Virago.

Women's Design Service (n.d.) 'Older Women and Education Group – future places, future spaces', Broadsheet 9, WDS.

Chapter 1

Anderson, B. (1991) *Imagined Communities*, London: Verso.

Anzaldúa, G. (1987) *Borderlands/La Frontera: The New Mestiza*, San Francisco: Spinster/Aunt Lute Press.

—— (1991) 'To(o) queer the writer – *Loca, escritora y chicana*', in B. Warland (ed.) *Inversions*, London: Open Letters.

Bammer, A. (1991) *Partial Visions: Feminism and Utopianism in the 1970s*, London: Routledge.

Bennington, G. (1994) 'Postal politics and the institution of the nation', in H. Bhabha (ed.) *The Location of Culture*, London: Routledge.

Berlant, L. and Freeman, E. (1993) 'Queer nationality', in M. Warner, *Fear of a Queer Planet: Queer Politics and Social Theory*, Minneapolis: University of Minnesota Press.

Bhabha, H. (1990) *Nation and Narration*, London: Routledge.

—— (1994) 'Dissemination: time, narrative, and the margins of the modern nation', in *The Location of Culture*, London: Routledge.

Butler, J. (1990) *Gender Trouble: Feminism and the Subversion of Identity*, London: Routledge.

Castle, T. (1993) *The Apparitional Lesbian: Female Homosexuality and Modern Culture*, New York: Columbia University Press.

Daly, M. (1978) *Gyn/Ecology: The Metaethics of Radical Feminism*, Boston: Beacon Press.

Dollimore, J. (1991) *Sexual Dissidence: Augustine to Wilde, Freud to Foucault*, Oxford: Clarendon University Press.

Gellner, E. (1983) *Nations and Nationalism*, Oxford: Blackwell.

Heng, G. and Devan, J. (1992) 'State fatherhood: the politics of nationalism, sexuality, and race in Singapore', in A. Parker *et al.* (eds) *Nationalisms and Sexualities*, New York: Routledge.

Hobsbawm, E. J. (1990) *Nations and Nationalism since 1780*, Cambridge: Cambridge University Press.

Jameson, F. (1977) 'Of islands and trenches: naturalisation and the production of Utopian discourse', *Diacritics* 7(2), 21 February 1977.

Johnston, J. (1973) *The Lesbian Nation: The Feminist Solution*, New York: Touchstone Books/Simon & Schuster.

Layoun, M. (1992) 'Palestine women, national narratives', in A. Parker *et al.* (eds) *Nationalisms and Sexualities*, New York: Routledge.

Lewis, E. (1915) *Edward Carpenter: An Exposition and an Appreciation*, London, quoted in G. L. Mosse, *Nationalism and Sexuality*, Madison: University of Wisconsin Press.

McClintock, A. (1995) *Imperial Leather: Race, Gender, Sexuality in the Colonial Contest*, New York: Routledge.

Maggenti, M. (1991) 'Women as queer nationals', *Out/Look* (Winter): 20–3.

Moraga, C. (1983) *Loving in the War Years*, Boston: South End Press.

Mosse, G. L. (1985) *Nationalism and Sexuality*, Madison: University of Wisconsin Press.

Parker, A., Russo, M., Sommer, D. and Yaeger, P. (eds) (1992) *Nationalisms and Sexualities*, New York: Routledge.

Phelan, S. (1989) *Identity Politics: Lesbian Feminism and the Limits of Community*, Philadelphia: Temple University Press.

—— (1994) *Getting Specific: Postmodern Lesbian Politics*, Minneapolis: University of Minnesota Press.

Pratt, M. B. (1984) 'Identity, skin, blood, heart', in *Yours in Struggle: Three Feminist Perspectives on Anti-Semitism and Racism*, Brooklyn, NY: Long Haul Press.

Radhakrishnan, R. (1992) 'Nationalism, gender and narrative', in A. Parker *et al.* (eds) *Nationalisms and Sexualities*, New York: Routledge.

Raiskin, J. (1994) 'Inverts and hybrids: lesbian rewritings of sexual and racial identities', in L. Doan, *The Lesbian Postmodern*, New York: Columbia University Press.

Rensan, E. (1990) 'What is a nation?', in H. Bhabha, *Nation and Narration*, London: Routledge.

Said, E. (1990) 'Reflections on exile', in R. Ferguson *et al.* (eds) *Out There – Marginalization and Contemporary Culture*, Boston: MIT Press.

Schulman, S. (1995) *Rat Bohemia*, New York: Dutton/Penguin Books.

Scott, J. H. (1990) 'From foreground to margin: female configurations and masculine self-representation in black nationalist fiction', in A. Parker *et al.* (eds) *Nationalisms and Sexualities*, New York: Routledge.

Sedgwick, E. K. (1991) *Epistemology of the Closet*, Hemel Hempstead: Harvester Wheatsheaf.

Seidman, S. (1993) 'Identity and politics in a post-modern gay culture: some historical and conceptual notes', in Michael Warner (ed.) *Fear of Queer Planet: Queer Politics and Social Theory*, Minneapolis: University of Minnesota Press, pp. 105–42.

Shugar, D. R. (1995) *Separatism and Women's Community*, Lincoln: University of Nebraska Press.

Warner, M. (ed.) (1993) *Fear of a Queer Planet: Queer Politics and Social Theory*, Minneapolis: University of Minnesota Press.

Weeks, J. (1995) *Invented Moralities: Sexual Values in an Age of Uncertainty*, Oxford: Polity Press.

Wilson, E. (1991) *The Sphinx in the City: Urban Life, the Control of Disorder, and Women*, London: Virago.

Wittig, M. (1986) *The Lesbian Body*, Boston: Beacon Press.

Chapter 2

Berg, L. D. and Kearns, R. A. (1996) 'Naming as norming? Race, gender and the identity politics of naming places in Aotearoa/New Zealand', *Environment and Planning D: Society and Space* 14(1): 99–122.

Census of Population and Dwellings (1991) *Waikato/Bay of Plenty Regional Report*, Wellington: Department of Statistics New Zealand.

Chavkin, W. (1992) 'Woman and fetus: the social construction of conflict', in C. Feinman (ed.) *The Criminalization of a Woman's Body*, New York: Haworth Press, pp. 193–202.

Collins English Dictionary (1979) Glasgow: William Collins.

Davis-Floyd, R. (1986) 'Birth as an American rite of passage', PhD thesis, Austin, University of Texas.

Fergusson, S. (1991) 'Myth and the creation of urban landscapes: "Centre Place"', research project (unpublished), University of Waikato.

Grosz, E. (1992) 'Bodies–cities', in B. Colomina (ed.) *Sexuality and Space*, Princeton, NJ: Princeton Architectural Press.

Jackson, P. (1993) 'Towards a cultural politics of consumption', in J. Bird, B. Curtis, T. Putnam, G. Robertson and L. Tickner (eds) *Mapping the Futures: Local Cultures, Global Change*, London: Routledge.

Johnson, L. (1989) 'Embodying geography – some implications of considering the sexed body in space', *New Zealand Geographical Society Proceedings of the 15th New Zealand Geography Conference*, Dunedin, August, pp. 134–8.

—— (1990) 'New courses for a gendered geography: teaching feminist geography at the University of Waikato', *Australian Geographical Studies* 28(1): 16–27.

Kristeva, J. (1980) 'Motherhood according to Giovanni Bellini', in her *Desire in Language*, trans. by Lion S. Roudiez, New York: Columbia University Press.

Lloyd, G. (1993) 'The man of reason: 'male' and 'female'', in *Western Philosophy*, London: Routledge.

Longhurst, R. (1997) '(Dis)embodied geographies', *Progress in Human Geography* 21(4): 486–501.

Longhurst, R. (1995) 'Geography and the body', *Gender, Place and Culture: A Journal of Feminist Geography* 2(1): 97–105.

Matrix Book Group (eds) (1984) *Making Space: Women and the Man-Made Environment*, London: Pluto.

Morgan, D. H. J. and Scott, S. (1993) 'Bodies in a social landscape', in S. Scott and D. H. J. Morgan (eds) *Body Matters*, London: Falmer Press, pp. 1–21.

Rose, G. (1993) *Feminism and Geography: The Limits of Geographical Knowledge*, Cambridge: Polity Press.

Spain, D. (1992) *Gendered Spaces*, Chapel Hill and London: University of North Carolina Press.

Spoonley, P. (1995) 'Constructing ourselves: the post-colonial politics of European/Pakeha', in M. Wilson and A. Yeatman (eds) *Justice and Identity: Antipodean Practices*, Wellington: Bridget Williams.

Weisman, L. K. (1992) *Discrimination by Design: A Feminist Critique of the Man-made Environment*, Urbana: University of Illinois Press.

Winchester, H. (1992) 'The construction and deconstruction of women's roles in the urban landscape', in K. Anderson and F. Gale (eds) *Inventing Places: Studies in Cultural Geography*, New York: Wiley.

Young, I. (1990) 'Pregnant embodiment', in *Throwing Like a Girl and Other Essays in Feminist Philosophy and Social Thought*, Bloomington and Indianapolis: Indiana University Press.

Chapter 3

Bethnal Green City Challenge (1994) *Action Plan 1994/5*, London: BGCC.

Butt, J. and Kurshida, M. (1996) *Social Care and Black Communities: a Review of Recent Research Studies*, London: HMSO.

Census for Ethnic Groups in Tower Hamlets 1991 in the Globe Centre's Isle of Dogs HIV/AIDS outreach project, 'Community Vision and Plan' 1996.

Department of the Environment (1996) *Regeneration Research Report: City Challenge Interim National Evaluation*, London: HMSO.

Mohila/Hawan Course for Working with Young People (1996) course handbook.

Robson, B., Russell, H., Dawson, J., Garside, P. and Parkinson, M. (1996) *Assessing the Impact of Urban Policy*, an interim national evaluation of City Challenge, London: HMSO, in Regeneration Research Report, Department of the Environment.

Salvat, Jilly (1996) 'Women in youth work training – Mohila/Hawan course for working with young people' (unpublished draft report, Goldsmiths' College, London).

Spitalfields Small Business Association (1991) grant application.

Women's Design Service (1992) 'Challenging women', Broadsheet 3, WDS.

Chapter 4

Backhouse, C. and Flaherty, D. H. (eds) (1992) *Challenging Times: The Women's Movement in Canada and the United States*, Montreal and Kingston: McGill-Queen's University Press.

Bell, David and Valentine, Gill (eds) (1995) *Mapping Desire: Geographies of Sexualities*, London: Routledge.

Butler, Judith (1990) *Gender Trouble: Feminism and the Subversion of Identity*, London and New York: Routledge.

Carroll, William K. (ed.) (1992) *Organizing Dissent: Contemporary Social Movements in Theory and Practice*, Toronto: Garamond Press.

Carty, Linda E. (ed.) (1993) *And Still We Rise: Feminist Political Mobilizing in Contemporary Canada*, Toronto: Women's Press.

Casella, Emilia (1992) ' "No reason" for Ellul inquiry Justice for Debra Coalition told', *The Hamilton Spectator*, 10 November: B1.

Davy, Denise (1992) 'Victims protest court "injustice" ', *The Hamilton Spectator*, 28 July: C1.

—— (1993) 'Firing an attempt to shut me up feminist claims', *The Hamilton Spectator*, 20 January: B1.

—— (1994) 'A mother's crusade', *The Hamilton Spectator*, 10 March: D1.

Deverell, Johan (1992) 'Women protest "travesty of justice" ', *The Toronto Star*, 10 November: A10.

Dobash, R. E. and Dobash, R. P. (1992) *Women, Violence and Social Change*, New York: Routledge.

Durocher, Constance (1990) 'Heterosexuality: sexuality or social system?', *Resources for Feminist Research* 19(3/4): 13–18.

Findlay, Sue (1988) 'Feminist struggles with the Canadian state', *Resources for Feminist Research* 17(3): 5–9.

Frye, Marilyn (1992) *Willful Virgin: Essays in Feminism 1976–1992*, Freedom, CA: Crossing Press.

Gold, Lee (1991) 'Are shelters obsolete?', *Canadian Woman Studies* 12(1): 44–5.

Grant, Ali (1996) 'Geographies of oppression and resistance: contesting the reproduction of the heterosexual regime', unpublished PhD thesis, McMaster University.

—— (1997) 'Dyke geographies: all over the place', in Gabriele Griffin and Sonya Andermahr (eds) *Straight Studies Modified: Lesbian Interventions in the Academy*, London: Cassell.

—— (forthcoming) 'And still the lesbian threat: or, how to keep a good woman a woman', *Journal of Lesbian Studies*.

Hamilton Spectator, The (1991) 'Assault centre head charged in paint attack', 5 December.

Holt, Jim (1991) 'To serve and protect', *The Hamilton Spectator*, 30 November: A1 and D1.

Lefaive, Doug (1992) 'Spray-paint fine too harsh women say', *The Hamilton Spectator*, 21 February: B1.

Longbottom, Ross (1992) '$500,000 promise survives controversial "lesbian" ad', *The Hamilton Spectator*, 27 November: B4.

Peters, Ken (1993a) ' "Ignorance" behind debate over lesbian ad', *The Hamilton Spectator*, 13 January: B1.

—— (1993b) 'The great divide', *The Hamilton Spectator*, 1 May.

Prokaska, Lee (1993a) 'Justice vigil into 2nd year', *The Hamilton Spectator*, 27 January: B1.

—— (1993b) 'Her quest for Debra', *The Hamilton Spectator*, 28 January: D2.

Rich, Adrienne (1986) *Blood, Bread, and Poetry: Selected Prose 1979–1985*, New York: Norton.

Statistics Canada (1992) Profile of census tracts in Hamilton, Part A, Ottawa: Industry, Science and Technology Canada. 1991 Census of Canada. Catalogue Number 95–341.

Sumi, Craig (1992) 'Women's shelter looks beyond ad controversy', *The Hamilton Spectator*, 26 November: C7.

Tait, Eleanor (1992) ' "Lesbian" ad jeopardizes funds for women's shelter', *The Hamilton Spectator*, 20 November: B6.

Timmins, Leslie (ed.) (1995) *Listening to the Thunder: Advocates Talk about the Battered Women's Movement*, Vancouver: Women's Research Centre.

Todd, Rosemary (1992) 'Women divided on barring men', *The Hamilton Spectator*, 18 September: B1.

Untinen, Leni (1995) 'Safety for my sisters', in Leslie Timmins (ed.) *Listening to the Thunder: Advocates Talk about the Battered Women's Movement*, Vancouver: Women's Research Centre, pp. 173–86.

Valentine, Gill (1993a) 'Desperately seeking Susan: a geography of lesbian friendships', *Area* 25(2): 109–16.

—— (1993b) 'Negotiating and managing multiple sexual identities: lesbian time-space strategies', *Transactions* (Institute of British Geographers) 18: 237–48.

—— (1993c) '(Hetero)sexing space: lesbian perceptions and experiences of everyday space', *Environment and Planning D: Society and Space* 11: 395–413.

Walker, Gillian A. (1990) *Family Violence and the Women's Movement: The Conceptual Politics of Struggle*, Toronto: University of Toronto Press.

Wine, Jeri Dawn and Ristock, Janice L. (eds) (1991) *Women and Social Change: Feminist Activism in Canada*, Toronto: Lorimer.

Wittig, Monique (1992) *The Straight Mind and Other Essays*, Boston: Beacon Press.

Yllö, Kersti and Bograd, Michele (eds) (1988) *Feminist Perspectives on Wife Abuse*, Newbury Park, CA: Sage Publications.

Chapter 5

Ardener, S. (1981) *Women and Space: Ground Rules and Social Maps*, London: Croom Hill.

Barker, F. and Jackson, P. (1985) *London: 2000 Years of a City and its People*, London: Macmillan.

Beckett, J. and Cherry, D. (n.d.) 'Sorties: ways out from behind the veil of representation', *Feminist Art News* 3(4): 3–5.

Bloomfield, B. C. (1993) *Dictionary of National Biography: Missing Persons*, Oxford: Oxford University Press.

Bolt, A. (ed.) (1932) *Our Mothers*, London: Victor Gollancz.

Borden, I., Kerr, J., Pivaro, A. and Rendell, J. (eds) (1996) *Strangely Familiar: Narratives of Architecture in the City*, London: Routledge.

Boys, J. (1984) 'Is there a feminist analysis of architecture?', *Built Environment* 10(1): 25.

Builder (1889) 57 (9 November).

Charles, E. (1898) RIBA Heinz Gallery, nomination papers, British Architectural Library (BAL) Manuscript & Archives Collection.

—— and Charles, B. (n.d.) architectural drawings, inscribed with their work/home address, BAL Drawings Collection.

Cherry, D. (1993) *Painting Women: Victorian Women Artists*, London: Routledge.

—— (1995) 'Women artists and the politics of feminism 1850–1900', in C. Campbell Orr (ed.) *Women in the Victorian Art World*, Manchester: Manchester University Press.

Conway, M. D. (1882) *Travels in South Kensington*, London: Trübner.

Darley, G. (1990) *Octavia Hill: A Life*, London: Constable.

Davidoff, L. and Hall, C. (1987) *Family Fortunes: Men and Women of the English Middle Class 1780–1850*, London: Hutchinson.

Davidoff, L., L'Esperance, J. and Newby, H. (1976) 'Landscape with figures: home and community in English society', in J. Mitchell and A. Oakley (eds) *The Rights and Wrongs of Women*, Harmondsworth: Penguin.

Davin, A. (1978) *Feminist History: A Sponsored Walk*, London: Community Press.

Englishwoman's Review (1876) 7 (15 May): 223–4.

—— (1882) 13 (15 December): 547–8.

Forty, A. (1989) 'The Mary Ward Settlement', *Architects' Journal* (2 August): 28–48.

Gandy, F., Perry, K. and Sparks, P. (1991) *Barbara Bodichon 1827–1891*, catalogue of centenary exhibition, Girton College, Cambridge.

Kelly's Post Office Directory (1850–1900).

Lefebvre, H. (1994) *The Production of Space*, trans. D. Nicholson-Smith, Oxford: Blackwell.

London Illustrated News (1860) 28 January (Westminster Archives).

Manton, J. (1987 [1965]) *Elizabeth Garrett Anderson: England's First Woman Physician*, London: Methuen.

Massey, D. (1994) *Space, Place and Gender*, Cambridge: Polity Press.

Mayhew, H. (1861) *London Labour and the London Poor*, Vol. IV; reprinted (1968), New York: Dover.

Melville, H. (1841) engraving after T. H. Sheperd, *London Interiors*, and *Graphic*, 16 January 1875, illus. in F. Barker, and P. Jackson (1974) *London: 2000 Years a City and Its People*, London: Macmillan, p. 303.

Nava, M. and O'Shea, A. (1996) *Modern Times*, London: Routledge.

Nead, L. (1988) *Myths of Sexuality: Representations of Women in Victorian Britain*, Oxford: Blackwell.

Neiswander, J. (1988) 'Liberalism, nationalism and the evolution of middle-class values: the literature on interior decoration in England', PhD thesis, University of London.

Pankhurst, R. (1979) *Sylvia Pankhurst: Artist and Crusader*, London: Paddington Press.

Pearson, L. F. (1988) *The Architectural and Social History of Cooperative Living*, London: Macmillan.

Pollock, G. (1988) 'Modernity and the spaces of femininity', in G. Pollock, *Vision & Difference*, London: Routledge, pp. 50–90.

Queen (1890) 88 (4 October).

—— (1898) 23 (December): 1081.

Rappaport, E. (1993) 'Gender and commercial culture in London 1860–1914', PhD thesis, Rutgers University.

Strachey, R. (1927) *Women's Suffrage and Women's Service*, London: National Society for Women's Suffrage.

Sutherland, J. (n.d. [*c*. 1990]) *The Mary Ward Centre 1890–1990*, published lecture.

Tickner, L. (1987) *The Spectacle of Women: Imagery of the Suffrage Campaign 1907–14*, London: Chatto & Windus.

Urry, J. (1994) *Consuming Places*, London: Routledge.

Vickery, A. (1993) 'Golden age to separate spheres? A review of the categories and chronologies of women's history', *Historical Journal* 36(3): 383–414.

Walker, L. (1995) 'Vistas of Pleasure: Women Consumers of Urban Space in the West End of London 1850–1900' in C. Campbell Orr (ed.) *Women in the Victorian Art World*, Manchester: Manchester University Press.

—— (1996) 'A West-End of one's own: Women's buildings and social spaces from Bloomsbury to Mayfair', notes of an architectural walk organized by the Victorian Society.

—— and Ware, V. (forthcoming) 'Political pincushions: decorating the abolitionist interior 1790–1860', in Inga Bryden and Janet Floyd (eds) *Reading the Interior: Nineteenth-Century Domestic Space*, Manchester: Manchester University Press; the paper on which this essay is based was first given in April 1995 at the conference 'Reading the nineteenth-century domestic space', King Alfred's College, Winchester.

Walkowitz, J. (1992) *City of Dreadful Delight: Narratives of Sexual Danger in Late-Victorian London*, London: Virago.

Wilson, E. (1985) *Adorned in Dreams: Fashion and Modernity*, London: Virago.

—— (1991) *The Sphinx in the City: Urban Life, the Control of Disorder, and Women*, London: Virago.
Young Woman (1895) 4.

Chapter 6

AAUW Report (1995) *How Schools Shortchange Girls: A Study of Major Findings on Girls and Education*, New York: Marlowe.
Aperture (1995) 'Shooting back from the reservation: photographs' (Summer): 42.
Bonnie, J. Leadbeater, R. and Way, N. (1996) *Urban Girls: Resisting Stereotypes, Creating Identities*, New York: New York University Press.
Brown L. M. and Gilligan, C. (1992) *Meeting at the Crossroads: Women's Psychology and Girls' Development*, New York: Ballentine.
Buss, S. (1994) 'City syntax from young people's angle of vision: meaning and action in the postmodern urban spatial environment of Los Angeles', unpublished PhD thesis, University of California at Los Angeles.
Dewdney, A. and Lister, M. (1988) *Youth, Culture and Photography*, Basingstoke: Macmillan Education.
Graff, H. J. (1995) *Conflicting Paths: Growing up in America*, Cambridge, MA: Harvard University Press.
Hubbard, J. (1994) *Shooting back from the Reservation: A Photographic View of Life by Native American Youth*, New York: New Press.
Kurian, G. T. (1995) *Datapedia of the U.S. 1790–2000: America Year by Year*, Lanham, MD: Bernan Press.
Leavitt, J. and Saegert, S. (1990) *From Abandonment to Hope: Community Households in Harlem*, New York: Columbia University Press.
Orenstein, P. (1994) *Schoolgirls: Young Women, Self-Esteem and the Confidence Gap*, New York: Anchor Books.
Pipher, M. (1995) *Reviving Ophelia: Saving the Selves of Adolescent Girls*, New York: Ballentine.

Chapter 7

Adam, P. (1987) *Eileen Gray: Architect/Designer*, New York: Harry N. Abrams.
Bentham, Jeremy (1995) *The Panopticon Writings*, ed. Miran Bozovic, London: Verso.
Blanchot, M. (1982) 'The two versions of the imaginary', in *The Space of Literature*, Lincoln: University of Nebraska Press.
Borden, J., Kerr, J., Pivaro, A. and Readell, J. (eds) (1996) *Strangely Familiar: Narratives of Architecture in the City*, London: Routledge.
Boys, Jos (1989) 'From Alcatraz to the OK Corral: images of class and gender', in J. Attfield and P. Kirkham (eds) *A View from the Interior: Gender and Design*, London: Women's Press.
Charley, J. (1996) 'Sentences upon architecture', in I. Borden *et al.* (eds) *Strangely Familiar: Narratives of Architecture in the City*, London: Routledge.
Coleman, Alice (1985) *Utopia on Trial: Vision and Reality in Planned Housing*, London: Hilary Shipman.
Colomina, Beatriz (ed.) (1992) *Sexuality and Space*, Princeton, NJ: Princeton Architectural Press.
Easton Ellis, Bret (1985) *Less than Zero*, London: Picador.

Foucault, Michel (1979) *Discipline and Punish: The Birth of the Prison*, trans. A. Sheridan, Harmondsworth: Penguin.

hooks, bell (1994) *Outlaw Culture: Resisting Representations*, New York: Routledge.

Hough, Michael (1977) 'No sense in trying to turn back the clock', *The Guardian*, 23 April.

L'amour fou: photography and surrealism (1986) London: Arts Council.

Lingwood, J. (1995) *House Rachel Whiteread*, London: Phaidon.

Markus, Thomas (1993) *Buildings and Power*, London: Routledge.

Moorhouse, Jocelyn (dir.) (1991) *Proof*, Australia.

Newman, Oscar (1983 [1972]) *Defensible Space: People and Design in the Violent City*, London: Architectural Press.

Noyse, P. (dir.) (1993) *Sliver*, USA.

Photographic Surveillance Techniques for Law Enforcement Agencies (1972) n.p.: Kodak.

Ryle, John (1996) 'Gaze of power', *The Guardian*, 12 January.

Soja, E. (1995) 'Heterotopologies', in S. Watson and K. Gibson (eds) *Post Modern Cities and Spaces*, Oxford: Blackwell.

Sontag, Susan (1983) *A Susan Sontag Reader*, Harmondsworth: Penguin.

Women's Design Service (1996) *Public Surveillance Systems*, London: WDS.

Chapter 8

Berg, E. *et al.* (1982) *Det lilla kollektivhuset. En modell för praktisk tillämpning* (The small collective house. A model to be implemented), Stockholm: Swedish Council for Building Research.

Hayden, D. (1976) *Seven American Utopias: The Architecture of Communitarian Socialism, 1790–1975*, Cambridge, MA: MIT Press.

—— (1981) *The Grand Domestic Revolution: A History of Feminist Designs for American Homes, Neighborhoods, and Cities*, Cambridge, MA: MIT Press.

Koyabe, I. (1994) 'Residents' participation in the design of housing: a study of the Swedish collective house Färdknäppen', report no. R7:1994, Stockholm: Department of Building Function Analysis, School of Architecture, Royal Institute of Technology.

Lundahl, G. and Sangregorio, I.–L. (1992) *Femton kollektivhus. En idé förverkligas* (Fifteen collective houses. An idea put into practice), Stockholm: Swedish Council for Building Research.

McCamant, K. and Durrett, C. (1994) *Cohousing: a Contemporary Approach to Housing Ourselves*, Berkeley, CA: Ten Speed Press.

Ottes, L. *et al.* (eds) (1995) *Gender and the Built Environment: Emancipation in Planning, Housing and Mobility in Europe*, Assen, Holland: Van Gorcum.

Sangregorio, I.–L. (1994) *På spaning efter ett bättre boende. Bygga och bo på kvinnors villkor* (On the lookout for better ways of housing ourselves. Building and living on women's terms), Stockholm: Swedish Council for Building Research.

—— (1995) 'Collaborative housing: the home of the future? Reflections on the Swedish experience', in L. Ottes *et al.* (eds), *Gender and the Built Environment: Emancipation in Planning, Housing and Mobility in Europe*, Assen, Holland: Van Gorcum.

Sullerot, E. (1965) *Demain les femmes*, Paris: Laffont-Gonthier.

Chapter 9

Ageyman, J. (1988) 'Ethnic minorities – an environmental issue?', *Ecos* 9(3): 2–5.

Burgess, J. (1994) 'The politics of trust: reducing fear of crime in urban parks', Comedia-Demos Working Paper 8, London.

—— (1995) 'Growing in confidence: a research report on perceptions of risk in recreational woodlands', Countryside Commission technical report CCP457, Cheltenham, Glos: Countryside Commission (CC Postal Sales, PO Box 124, Walgrave, Northampton NN6 9TL).

—— (1996) 'Focusing on fear: the use of focus groups in a project for the Community Forest Unit, Countryside Commission', *Area* 28: 130–5.

—— Harrison, C. M. and Limb, M. (1988) 'People, parks and the urban green: a study of popular meanings and values for open spaces in the city', *Urban Studies* 25: 455–73.

Carr, S., Francis, M., Rivlin, L. G. and Stone, A. M. (1992) *Public Space*, Cambridge: Cambridge University Press.

Cooper-Marcus, C. and Francis, C. (1990) *People Places: Design Guidelines for Urban Open Space*, New York: Van Nostrand Reinhold.

Evans, D. J., Fyfe, N. R. and Herbert, D. (eds) (1992) *Crime, Policing and Place: Essays in Environmental Criminology*, London: Routledge.

Ferraro, K. F. (1996) 'Women's fear of victimisation: shadow of sexual assault?', *Social Forces* 75: 667–723.

Gardner, C. (1994) 'Reclaiming the night: night-time use, lighting and safety in Britain's parks', Comedia, The Future of Urban Parks and Open Spaces series, Working Paper 7.

Garofalo, J. (1981) 'The fear of crime: causes and consequences', *Journal of Criminal Law and Criminal Policy* 72(2): 839–57.

Geason, S. and Wilson, P. (1989) *Designing out Crime: Crime Prevention through Environmental Design*, Canberra: Australian Institute of Criminology.

Grant, A. (1989) 'Planning for sexual assault prevention: women's safety in High Park, Toronto', Toronto: METRAK (158 Spadina Road, Toronto, Ontario M5R 2T8).

Greenhalgh, L. and Worpole, K. (1995) *Park Life: Urban Parks and Social Renewal*. London: Comedia/Demos.

—— (1996) *People, Parks and Cities: a Guide to Current Good Practice in Urban Parks*, London: HMSO.

Harrison, C. M., Burgess, J., Millward, A. and Dawe, G. (1995) 'Accessible natural greenspace in towns and cities: a review of appropriate size and distance criteria', English Nature Research Reports No. 153, Peterborough.

—— Limb, M. and Burgess, J. (1987) 'Nature in the city: popular values for a living world', *Journal of Environmental Management* 25: 347–62.

Herbert, D. T. (1993) 'Neighbourhood incivilities and the study of crime in place', *Area* 25(1): 45–54.

Home Office Standing Conference on Crime Prevention (1989) *Report of the Working Group on the Fear of Crime*. London: Home Office.

Hough, M. (1995) 'Anxiety about crime: findings from the 1994 British Crime Survey', London: Home Office Research and Planning Unit, Report 147.

Lee, T. (1991) 'Attitudes towards and preferences for forestry landscapes', University of Surrey, unpublished report for the Forestry Authority and Countryside Commission (enquiries to the Forestry Authority, 231 Corstorphine Road, Edinburgh EH2 7AT).

McNeill, S. (1987) 'Flashing: its effect on women', in J. Hanmer and M. Maynard (eds) *Women, Violence and Social Control*, London: Macmillan.

Malik, S. (1992) 'Colours of the countryside – a whiter shade of pale', *Ecos* 13(4): 33–40.

Mayhew, P. and Maung, N. A. (1993) 'Surveying crime: findings from the 1992 British Crime Survey', London: Home Office Research and Statistics Department, No. 2.

Merry, S. (1981) 'Defensible space undefended: social factors in crime control through environmental design', *Urban Affairs Quarterly* 16(4): 397–422.

Mirrlees-Black, C., Mayhew, P. and Percey, A. (1996) 'The 1996 British Crime Survey, England and Wales', London: Government Statistical Service, Issue 19/96.

Newman, O. (1972) *Defensible Space: People and Design in the Violent City*, London: Architectural Press.

Pain, R. (1991) 'Space, sexual violence and social control: integrating geographical and feminist analyses of women's fear of crime', *Progress in Human Geography* 15(4): 415–31.

—— (1995) 'Elderly women and fear of violent crime – the least likely victims: a reconstruction of the extent and nature of risk', *British Journal of Criminology* 35: 584–98.

Painter, K. (1991) 'An evaluation of better street lighting on crime and fear: a review', London: Crime Prevention Unit, Home Office, Paper 29.

—— (1992) 'Different worlds: the spatial, temporal and social dimensions of female victimisation', in D. J. Evans, N. R. Fyfe and D. Herbert (eds) *Crime, Policing and Place: Essays in Environmental Criminology*, London: Routledge, pp. 164–95.

Pawson, E. (1993) 'Rape and fear in a New Zealand city', *Area* 25(1): 55–63.

Safe City Committee of the City of Toronto (1992) 'A working guide for planning and designing safer urban environments', Toronto: Safe City Committee and the Planning and Development Committee.

Schroeder, H. W. and Anderson, L. M. (1984) 'Perceptions of personal safety in urban recreation sites', *Journal of Leisure Research* 16: 178–94.

Smith, S. (1986) *Crime, Space and Society*, Cambridge: Cambridge University Press.

Soothill, K. and Walby, S. (1991) *Sex Crime in the News*, London: Routledge.

Stanko, E. A. (1987) 'Typical violence, normal precaution: men, women and interpersonal violence in England, Wales, Scotland and USA', in J. Hanmer and M. Maynard (eds) *Women, Violence and Social Control*, London: Macmillan, pp. 122–34.

—— and Hobdell, K. (1993) 'Assault on men: masculinity and male victimization', *British Journal of Criminology* 33: 400–15.

Storey, K. (1991) 'The safety of public open space – three arguments for design', *Landscape Architectural Review* (July): 13–15.

Talbot, J. F. and Kaplan, R. (1984) 'Needs and fears, the responses to trees and nature in the inner city', Journal of Arboriculture 10(8): 222–8.

Valentine, G. (1989) 'The geography of women's fear', *Area* 21(4), 385–90.

—— (1990) 'Women's fear and the design of public spaces', *Built Environment* 16(4): 288–303.

—— (1992) 'Images of danger: women's sources of information about the spatial distribution of male violence', *Area* 24(1): 22–9.

—— (1997) 'Angels and devils: moral landscapes of childhood', *Society and Space* 14: 505–630.

Walker, J. (1993) 'Woods for Walsall', *Landscape Design* 216: 37–8.

Williams, P. and Dickinson, J. (1993) 'Fear of crime: read all about it? The relationship between newspaper crime reporting and fear of crime', *British Journal of Criminology* 33(1): 33–56.

Chapter 10

Bondi, L. (1993) 'Locating identity politics', in M. Keith and S. Pile (eds) *Place and the Politics of Identity*, London: Routledge.

Butler, J. (1990) *Gender Trouble: Feminism and the Subversion of Identity*, London: Routledge.

—— (1992) 'Contingent foundations: feminism and the question of postmodernism', in J. Butler and J. Scott (eds) *Feminists Theorise the Political*, London: Routledge.

Gatens, M. (1990) 'A critique of the sex/gender distinction', in S. Gunew (ed.) *A Reader in Feminist Knowledge*, London: Routledge.

Hall, S. (1992) 'The question of cultural identity', in S. Hall, D. Held and T. McGrew (eds) *Modernity and its Futures*, Cambridge: Polity Press.

—— (1996) 'Introduction: who needs identity?', in S. Hall and P. Du Gay (eds) *Questions of Cultural Identity*, London: Sage Publications.

Jagose, A. (1994) *Lesbian Utopics*, London: Routledge.

Keith, M. and Pile, S. (eds) (1993) *Place and the Politics of Identity*, London and New York: Routledge.

King, K. (1994) *Theory in its Feminist Travels – Conversations in U.S. Women's Movements*, Bloomington: Indiana University Press.

Lesbians On The Loose, November 1991–November 1995, Sydney: Francis Rand.

Pile, S. and Thrift, N. (1995) 'Mapping the subject', in S. Pile and N. Thrift (eds) *Mapping the Subject: Geographies of Cultural Transformation*, London: Routledge.

Rose, G. (1993) *Feminism and Geography: The Limits of Geographical Knowledge*, Cambridge: Polity Press.

Soja, E. and Hooper, B. (1993) 'The spaces that differences make: some notes on the geographical margins of the new cultural politics', in M. Keith and S. Pile, (eds) *Place and the Politics of Identity*, London: Routledge.

Women Out Loud (1994) 'Cracks in the Lesbian Nation', Radio National, Australian Broadcast Commission, 17 September.

Young, I. M. (1990) 'The ideal of community and the politics of difference', in L. J. Nicholson (ed.) *Feminism/Postmodernism*, London: Routledge.

Chapter 11

Bilby, K. (1995) 'Jamaica', in P. Manuel (with Kenneth Bilby and Michael Largey) *Caribbean Currents: Caribbean Music from Rumba to Reggae*, London: Latin American Bureau.

Brinkworth, L. (1992) 'Why are the sisters taking up the slack?', *The Guardian*, 25 June: 21.

Burston, P. (1995) 'Faggamuffins' night out', *The Independent*, 1 February: 22.

Cooper, C. (1993) *Noises in the Blood: Orality, Gender and the 'Vulgar' Body of Jamaican Popular Culture*, London: Macmillan.

—— (1994) ' "Lyrical Gun": metaphor and role play in Jamaican dancehall culture', *The Massachusetts Review* XXXV (3/4): 427–9.

—— (1995) 'Lady Saw's reward – slackness upfront', *The Jamaican Observer* (n.d.).

Ellis, P. (ed.) (1986) *Women of the Caribbean*, London: Zed Press.

Julien, I. (director) (1994) *The Dark Side of Black*, Black Audio/Normal Production for BBC TV, April, BBC2 (UK).

O'Brien, L. (1995) 'The making of a black Madonna', *The Guardian*, 13 October: 12–13.

Rose, T. (1994) *Black Noise: Rap Music and Black Culture in Contemporary America*, Hanover, NH: University Press of New England.

Sawyer, M. (1995) 'Lady sings it blue', *The Observer*, 19 February: 32–4.

Skeggs, B. (1993) 'Refusing to be civilised: "race", sexuality and power', in H. Afshar and M. Maynard (eds) *The Dynamics of 'Race' and Gender*, London: Taylor & Francis.

Skelton, T. (1989) 'Women, men and power: gender relations in Montserrat', unpublished PhD thesis, University of Newcastle upon Tyne.

—— (1995a) ' "Boom, Bye, Bye": Jamaican ragga and gay resistance', in D. Bell and G. Valentine (eds) *Mapping Desire: Geographies of Sexualities*, London: Routledge.

—— (1995b) ' "I sing dirty reality, I am out there for the ladies," Lady Saw: women and Jamaican ragga music, resisting patriarchy', *Phoebe: Journal of Feminist Scholarship, Theory and Aesthetics*, Oneonta, NY: State University of New York.

Zabihyan, K. (director/producer) (1995) *Yardies*, Observer Films, broadcast 21 February, ITV (UK).

Chapter 12

Bourdieu, P. (1977) *Outline of a Theory of Practice*, Cambridge Studies in Social Anthropology, Cambridge: Cambridge University Press.

Cockburn, C. (1985) *Machinery of Dominance: Women, Men and Technical Know-how*, London: Pluto Press.

Dinnerstein, D. (1987) *The Rocking of the Cradle and the Ruling of the World*, London: Women's Press.

Easlea, B. (1981) *Science and Sexual Oppression: Patriarchy's Confrontation with Woman and Nature*, London: Weidenfeld & Nicolson.

Halford, S. and Savage, M. (1995) 'Restructuring organisations, changing people: gender and restructuring in banking and local government', *Work, Employment and Society* 9(1): 97–122.

Hall, P. (1985) 'The geography of the fifth Kondratieff', in P. Hall and A. Markusen (eds) *Silicon Landscapes*, London: Allen & Unwin, pp. 1–19.

Hartsock, N. (1985) *Money, Sex and Power*, Boston: Northeastern University Press.

Henry, N. and Massey, D. (1995) 'Competitive times in high tech', *Geoforum* 26(1): 49–64.

Ho, M.-W. (1993) *The Rainbow and the Worm: the Physics of Organisms*, London: World Scientific.

Jay, N. (1981) 'Gender and dichotomy', *Feminist Studies* 7(1) (Spring): 38–56.

Keller, E. F. (1982) 'Feminism and science', *Signs: Journal of Women in Culture and Society* 7(3): 589–602.

—— (1985) *Reflections on Gender and Science*, New Haven, CT: Yale University Press.

Kidder, T. (1982) *The Soul of a New Machine*, Harmondsworth: Penguin.

Lefebvre, H. (1991) *The Production of Space*, trans. D. Nicholson-Smith, Oxford: Blackwell.

Lloyd, G. (1984) *The Man of Reason: 'Male' and 'Female' in Western Philosophy*, London: Methuen.

Massey, D. (1996) 'Politicising space and place', *Scottish Geographical Magazine* 112(2): 117–23.

—— (forthcoming) 'Economic/non-economic', in R. Lee and J. Wills (eds) *Geographies of Economies*, London: Arnold.

—— Quintas, P. and Wield, D. (1992) *High-tech Fantasies: Science Parks in Society, Science and Space*, London: Routledge.

Moore, H. (1986) *Space, Text and Gender*, Cambridge: Cambridge University Press.

Noble, D. (1992) *A World without Women: the Christian Clerical Culture of Western Science*, New York: Alfred A. Knopf.

O'Brien, M. (1981) *The Politics of Reproduction*, London: Routledge & Kegan Paul.

Sartre, J.-P. (1943) *Being and Nothingness*, trans. H. E. Barnes, London: Methuen.

Segal Quince & Partners (1985) *The Cambridge Phenomenon*, Cambridge: Segal Quince & Partners.

Turkle, S. (1984) *The Second Self: Computers and the Human Spirit*, London: Granada.

Wajcman, J. (1991) *Feminism Confronts Technology*, Cambridge: Polity Press.

Chapter 13

Amory, D. (1996) 'Club Q: dancing with (a) difference', in E. Lewin (ed.) *Inventing Lesbian Cultures in America*, Boston: Beacon.

Anzaldúa, G. (1987) *Borderlands/La Frontera: The New Mestiza*, San Francisco: Spinster/Aunt Lute Press.

Baym, N. (1995) 'The emergence of community in computer mediated communication', in S. G. Jones (ed.) *Cybersociety: Computer Mediated Communication and Community*, London: Sage.

Benedikt, M. (ed.) (1991) *Cyberspace: First Steps*, Cambridge, MA: MIT Press.

Correll, S. (1995) 'The ethnography of a lesbian bar: the lesbian cafe', *Journal of Contemporary Ethnography* 24(3): 270–98.

D'Emilio, J. (1992) 'Gay politics, gay community: San Francisco's experience', *Making Trouble: Essays on Gay History, Politics and the University*, New York: Routledge.

De Monteflores, C. and Shultz, S. (1978) 'Coming out: similarities and differences for lesbians and gay men', *Journal of Social Issues* 34: 59–72.

Eder, D., Staggenborg, S. and Sudderth, L. (1995) 'The national women's music festival: collective identity and diversity in a lesbian-feminist community', *Journal of Contemporary Ethnography* 23(4): 485–515.

Faderman, L. (1991) *Odd Girls and Twilight Lovers: A History of Lesbian Life in Twentieth-Century America*, New York: Penguin.

Ferguson, A., Zita, J. N. and Pyne Addelson, K. (1982) 'On "compulsory heterosexuality and lesbian existence": defining the issues', in N. Keohane, M. Z.

Rosaldo and B. C. Gelphi (eds) *Feminist Theory: A Critique of Ideology*, Brighton: Harvester.

Franzen, T. (1993) 'Differences and identities – feminism and the Albuquerque lesbian community', *Signs: Journal of Women in Culture and Society* 18(4) (Summer): 891–906.

Gibson, W. (1984) *Neuromancer*, New York: Ace.

Hall, K. (1996) 'Cyberfeminism', in S. Herring (ed.) *Computer-Mediated Communication: Linguistic, Social and Cross-Cultural Perspectives*, Amsterdam: John Benjamins.

Hine, C. (1994) *Virtual Ethnography*, CRICT discussion paper no. 43 (May), Uxbridge, Mx: Centre for Research into Innovation, Culture and Technology (CRICT).

Jagose, A. (1993) 'Way out: the category "lesbian" and the fantasy of the utopic space', *Journal of the History of Sexuality* 4(2): 264–87.

Kendall, L. (1996) 'MUDder? I hardly know 'er! Adventures of a feminist MUDder', in L. Cherny and E. R. Weise (eds) *Wired Women: Gender and New Realities in Cyberspace*, Seattle: Seal.

Kreiger, S. (1982) 'Lesbian identity and community: recent social science literature', in E. B. Friedman *et al.* (eds) *The Lesbian Issue: Essays from Signs*, Chicago: University of Chicago.

Kroker, A. and Weinstein, M. A. (1994) *Data Trash: the Theory of the Virtual Class*, New York: St Martin's Press.

Lemon, G. and Patton, W. (1997) 'Lavender blue: issues in lesbian identity development with a focus on Australian lesbian community', *Women's Studies International Forum* 20(1) Jan.–Feb.: 113–27.

Phelan, S. (1989) *Identity Politics: Lesbian Feminism and the Limits of Community*, Philadelphia: Temple University Press.

—— (1994) *Getting Specific: Postmodern Lesbian Politics*, Minneapolis: University of Minnesota Press.

Plant, S. (1995) 'The future looms: weaving women and cybernetics', *Body and Society* 1(3–4): 45–64.

—— (1996) 'On the matrix: cyberfeminist simulations', in R. Sheilds (ed.) *Cultures of Internet: Virtual Spaces, Real Histories, Living Bodies*, London: Sage.

Ponse, B. (1978) *Identities in the Lesbian World: The Social Construction of Self*, Westport, CT: Greenwood.

Reid, E. (1995) 'Virtual worlds: culture and imagination', in S. G. Jones (ed.) *Cybersociety: Computer Mediated Communication and Community*, London: Sage.

Rheingold, H. (1993) *The Virtual Community: Homesteading on the Electronic Frontier*, Menlo Park, CA: Addison-Wesley.

Rich, A. (1980) 'Compulsory heterosexuality and lesbian existence', *Signs: Journal of Women in Culture and Society* 5(4) (Summer) 631–60.

Stacey, J. (1991) 'Promoting normality: section 28 and the regulation of sexuality', in S. Franklin, C. Lury and J. Stacey, *Off Centre: Feminism and Cultural Studies*, Cultural Studies Birmingham series, London: HarperCollins Academic, pp. 284–304.

Stein, A. (ed.) (1993) *Sisters, Sexperts, Queers: Beyond the Lesbian Nation*, New York: Plume.

Stone, A. R. (1991) 'Will the real body please stand up? Boundary stories about virtual cultures', in M. Benedikt (ed.) *Cyberspace: First Steps*, Cambridge, MA: MIT Press.

Lash, S. and Urry, J. (1994) *Economics of Signs and Space*, London: Sage.

Lawrence, E. (1982) 'Just plain common sense: the "roots" of racism', in Centre for Contemporary Cultural Studies (comp.) *The Empire Strikes Back: Race and Racism in 70s Britain*, London: Hutchinson.

McCorquodale, D., Ruedi, K. and Wigglesworth, S. (eds) (1996) *Desiring Practices: Architecture, Gender and the Interdisciplinary*, London: Black Dog Publishing.

MacKenzie, S. (1989) *Visible Histories: Women and Environments in a Postwar British City*, Montreal: McGill-Queen's University Press.

Massey, D. (1985) *Spatial Divisions of Labour: Social Structures and the Geography of Production*, London: Macmillan.

—— (1994) *Space, Place and Gender*, Cambridge: Polity Press.

—— (1996) 'Masculinity, dualisms and high technology', in N. Duncan (ed.) *Bodyspace: Destabilizing Geographies of Gender and Sexuality*, London and New York: Routledge, pp. 109–126.

Matrix Book Group (eds) (1984) *Making Space: Women and the Man-made Environment*, London: Pluto.

Morris, M. (1992) 'The man in the mirror: David Harvey's "Condition of Post-Modernity" ', *Theory, Culture and Society* 9: 253–79.

Palmer, J. and Dodson, M. (eds) (1996) *Design and Aesthetics*, London: Routledge.

Perkin, S. (1989) *The Rise of Professional Society*, London: Routledge.

Pile, S. (1996) *The Body in the City: Psychoanalysis, Space and Subjectivity*, London: Routledge.

Roberts, M. (1991) *Living in a Man-made World: Gender Assumptions in Post-war Housing Design*, London: Macmillan.

Rose, G. (1993) *Feminism and Geography: The Limits of Geographical Knowledge*, Cambridge: Polity Press.

—— (1996) 'As if the mirrors had bled', in N. Duncan (ed.) *Bodyspace: Destabilizing Geographies of Gender and Sexuality*, London and New York: Routledge, pp. 56–74.

Rowbotham, S. (1973) *Woman's Consciousness, Man's World*, Harmondsworth: Penguin.

Soja, E. (1989) *Postmodern Geographies*, London and New York: Verso.

Soja, E. and Hooper, B. (1993) 'The space that difference makes', in M. Keith and S. Pile (eds) *Place and the Politics of Identity*, London and New York: Routledge, pp. 183–206.

Valentine, G. (1996) '(Re)Negotiating the "heterosexual street" ', in N. Duncan (ed.) *Bodyspace: Destabilizing Geographies of Gender and Sexuality*, London and New York: Routledge, pp. 146–55.

Warren, M. (1993) *Economics of the Built Environment*, Oxford: Butterworth-Heinemann.

Werkele, G. *et al.* (eds) (1980) *New Space for Women*, Boulder, CO: Westview.

Wilson, E. (1991) *The Sphinx in the City: Urban Life, the Control of Disorder, and Women*, London: Virago.

Women and Geography Study Group of the IBG (1984) *Geography and Gender: an Introduction to Feminist Geography*, London: Hutchinson.

Zukin, S. (1993) *Landscapes of Power*, Berkeley, CA: University of California Press.

Index

This book is dedicated to my
five pillars of wisdom:
Hope Dellon
Hannah O'Grady
Barbara Lowenstein
Mary South
Krystyna Green